Animal (De)liberation: Should the Consumption of Animal Products Be Banned?

Jan Deckers

]u[

ubiquity press
London

Published by
Ubiquity Press Ltd.
6 Windmill Street
London W1T 2JB
www.ubiquitypress.com

First published 2016

Cover design by Amber MacKay
Cover illustration by Els Van Loon

Printed in the UK by Lightning Source Ltd.
Print and digital versions typeset by Siliconchips Services Ltd.

ISBN (Hardback): 978-1-909188-83-9
ISBN (Paperback): 978-1-909188-84-6
ISBN (PDF): 978-1-909188-85-3
ISBN (EPUB): 978-1-909188-86-0
ISBN (Mobi/Kindle): 978-1-909188-87-7

DOI: http://dx.doi.org/10.5334/bay

The full text of this book has been peer-reviewed to ensure high academic standards. For full review policies, see http://www.ubiquitypress.com/

Suggested citation:
Deckers, J 2016 *Animal (De)liberation: Should the Consumption of Animal Products Be Banned?* London: Ubiquity Press. DOI: http://dx.doi.org/10.5334/bay. License: CC-BY 4.0

To read the free, open access version of this book online, visit http://dx.doi.org/10.5334/bay or scan this QR code with your mobile device:

For Els Van Loon,

*with gratitude, in the hope that this book may go some way
towards answering your call to pass on my joy in the lives of animals,
and that all may be liberated from human domination*

Contents

Acknowledgements

As everyone makes decisions about what to eat on a daily basis, the topic of this book is important. This is why I have chosen to facilitate wide distribution by publishing this work as an Open Access book under a Creative Commons Attribution Licence. I am very grateful to Ubiquity Press, and particularly to Frank Hellwig and Anastasia Sakellariadi, for their support in this project, and to the institutions that provided the grants that helped in the development and the publication of this book. A grant was received from the Wellcome Trust [104137/Z/14/Z] to fund a conference, held in September 2014, which featured the work of many scholars from a wide range of countries who work in areas related to the topic of this book. The Trust also funded the publication costs of this book. Other grants were received from the Economics and Social Research Council (ESRC), which funded the 'Deliberating the Environment' research project [RES 151250014], and from Beacon North East, which funded another conference on the book's theme in 2011. My gratitude also goes to those who participated in these conferences, as well as to my collaborators on the ESRC project, Derek Bell, Mary Brennan, Tim Gray, and Nicola Thompson. I also thank those whose views were analysed in this book, including a group of people from Newcastle-upon-Tyne, a city in the north-east of England; staff and students at Newcastle University; and everyone who contributed to the film 'Slaughterhouse—The Task of Blood', a film produced and directed by Brian Hill from Century Films, which was broadcast on the British Broadcasting Corporation's BBC Two on 4 July 2005.

Writing this book has not been easy. This is why I also express my gratitude to Jo and Stella, who have supported me brilliantly, and who have tolerated my company during the good and the bad times. The support that I received from many colleagues at Newcastle University and from the University's library, as well as from those who work in the Centre for Values, Ethics, and the Law in Medicine at the University of Sydney, has also been much appreciated. Many thanks also to two anonymous referees and to Alejandra Mancilla and John Lazarus for their helpful comments, to Nourane Clostre for the many wonderful suggestions that I owe to her brilliant proof-reading skills, to Jen Fleming for lending me a nice laptop, and to Kathrin Herrmann for storing copies of successive drafts. I am particularly grateful for the detailed feedback I received from Linnea Laestadius (University of Wisconsin-Milwaukee), with whom I collaborated on some of the book's themes and issues, facilitated by a British Council Researcher Links Travel Grant.

I also express my gratitude to Springer Science+Business Media B.V. for granting me the kind permission to use and build on the ideas first developed in my article 'What policy should be adopted to curtail the negative global health impacts associated with the consumption of farmed animal products?' (Deckers 2010); some of the ideas in section 3.5 have also been developed, with kind permission again, from my article 'In defence of the vegan project' (Deckers 2013b).

The writing of this book would not have been possible without all the support that I have received from the numerous teachers who have taken it upon themselves to try to educate me at the Gemeentelijke Basisschool in Nieuwmoer, the College Essen, the Catholic University of Leuven, and the University of St Andrews. I would like to express my gratitude to all of them, except to those very few individuals who were rather nasty. Out of courtesy, I shall not mention their names. I shall, however, mention the name of my favourite teacher, Els Van Loon, to whom this book is dedicated. I am also greatly appreciative of those who have supported my education by financial and other means, including the Government of Belgium, the VZW Studieondersteuning, the Student Awards Agency for Scotland, the Faculty of Divinity and the Department of Moral Philosophy at the University of St Andrews, and particularly my parents, Maria and Wilfried.

Introduction

This book is about animals, and more particularly about the most common manner in which most people relate to other animals: by eating them. The vast majority of people eat animals, but some do not do so. I used to eat animals almost every day until twenty-five years ago, when I stopped doing so, with the exception of fish who had not been farmed, whom I carried on eating now and again. My rationale for continuing to eat some fish was that, unlike many other animals, fish who had not been farmed might have had relatively good lives, and, given that they die naturally anyway, I thought it would be acceptable to 'kill them for food', by which I mean—throughout this book—the killing of animals in order to eat them. This state of semi-vegetarianism continued for a few years, until I also started questioning the very practice of killing animals for food. As I adopted the view that it was better to avoid killing animals for food where there was no need for us to do so, I became a vegetarian. Having later adopted the view that it was not consistent to be only a vegetarian in light of the fact that the production of vegetarian food is inextricably linked, at least in the vast majority of situations, with the intentional killing of animals for food, I then became a vegan fifteen

How to cite this book chapter:
Deckers, J 2016 *Animal (De)liberation: Should the Consumption of Animal Products Be Banned?* Pp. 1–12. London: Ubiquity Press. DOI: http://dx.doi.org/10.5334/bay.a.
License: CC-BY 4.0

years ago. I define a vegan as someone who abstains from the consumption of substances that are part of, or have been created by, animals, with the exception of human milk and honey. Veganism is also sometimes referred to as 'total vegetarianism', but I define a vegetarian diet in this book as a diet that, whilst not including animal flesh, includes other animal products in addition to those mentioned in my previous sentence, for example milk from other animals or eggs.

Whilst this text might be perceived to be the exercise of a scholar who tries to understand his dietary choice, this is not the full story. I also have an interest in ethics, the quest for and the articulation of values that ought to be universally endorsed (Jamieson 1990; Daniels 1979; Rawls 1971). At this moment in time, I feel very strongly that veganism is the right choice for me. Even if I do not think that it is the right choice for all human beings, I think that it ought to be for those who are in morally similar situations to mine. To me, veganism is not a matter of taste. It matters, and I do not think it merely matters to me. What one decides to eat matters to many other people too, and it may matter also to those who are eaten. When I talk about ethics, I talk about what ought to matter, not just for me, but also for other human moral agents, and this raises the question whether the adoption of a vegan diet ought to be universally endorsed. Put more forcefully, it raises the question whether the consumption of animal products ought to be banned.

One reason why the answer that will be given to this question may not move everyone to appropriate action is that our dominant culture works hard to hide from public view the reality of the animals whose products are being eaten. One way in which this is done is by keeping the places where living animals are transformed into products away from places where many people tend to congregate. Though not all slaughterhouses may keep their doors closed, many are situated in areas where people will not go unless they deliberately want to visit them, and I have not seen any with glass walls. To some degree, the animals who are killed in slaughterhouses may even be hidden from those who kill them as well, depending on the extent to which the killing process is mechanised. In slaughterhouses, the real animals who were once alive and kicking are turned from concrete living beings into abstract products and concepts. Adams (1990, 40) has commented as follows: 'Through butchering, animals become absent referents. Animals in name and body are made absent *as animals* for meat to exist' [emphasis in original].

Indeed, not only are animals made abstract by being butchered, but their concrete bodies are also fragmented and then lumped together again into the concept of 'meat'. Not only have abstract nouns such as 'meat', 'livestock', 'pork', 'beef', and 'chicken' been created and mobilised to express human separation from and domination of other animals, but the terms that are used to describe the killing of other animals and the killing of humans are also separated neatly, which is partly why the word 'slaughter', for example, has a very different connotation from the word 'murder' (Jepson 2008). Some concepts are also notable for their absence, which is what moved Joy (2010, 28–30) to launch the concept of 'carnism'. The view that it is fine to consume flesh has been so deeply ingrained in many cultures that only the aberrant ideologies of vegetarianism and veganism required labelling: Joy's concept reacts to this, as it is more appropriate to refer to someone who believes that it is justifiable to eat flesh as a 'carnist' than as an omnivore, given that the latter term refers merely to a biological propensity.

Animals are also hidden from view in bioethics, a discipline that has frequently focused exclusively on human health care interests without regard for the interests of other species (Wolfe 2010, 56). However, when the word 'bioethics' is understood properly, it must be taken to refer to the application of ethics to all biological organisms. The reduction of bioethics to a narrow conception of human health care ethics stems from a strong anthropocentric view that reducing the nonhuman world to a collection of objects for our ends can be an adequate means to human health care. As the objectification of other animals for human food and the ideology of carnism are regarded as the norm, it is simply assumed that they do not need a defence—even if there are signs that this is now changing (see e.g. Scruton 2000). What most, if not all, people, carnist or otherwise, do agree on, however, is that human health—however badly it might be conceived of—ought to matter, which takes me to the first specific question of this book: might a vegan diet be healthy, or even healthier than a non-vegan one? This question is important as many people refrain from adopting vegan diets in the belief that they are nutritionally inadequate. If this were so, any moral theory that claims that veganism ought to be adopted by a lot of people would seem to be standing on very shaky ground. If it could be shown, however, that a well-chosen vegan diet might be healthier than alternative diets, it would provide an additional reason for adopting it.

In the main text of this book I assume that a vegan diet can be healthy. Accordingly, the objection that vegan diets ought never to be recommended on the grounds that they would necessarily compromise the health of those who adopt them is unsound. The assumption that a vegan diet can be healthy is based on my exploration of the nutrition literature, as there may be little debate that good human health cannot be achieved unless human diets are nutritionally adequate, regardless of all the other things that I shall consider to be necessary for diets to be healthy. As the nutrition literature is complicated and may distract from the moral argument in spite of its importance for that very same moral argument, my narrow, nutritionally-based answer to the first question of importance in this book has been reserved for the book's appendix, which provides a detailed overview of the academic literature on vegan nutrition. A similar appendix was provided in the first edition of Singer (1975)'s *Animal Liberation*, but no longer featured in the second edition due to his view that the 'nutritional adequacy of a vegetarian diet is not in dispute' (Singer 1990, 258). As I shall argue that even within the theory adopted by Singer most vegetarian diets are beset with the same moral problems as those that are associated with many omnivorous diets, the question of real importance, however, is whether there is no debate about the nutritional adequacy of a *vegan* diet. (Incidentally, this is not the only point where Singer (1990) and I differ.) From my personal experience, which is also informed by the research findings reported in chapter four (section 4.3.3), the belief that a vegan diet can be nutritionally adequate is much disputed. Indeed, a major obstacle to vegan diets being adopted more widely is the belief that they are nutritionally inadequate, or at least sub-optimal.

The view that any theory that jeopardises human health does not stand much of a chance of being universally adopted may not be contested. What may be more controversial is my claim, defended in an earlier work (Deckers 2011a), that health should be the only thing that ought to matter in bioethics. Hedonists might object that happiness, rather than health, is the crucial thing that ought to matter. Accordingly, they might argue that a life spent in merriment is better than a boring life in good health. I concede that they have a point and that the pursuit of happiness is not a bad thing, even if it might undermine one's physical health. However, provided that we understand the concept of health holistically, including both physical and psychological health—with happiness contributing to the latter—the objection does not undermine the theory that health, or well-being, is the only thing that we ought to be concerned with. Indeed, the concept of holistic health could also be replaced by that of welfare, provided that the latter is not interpreted in terms of a subjective feeling, but in terms of something that can be deemed to be good even if it is not consciously experienced as such. Accordingly, someone who feels great or someone who does not feel anything at all might still not fare well. In this respect, my concern with welfare does not preclude a concern with killing, which contrasts with the views of many members of the 'animal welfare science community' (Haynes 2008; see also K. Schmidt 2011).

Whereas the definition of health used in the appendix is very narrow in considering merely the nutritional health or otherwise of vegan diets, the main text of this book adopts a very expansive notion of health. If such a wide definition is adopted, I believe that this book's theory can also accommodate the key issues that both capability theorists and rights theorists are concerned with. In the capabilities approach adopted by Nussbaum (2006, 76), for example, the importance of 'flourishing' is repeated over and over again, suggesting that a flourishing or healthy life is at the core of her list of capabilities: life; bodily health; bodily integrity; senses, imagination, and thought; emotions; practical reason; affiliation; (a relationship with) other species; play; and political and material control over one's environment. Similarly, in the rights approach adopted by Caney (2008), it could be said that the human rights that he engages with, for example the rights to subsistence, property, and freedom from enforced relocation, are important precisely because they contribute to good health. Other human rights, such as, for example, the right to free speech or the right to privacy, are also important precisely because human health would be jeopardised if these rights were not protected.

In spite of its importance, we should also recognise that human beings do not have a right to health (Hessler and Buchanan 2002). This is so because, although human health is influenced by controllable social factors, our health is also influenced by things that are beyond our control. As some genetic and environmental factors cannot be controlled, some people just happen to be relatively healthy, whilst others happen to be fairly unhealthy, in spite of the fact that both groups may receive appropriate health care. If we do not have a right to health, perhaps it could be said that we should be granted a right to health care. In order for this to be possible, it is worth consulting what Raz (2010) has said about human rights. In his view, 'their existence depends on there being interests whose existence warrants holding others subject to duties to protect and promote them' (Raz 2010, 335). I may have an interest in flying to the moon, but the existence of this interest does not warrant that others should feel obliged to provide me with the means to do so. This is why Caney (2008, 538–539) has emphasised, inspired by Raz, that those interests that are sufficiently or vitally important, rather than trivial, and that can be accompanied by duties that are not 'unreasonably demanding' make good candidates for grounding rights.

This book shares with Raz (2010) and Caney (2008) a commitment to an interest-based theory, and focuses on our duties to protect and promote important interests. Whereas I shall sometimes spell out which rights are safeguarded by those duties, at other times I connect the duties of human moral agents directly to significant moral interests without mentioning the rights that may or may not be associated with them. Given that what may be reasonable in one context may be unreasonable in another, I do not adopt the view that rights must always be respected, but that talking about rights may nevertheless be useful to highlight important interests that must be attended to unless doing so conflicts with one's duty. Some interests are clearly better candidates to deserve the protection afforded by duties than others. My interest in flying to the moon is not vital to me. Even if I might claim otherwise (perhaps because of my delusion), it would be unreasonable to expect that others should be obliged to provide me with the means, for example a rocket, to satisfy what ought to be no more than a trivial interest for me.

This book adopts the view that, in every situation, human moral agents must act in such a way that they prioritise their more important over their less important interests. In situations where we do not aim to achieve the highest good, less important interests would be granted precedence over more important interests, which would be wrong. This book breaks new ground by arguing that the most important interest that human moral agents ought to consider in relation to the consumption of animal products is their interest in their own health, holistically conceived. As there is no greater interest than this, all moral agents have an unconditional duty to strive for their holistic health. This does not imply that all moral agents also have unconditional rights to health care: moral agents may have the wrong ideas about what contributes to their holistic health—for example, some may intend to kill other human beings for a goal that they wrongly claim to be necessary to obtain holistic health. In some circumstances, for example out of self-defence, it may be necessary to deny such people a right to health care; for example where injuring or even killing them may be necessary to thwart their plans. Nevertheless, I have argued elsewhere that all human beings, including those who may not be able to act morally because of a severe impairment, have a non-trivial interest in health care and that there are many situations where it is not too demanding on others to care for their well-being (Deckers 2011a). Whilst there is debate about what this right might entail and when it might be trumped (see e.g. Ruger 2006; Lautensach 2015), I like the fact that many nations show some support for the principle that limited health care resources should be available for all human beings, grounded in the human right to health care. All human beings therefore ought to possess a *prima facie* right to health care. The words '*prima facie*' are important here: duty-bearers are not always obliged to act on a particular duty, but they must do so unless their concern with holistic health demands that they prioritise another duty.

Whereas I adopt the view that moral agents have an unconditional holistic health care duty towards themselves, this does not imply that their personal physical health must necessarily be paramount, since human moral agents cannot promote their holistic health without caring for their moral health. By a concern for one's 'moral health' I mean cultivating the right virtues, values, and attitudes without which it would not be possible to act morally. Accordingly, tending to one's holistic health does not rule out the possibility that significant or even ultimate physical health sacrifices may be required to protect these moral qualities. I shall argue that other theories in animal ethics have either placed insufficient importance on this duty or misunderstood its content, resulting in problematic moral theories related to the consumption of animal products.

If we accept the view that, in order to fulfil their holistic health care duties, human moral agents must consider not only how their actions affect themselves, but also how they affect other human beings, we must explore not only how diets, vegan or otherwise, affect those who adopt them, but also how they affect others. Whilst moral philosophy has traditionally focused mainly on relationships between human beings in the here and now, in abstraction from their wider temporal and spatial contexts, the harms associated with localised activities may have global consequences, some of which are delayed. Examples are the activities that may contribute to the health risks associated with climate change. In this light, bioethicists increasingly recognise that we must consider not only the interests of human beings who live nearby or who are living now, but also the interests of people who live further away, both in space as well as in time (Gardiner 2001; Bell 2011). When we scrutinise our dietary choices, we must therefore also consider how they might affect the interests of people who live far away, as well as those of future generations.

Our choices also impact upon other animals. A growing number of bioethicists have argued that not only humans, but also some other animals have interests, and that these interests must be taken seriously (Singer 1990; DeGrazia 1996; Cochrane 2012). Accordingly, this book also explores whether the consumption of animal products can be justified in light of any duties we may have to other organisms. Elsewhere I have developed a moral theory based on duties related to positive and negative Global Health Impacts (GHIs), where the concept of GHI was introduced as a unit of measurement to evaluate the effects of human actions on the health of all biological organisms (Deckers 2011a). If health is the only thing that matters morally, it follows that, when we consider the moral quality of any particular action, we must assess its potential health impacts. The word 'global' has been added to emphasise three things. Firstly, it highlights that the concept of health should be understood broadly when we assess the health impacts of our (proposed) actions. It underlines a holistic understanding of health, encapsulating all things that are conducive to flourishing. Secondly, it stresses that the consequences of our actions upon the health of the global population of human beings, including those who have not yet been born, should be considered. And thirdly, the word 'global' also refers to the need to consider the effects of our actions upon all the nonhuman organisms that live on our globe.

Our holistic health care duty can also be understood as a duty to act in ways that maximise positive GHIs. An alternative formulation of this duty is a duty to minimise negative GHIs. The reason why these expressions are interchangeable relates to my use of the concepts of 'act' and 'actions' in this book. These are used to refer to both positive actions (commissions) and negative actions (omissions), where GHIs can be produced through either. This is an important point. It highlights that the duty to minimise negative GHIs is not a duty to act as little as possible out of fear that doing something would produce negative GHIs. Whenever we decide not to act, we must also consider the opportunity costs, which is why a decision not to act can produce more negative GHIs than a decision to act. Similarly, an action may fail to maximise positive GHIs by producing more negative GHIs compared to inaction.

In order to minimise negative GHIs or to maximise positive GHIs, moral agents must prioritise their greatest (morally relevant) interest or act in accordance with their (highest) duty in any particular situation. The relative wrongness of an action is therefore determined by the degree to which its negative GHIs exceed the smallest quantity of negative GHIs that might be produced by the action that fulfils one's duty. This duty-based theory is consequentialist: a particular duty must be ignored where the negative GHIs of fulfilling it are greater than the negative GHIs of fulfilling one's highest duty, where the latter is grounded in the most important interest. This may result, for example, in a duty to improve the health of one given child rather than the health of two other children where it is clear that this is one's overriding duty, for example because the former child happens to be one's own and the latter are unrelated

(Cottingham 1986). By not prioritising one's overriding duty, unacceptable negative GHIs are produced. This is why, strictly speaking, those duties that lose out are not really duties, but competing moral considerations, in the same way that, strictly speaking, rights are not rights in situations where morality demands that they are ignored. I shall nevertheless use the concepts of rights and duties to refer also to these overridden interests to highlight that, in many situations, it would be good to abide by them and thus to recognise their *prima facie* claims on us, even if they might be overridden in specific situations.

How the concept of GHIs may operate in a moral theory can be illustrated using a straightforward example. If my daughter has a right to education and if we assume that she is not schooled at home, it is my duty, as a parent, to live in such a way that I allow her to exercise her fundamental interest in education. If I am unable to fulfil this duty because I decide to intoxicate myself through the consumption of large quantities of alcohol, it might be said that I would act wrongly through my failure to maximise positive GHIs. However strong my interest in drinking alcohol might be, the satisfaction of this interest ought not to jeopardise my duty to produce a particular positive GHI, which in this case would be to facilitate my child's right to receiving an adequate education. If the reason for not taking her to school related to a conflict with my duty to take a relative to hospital for an urgent medical reason, however, her right would have been ignored, but justifiably so, namely to tend to one's highest duty. I would fail to prioritise the greatest interest (fail to maximise positive GHIs or to minimise negative GHIs) if I prioritised my daughter's education in this situation.

In light of this moral framework, the general question addressed in this book is whether or not human beings who consume particular animal products in particular situations fail to minimise negative GHIs. Put differently, this book aims to shed light on situations where consuming animal products does and where it does not violate human moral agents' duties to prioritise their greatest moral interest in any given situation. A charge that has been pressed against many people who adopt omnivorous diets is that they contribute to a 'food crisis' (Singer 2009, 122), or to 'world hunger' (Marcus 2001, 153–169; Webb 2010). Many vegan diets, by contrast, have been hailed for protecting the health care interests of human beings (ADA 1997; Marcus 2001; Lanou 2009). This takes me to the second specific question of this book: Does the consumption of animal products jeopardise the human right to health care by causing zoonoses (diseases that can spread from other to human animals) and resource shortages? In my first chapter, a survey of some of the negative GHIs associated with dietary choices will reveal that these choices can result in severe consequences for the health of human beings, warranting a positive answer to this question in some situations and a moral imperative for dietary change. The GHIs that are discussed here, however, do not include any that may be associated with how other organisms ought or ought not to be treated by us. Rather, they are limited merely to how the consumption of animal products affects human beings through the emergence and spread of zoonoses as well as through its effects on land, water, fossil fuels, and atmospheric resources, regardless of how these issues affect the lives of nonhuman beings.

For analytic purposes, therefore, the first chapter ignores any questions related to whether moral agents should embrace particular duties towards the nonhuman world: chapter one is more empirical than philosophical. The balance is tilted in chapter two, where it will be argued that our duty to strive for holistic health cannot be fulfilled unless moral agents embrace particular duties towards nonhuman entities. In recognition of the interests of other animals, some bioethicists have argued that some animals should be granted particular rights, such as the right to be protected from the human infliction of pain or suffering (Singer 1990) or the right to treatment that respects the animal's inherent value (Regan 1983). Whereas Singer has opposed being classed as a rights theorist (Singer 1987), what is at the core of his work is the recognition that some animals have interests and that they deserve our moral consideration in light of these, which is why we may also say that they have certain *prima facie* rights against us, regardless of whether these might be trumped by the greater good (see also Llorente 2009). A different rights theorist is Francione (2010a): as Francione (2010a, 74) adopts the view that nonhuman animals have absolute rights not to be used for a wide range of human purposes, including for dietary purposes, he argues that veganism is a 'nonnegotiable moral baseline'. If this is a valid view, anyone who ever eats animal products, in any imaginable situation, would fail to minimise negative GHIs.

I explore theories about animal rights in chapter two. In doing so, I develop a new theory on the consumption of animal products, arguing that the duty to strive for holistic health demands that human moral agents adopt particular duties not only towards other animals, but also towards themselves. I have mentioned already that the latter duties have not been considered adequately in other theories. Whereas a new moral theory is proposed, I also appreciate that people's views on which actions should be considered to be duties and on how to weigh their relative importance may vary widely. The duties that are argued for in this book are based on my deliberations on my feelings, some of which relate to experiences that I have had in my life of looking after and killing other animals, particularly pigeons, whom I used to race for many years. The word 'feelings' is used here deliberately, as this theory is very much in agreement with Hume (1978, 470)'s view that 'morality ... is more properly felt than judg'd of' (although I do not wish to claim that judgements are based on anything other than feelings). Though this does not imply that all feelings are moral feelings, I believe that our feelings must nevertheless be taken seriously, and it is my view that any moral theory that suggests otherwise would not only lack a basis from which to do so, but also merely substitute some feelings with other feelings. To give adequate consideration to our interest in holistic health, I feel very strongly that a number of interests must be highlighted, where some of these have either been ignored or downplayed by moral agents and theorists who have considered this topic.

One interest that I value highly is logic, which is why I think that we should try to live consistently. A vegetarian who consumes eggs from hens who are killed when they are considered 'spent', but who opposes their being killed in these circumstances, for example, is not living consistently by supporting an activity that they object to. Another feeling that I cherish is one that Steiner (2008) has highlighted to have a crucial role in moral theory, the feeling of kinship with animals, which sits at the heart of my commitment to 'animalism'. Our 'animalist' interest is an interest in attributing greater moral significance to either dead or living animals than to other biological organisms. It will be argued that the moral implications of this interest for the consumption of animal products, however, result in significant differences from the views of other scholars (e.g. Singer 1990; Francione 2008; Cochrane 2012). This is also because my theory argues for the importance of recognising a related 'evolutionist' interest, or an interest in attributing greater moral significance to those animals biologically closer to us.

Whereas my theory is new in arguing how these interests should be integrated, it also recognises the importance of interests that have been highlighted by other scholars, including moral agents' interests in avoiding actions that either intentionally inflict or pose relatively high risks of inflicting pain, suffering, and death upon animals (e.g. Palmer 2010; Regan 1983; S. Davis 2003; Schedler 2005). It also draws on the work of others in exploring the relevance of different organisms' capacities to enjoy rich experiences (e.g. Birch and Cobb 1984). A final interest that I consider to have been neglected is the safeguarding of the integrity of nature. Whilst this interest is relevant where we decide whether or not to allow other animals to live independently, I consider its relevance especially in relation to biotechnological projects that seek to alter animals through conventional breeding technologies and through genetic engineering, as well as in relation to projects that seek to develop in-vitro flesh for human consumption. By weighing these interests against one another, chapter two culminates in a defence of a new moral theory on the consumption of animal products: qualified moral veganism.

My commitment to veganism is qualified as my theory does not demand that human beings abstain from eating animal products in all situations. It is a moral rather than a dietary position that can be adopted by everyone, even by those who ought not to adopt vegan diets for justifiable personal, social, or ecological reasons. It is a vegan theory in the sense that vegan diets ought to be the default diets for the majority of the human population.

Chapter three is about politics. Few people appear to adopt qualified moral veganism. My view about laws, however, is that they should protect important moral values—for example those that might not be protected adequately because of the well-known free-rider problem (Hardin 1968). This also questions their validity where they fail to do so (see e.g. Bankowski 2001), raising the question of how legal change might be brought about to secure the important moral values that qualified moral veganism tries to protect. In pluralistic societies, people are bound to have widely diverging views about what constitutes the moral good, what counts as a positive or a negative GHI, and how we should assess GHIs' magnitudes. Some might argue that the intentional killing of an animal for food, for example, is an act that always produces unacceptable negative GHIs, whereas others might argue that it is always justifiable. In light of this pluralism, some might argue that we should adopt a *laissez-faire* approach whereby we allow everyone to decide for themselves how they wish to live their lives. The problem with this approach is that it does not protect us against those who tarnish important moral values through unwitting or unwilling failures to embrace particular duties. Though it is fair to say that the introduction of laws may not necessarily protect moral values either, as many people still trespass against them, I nevertheless adopt the view that laws that are based on fair democratic procedures ought to be granted some respect as they may help to provide some orientation to people about what really ought to matter in this complex world. Whilst I believe that some laws are unjust and that they may thus contribute to the cultivation of the wrong attitudes, it does not undermine my belief that a society with democratically agreed laws is preferable to a society without such laws.

Those who adopt qualified moral veganism could pursue at least three political strategies to advance their cause. The first is to create or support educational campaigns in the hope that more people will adopt such a position; the second is to advocate the creation of better pricing systems that would result in products and services with relatively high negative GHIs being priced more highly than those with relatively low negative GHIs; and the third is to introduce a qualified ban on the consumption of animal products. The vegan project aims to bring about legal reform in the different nations of this planet to introduce qualified bans on the consumption of animal products and to promote the adoption of vegan diets for the majority of the human population. I shall engage with three objections that have been raised against this project. The first is that it would be pointless in view of the fact that many people are not prepared to embrace it. The second is that the vegan project should be rejected as it would jeopardise human food security unjustifiably. The third rejects the vegan project on the basis that it would alienate us from the natural world.

In spite of the fact that moral agents must take their duties seriously, few moral agents appear to adopt qualified moral veganism. This might stem from the possibilities either that people fail to act in accordance with their duties, either willingly or unwittingly, or that they fail to accept that they have a duty to adopt such a position. In chapter four I explore what other people think about qualified moral veganism by evaluating a number of discussions that others have had on the topic. Whilst chapters two and three engage with some academic criticisms of qualified moral veganism, chapter four evaluates the values of people who are not specialised in animal ethics on the issues raised by the consumption of animal products when they are stimulated to think about them.

Scholars are frequently criticised for locking themselves into the ivory towers of academia, and 'ethicists' are no exception. Chapter four is an attempt to get out and to explore carefully whether we can learn anything from how non-specialists reason about these issues or whether their perspectives might be challenged in the light of the moral claims defended in the earlier chapters. Several studies have found that many people are reluctant to think about the human use of other animals when they make food choices, and that they hold contradictory views about the human use of other animals (Plous 1993; Macnaghten 2004; Wolfson and Sullivan 2004; NCOB 2005; N. Williams 2008). The sheer fact that many people are unclear about what really ought to matter when we make dietary choices is highly significant for a scholar in ethics. It provides food for deliberation. In the 'Deliberating the Environment' study that I conducted with some of my colleagues at Newcastle University, several participants recognised that they held conflicting views. The results of this study are reported and discussed in chapter four, which engages with data from this study as well as data gathered elsewhere. It features the views of the following: academic staff and philosophy students from Newcastle University; people from relatively deprived parts of Newcastle-upon-Tyne (a city in the north-east of England); and slaughterhouse workers from Oldham (a town in the northwest of England). The University staff came together with local residents in a series of one-to-one deliberative exchanges, facilitated by a researcher. A 'deliberative exchange' was defined as a facilitated discussion between two people from different backgrounds (Bell et al. 2005; Gundersen 1995), but it could also be defined more broadly as an exchange of views between two people that may or may not be facilitated by a third person.

The facilitated deliberative exchange was found to be a valuable tool to promote interaction and learning between people (Bell et al. 2005). The interest that has been shown in this method of interacting is situated within the context of a growing interest amongst political scientists in the study of alternative modes of political engagement that focus on deliberation, including focus groups, citizens' juries, and deliberative exchanges. These examples of 'deliberative democracy' aim to promote deep listening, reflection, and evaluation, in an attempt to transcend the adversarial modes of engagement that characterise much political praxis. My focus in this book is on the deliberative exchanges that took place on the topic of 'animals and biodiversity'. Though none of the people whose views I shall engage with were asked specifically whether they agreed with qualified moral veganism, my deliberation on their views reveals that the ways in which these people tried to justify the killing of animals for food and their consumption of animal products fail to provide sufficient grounds to reject qualified moral veganism. My analysis also provides some evidence for the view that what is needed might not quite be what Steiner (2013, 162) has called for, namely 'a kind of soul conversion that can change the sensibilities of people', but merely a willingness to deliberate on one's values and to act in accordance with one's sensibilities, which may be suppressed through inappropriate socialisation.

CHAPTER ONE

The Consumption of Animal Products and the Human Right to Health Care

1.1 Introduction

As human beings cannot stay healthy for long without adequate food, many people may agree that the human right to health care should include a right to adequate food. Having sufficient food that is adequate is a very basic human need, which is why the human interest in food is an excellent candidate for grounding a human right. This right has been defended by many, including the United Nations (UN CESCR 1999; De Schutter 2011).

If we accept that every human being's right to health care includes a right to food, it might be argued that there are situations where this right can only be protected by using other animals for food. As many animal products are relatively dense in nutrients compared to other foods, some groups of people who might particularly benefit from the consumption of animal products are very young children with limited stomach capacities relative to their energy demands and people living with the human immunodeficiency virus (HIV) or acquired immunodeficiency syndrome (AIDS), who may have increased nutritional requirements but reduced appetites (Randolph et al. 2007; Roubenoff 2000). These are just some examples of groups of people who might be more vulnerable in situations where they were denied the option of consuming animal products. Some populations would also be vulnerable, for example some Inuit who live at high northern latitudes and who may lack not only sufficient plant foods to feed themselves, but also the means to acquire them from elsewhere. The consumption of animal products may also be vitally important to many people who live in Asia, where much human population growth in the near future is expected to occur. To meet the challenge of feeding this growing population, it has been argued that, in many areas with relatively adverse environmental conditions, using animals may be indispensable (Devendra 2007;

How to cite this book chapter:
Deckers, J 2016 *Animal (De)liberation: Should the Consumption of Animal Products Be Banned?* Pp. 13–50. London: Ubiquity Press. DOI: http://dx.doi.org/10.5334/bay.b. License: CC-BY 4.0

Sharma et al. 2012). Some significant advantages that are conferred by the use of animals for human food are that some animals can eat plants, such as grass, that human beings cannot digest, and that some animals are better able to cope with drought compared to plants, for example due to their greater mobility (Morton and Kerven 2013).

In addition, animals can be used to provide food not only directly, but also indirectly, by providing important services, for example by producing excrements that can be used as manure or fuel or by providing draught power and means of transportation that could save on human labour and fossil fuel consumption. In India, for example, over 55% of the total land that was cultivated in 2009 used animals for draught power (Phaniraja and Panchasara 2009). Research in Africa by Iannotti et al. has also shown that the acquisition and use of chickens to produce eggs is 'one of the few and first mechanisms for asset accumulation in poor households' (2014, 355). The authors add that programmes aimed at stimulating the keeping of chickens by poor people may be 'an uncracked part of the solution' to 'undernutrition ... in many parts of the world' (Iannotti et al. 2014, 366). Accordingly, any strategy that considers reducing the human use of other animals must be careful not to undermine some people's rights to food, an issue that I shall return to in section 3.5.2.

Although the stipulation of a right to food is not free from problems—including the problem of what the correlative duties are of those who must ensure that every human being is able to obtain sufficient food—many ethical theories accept that any personal liberties that may be possessed by some individuals ought to be restricted by the (negative) duty to avoid significant harm to some other individuals (Mill 1859; Raz 2010). In this light, some scholars have questioned the consumption of animal products, claiming that the fact that some people consume animal products causes hunger for other human beings (Rifkin 1993; Lewis 1994; Popkin and Du 2003; Webb 2010). Singer, for example, has claimed that the fact that a lot of food that could be eaten by humans is fed to farmed animals is the primary cause of 'the food crisis' (2009, 122), and Weis has similarly claimed that 'the meatification of diets' is 'a vector of global inequality, environmental degradation, and climate injustice' (2013, 81–82). Whereas the authors of an influential report—'the LEAD study'—entitled 'Livestock's Long Shadow', published by the Livestock, Environment, and Development Initiative (LEAD), a group co-ordinated by the Food and Agriculture Organization of the United Nations (FAO), grant that the farmed animals' sector is a major cause of environmental degradation, they cautiously reject the idea that this might be associated with injustice towards those who lack adequate food, writing: 'it is probably true that livestock do not detract food from those who currently go hungry' (Steinfeld et al. 2006, 270). What is undisputed, however, is that the increase in the human consumption of animal products over the last 50 years has been unprecedented. Most notably, the consumption of animals' body parts has increased by more than fourfold. Rather than speak of the number of animals whose bodies are being used for human consumption, dominant metrics refer to this rise in terms of an increase in tonnage, lumping the bodies of different animals together in a common unit. According to the FAO (2014), tonnage increased from 71,357,169 tonnes in 1961 to 262,919,740 tonnes in 2006 and to 302,390,507 tonnes in 2012, the latest year for which data are available at the time of writing.

About 30% of all animal-flesh consumption occurs in countries that account for no more than 12% of the world population. Ranked from higher to lower levels of total consumption, these are: the USA, Australia, New Zealand, Argentina, Canada, and Western European countries (where consumption data are combined) (Weis 2013). Although the consumption of animal products has now stagnated at high levels in many relatively rich countries, in many less affluent countries it has risen and is continuing to rise rapidly (Steinfeld et al. 2006, 15–16). China and Brazil in particular have seen rapid increases over the last 50 years, the former having seen a 15-fold and a 31-fold and the latter a 2.5-fold and an 11-fold increase in, respectively, total consumption and production of animal flesh (Weis 2013). A nutrition transition towards diets that are relatively rich in animal products has been and is taking place, which has been claimed to have contributed to recent food price increases (Popkin 2009). This transition is associated with an unprecedented rise in what has been called 'domesticated zoomass'—the weight of domesticated animals, which is estimated to have grown from 180 million tonnes in 1900 to 620 million tonnes in 2000, with what has been referred to as 'bovine biomass' having the largest share, with a share of 450 million tonnes (Smil 2002, 618).

Lipton (2001) has reported that, as demand for animal products frequently comes mainly from those who are relatively affluent, rising levels of affluence in relatively poor countries have led to an increasing amount of grain and land being used to feed farmed animals. Consequently, relatively poor people may suffer not only from the fact that the farmed animals' sector displaces parts of other food sectors, but also from being displaced themselves. This risk of being displaced has increased in recent times due to what Webster (2013, 10) has referred to as 'the second industrial revolution' in the farmed animals' sector's recent history—the first one being the capitalist transition from common to enclosed land. This second revolution, which started around 70 years ago, has resulted in the farm no longer depending on the land it occupies for its inputs. Rather, these can now be sourced from an increasingly globalised world where inputs are merely confined by capital and by the farm's ability to process them.

Consequently, many indigenous communities, for example in Australia and in the Cerrado of Brazil, have been displaced by land appropriation for the expansion of the farmed animals' sector (Aldrich et al. 2012; White et al. 2012; MacDonald and Simon 2011, 11–14; Stoll-Kleemann and O'Riordan 2015, 41). What Australia and Brazil also have in common is that their farmed animals' sectors are increasingly owned by a small number of large corporations with high levels of vertical integration (concentration of different stages of the production process) that allow these corporations to exercise a very high degree of control over the food system (MacDonald and Simon 2011; Loughnan 2012). These centralising tendencies are by no means absent in other nations. Many people who work for these large corporations, for example in slaughterhouses and in other settings where the farmed animals' sector relies on labour that is modelled on the repetitive, monotonous, and highly specialised work that is typical of many factories, belong to the lowest strata of society, and many are paid badly (Joy 2010, 85). Dillard (2008), for example, reports that in the USA most slaughterhouse workers are paid relatively poorly to work in conditions where they are likely to endure both physical and psychological harm. Many studies report similar concerns. A study in Denmark, for example, reported high levels of physical and mental problems amongst slaughterhouse workers (Kristensen 1991), whilst a study in Turkey identified increased psychological problems amongst butchers compared to office workers (Emhan et al. 2012). In many countries, large farms ('megafarms') and slaughterhouses are also situated in relatively deprived areas, creating significant health concerns caused by localised pollution (Fitzgerald 2010).

Against this backdrop, the objectives of this chapter are: firstly, to explore whether there are situations where the consumption of animal products jeopardises human rights to health care unjustifiably; and secondly, to address how human diets might be changed to address situations where it does so. As I shall argue in the appendix to this book, some people who consume particular animal products jeopardise their own health in some situations where they eat (too many) foods that are unhealthy, which imposes negative impacts on others, for example on taxpayers who pay for public health services. However, these are by no means the only ways in which human others are affected. In the preceding paragraph I have already reported facts that may trigger the question whether those who consume animal products impose unacceptable health risks on relatively poor people who may have little choice in deciding whether or not to work in conditions that are likely to compromise their physical and mental health. The same question might be asked when we consider the causal links between the human consumption of animal products and the creation and spread of zoonoses. Unlike diseases that may be caused directly by the consumption of animal products, many zoonoses also impact upon those who abstain from consuming animals.

After having described common zoonoses that have been associated with the consumption of animal products, this chapter will then consider whether the large quantities of resources that are used in the process of feeding the vast and increasing number of animals on the planet pose human health concerns. The land, water, and energy that are used to produce such a large quantity of animal products could frequently be used more efficiently if it was used to grow foods for direct human consumption. Even if the land, water, and energy requirements of different diets vary from place to place, depending (amongst other factors) on climate, water cycles, and the quality of the land, of the water, and of the technologies that are available, diets that include animal products generally require more resources. Some of the key issues that will be considered are the impacts on human health associated with land use and degradation, water use and pollution, and fossil fuel use and atmospheric pollution. Though these issues are interconnected, they will be separated for analytic reasons. A meta-analysis of different studies on these impacts has pointed out that studies have focused predominantly on global impacts that are relatively easy to quantify, such as emissions of greenhouse gases, and that localised impacts have been neglected because they are frequently much more difficult to quantify (Pluimers and Blonk 2011). This explains why this overview is biased towards issues that are of global concern.

Whereas it will become clear in chapter two that the consumption of animal products produces many other negative GHIs apart from those that are discussed here and that it therefore presents other concerns related to the human right to health care, the overview that will be provided in this chapter may be sufficient to raise serious concern even amongst those who fail to recognise the (moral importance of the) interests discussed in chapter two.

1.2 Zoonoses

The vast majority of human diseases spread between different species of animals (Woolhouse and Gowtage-Sequeria 2005; Torres-Vélez and Brown 2004; Grace 2015). Whereas some of these, for example tapeworms, primarily affect the bodies of those who consume animal products, others can affect everyone, regardless of whether or not they consume animal products themselves. The causes underlying the emergence and the re-emergence of zoonoses are complex. Whereas a detailed overview of these is provided by Ka-Wai Hui (2006), at least four reasons show that the consumption of animal products poses a significant concern. Firstly, the scale of the farmed animals' sector is unprecedented, increasing risk due to the sheer size of the animal population. Secondly, many animals display a high level of genetic uniformity as breeders select for a small number of traits, for example large muscle mass, resulting in a loss of resilience amongst populations and an increased susceptibility to infection. Thirdly, the vast majority of farmed animals are kept in confined spaces, increasing the risks of various infections due to increased contact, stress, and exposure to pathogens. Fourthly, animals are transported faster and over greater distances than ever before, increasing the spread of pathogens and reducing our ability to control it.

Many zoonoses stem from the ways in which farmed animals are treated by human beings. Cows are herbivorous animals, but many cows used to be fed with ground-up remains of slaughtered sheep and other cows, which led to bovine spongiform encephalopathy (BSE), which has also been called—ironically and derogatorily—'mad cow disease'. The causal agent of BSE, a prion, was subsequently transmitted to humans, causing new variant Creutzfeldt-Jakob Disease (nvCJD). Problems also stem from the ways in which human beings manage animal manure, of which there is no shortage. Manure provides a great vehicle for the spread of many pathogens which could subsequently present human health hazards (Kanaly et al. 2009, 23), for example *Cryptosporidium parvum*, *Vibrio cholerae*, *Enterococcus* spp., *Escherichia coli* serotype O157:H7 (or other faecal coliform bacteria that are pathogenic), staphylococci, and streptococci.

To fight disease, the farmed animals' sector uses a large quantity of different kinds of drugs. Particular concerns have been expressed over the large-scale use of antibiotics (Graham et al. 2016). Many antibiotics are used not because the animals are ill, but simply to prevent disease, or the spread of it, as well as to promote growth (by changing the bacteria in the animals' digestive systems so that more nutrients are absorbed) (Anomaly 2009; Price et al. 2015; Meek et al. 2015). The Union of Concerned Scientists (UCS), a non-profit organisation based in the USA, has estimated that the amount of antibiotics that are used by the farmed animals' sector in the USA merely to prevent disease is eight times greater than that of antibiotics used to treat human disease (UCS 2001). Globally, it has been estimated that about half of all antibiotics that are produced are given to farmed animals (Steinfeld et al. 2006, xx, 273). This promotes the development of drug resistant strains of pathogenic bacteria, of which box 1 provides some examples.

Antibiotic-resistant strains of *Salmonella*—the main pathogen involved in food-related deaths in humans—and of *E. coli* and *Campylobacter* have been found in many farmed animal products (Marshall and Levy 2011). Other zoonotic pathogens that are resistant to a whole array of drugs are quinolone-resistant *Campylobacter jejuni* and various tetracycline-resistant bacteria (Levy et al. 1976; K. Smith et al. 1999; Hermans et al. 2012); quinolone-resistant *Salmonella enterica* (Chiu et al. 2002; Mølbak et al. 1999; Dechet et al. 2006); and ceftriaxone-resistant *Salmonella enterica* (Fey et al. 2000).

As many people's bowels contain vancomycin-resistant *Enterococcus*, which can cause a range of infections in humans, this pathogen in particular presents a very serious health concern. It developed its resistance by the use of avoparcin on chicken farms (Bates et al. 1994; Aarestrup et al. 2000; Garcia-Migura et al. 2005; Sørensen et al. 2001). Vancomycin-resistant genes have also spread to some populations of the more common and more troublesome methicillin-resistant *Staphylococcus aureus* (MRSA). *Staphylococcus aureus* is a bacterium that can either transiently or permanently colonise the nasal cavity wherefrom it can migrate to infect other body parts, causing necrotising fasciitis, a severe infection of the skin (Bonten et al. 2001; Ferber 2002). Many strains of MRSA are actually multi-drug resistant, as about 90% of *Staphylococcus aureus* strains are resistant to penicillin and other penicillin-related antibiotics. MRSA is a very serious human health concern as about half of all nosocomial (hospital-acquired) infections have been reported to be MRSA infections (Aiello et al. 2006). Until recently, MRSA was only known to be a nosocomial pathogen, but in recent years the incidence of community-acquired MRSA has been increasing and transmission from farmed animals has been documented, for example in Dutch slaughterhouse workers (Gilbert et al. 2012; Huijsdens et al. 2006; Voss et al. 2005; Armand-Lefevre et al. 2005; van Belkum et al. 2008; Marshall and Levy 2011). In light of these connections, some scholars have started to speak of 'livestock-associated MRSA' (T. Smith and Pearson 2011). A Dutch study found that MRSA was carried by nearly 27% of pig farmers, while only 0.19% of individuals without contact with farmed animals were found to be carriers (van Cleef et al. 2010). A different study found that many veterinarians in Denmark and Belgium also carry the pathogen (Garcia-Graells et al. 2012).

Box 1: Examples of drug resistant bacteria in relation to the use of antibiotics in the farmed animals' sector

Vector-borne illnesses are diseases that are caused by infections that are transmitted to people by arthropods (insects and arachnids). Many vector-borne diseases, as well as viral diseases, have either emerged or become more severe because of human environmental changes, including deforestation and the reduction of biodiversity. The farmed animals' sector is a major contributor to these changes, and box 2 provides some examples of how some diseases may have either emerged or increased in prevalence because of it.

Examples of vector-borne diseases that have become more prevalent due to human deforestation are malaria and leishmaniasis (GECHH 2007, 50). Deforestation may open up new windows of opportunity for some of these vectors if what is known as the 'dilution effect' applies (Ostfeld 2009). This effect relates to the fact that vectors feed from a wider range of species in areas that are relatively rich in biodiversity, where some hosts are less likely to transmit the disease compared to the host that may be dominant in a more impoverished ecosytem.

A good example of a zoonotic viral disease that may have emerged for similar reasons is the Machupo virus. In the early 1960s, many forests were cleared in Bolivia to create agricultural land, and this was accompanied

(Box continued on next page)

(Box continued from previous page)

by the spraying of DDT to control the malaria mosquito. Forest clear-ance led to the migration of *Calomys* mice to arable land, while the DDT poisoned cats, their predators. The consequent increase in the mouse population was accompanied by an increase in the viruses they carried, resulting in the emergence of a new zoonotic viral fever, the Bolivian (Machupo) haemorrhagic fever, which killed around one seventh of the population who lived in the town of San Joaquín in northern Bolivia (GECHH 2007). Similar causal mechanisms underlie the emergence of Argentine haemorrhagic fever and Lassa fever (Ka-Wai Hui 2006).

Box 2: Examples of vector-borne and viral diseases that may have become more prevalent because of environmental changes caused in part by the farmed animals' sector

Concerns with the emergence of zoonoses are not limited to the farmed ani-mals' sector, but extend also to other animal products that are consumed by human beings. One of the most well-known zoonoses is HIV/AIDS: HIV-1 is thought to have emerged from SIVcpz, a simian immunodeficiency virus (SIV) found in a sub-species of chimpanzee (*Pan troglodytes troglodytes*) (Peeters et al. 1989); HIV-2 is thought to stem from SIVsmm, an SIV found in the sooty mangabey (*Cercocebus atys*) (Marx et al. 1991; Ka-Wai Hui 2006). Both HIV strains are likely to have emerged from human contact with the blood of infected chimpanzees and sooty mangabeys, possibly through butchering practices (Chitnis et al. 2000).

Finally, influenzas (flus) are viral diseases that have regained prominence in recent years. Flu viruses are categorised in A, B, and C types. B and C types are relatively mild and undergo changes through antigenic drift, the normal process of flu viruses' genetic mutation. The A type flu viruses, however, also undergo changes through antigenic shift, which involves a rapid change caused by genetic mixing between different subtypes, resulting in the creation of flus that can be relatively severe as human beings may not have come into contact with these new strains before. Though not many people have been killed by recent outbreaks, flus have had a devastating effect on many people in the 20th century through three pandemics: the 1918 ('Spanish influenza') H1N1 virus, the 1957 ('Asian influenza') H2N2 virus, and the 1968 ('Hong Kong influenza') H3N2 virus pandemics. The first one of these was particularly memorable, as it has been estimated to have killed up to 40 million people in 1918–20, or about 3% of the world population. Research has shown that the emergence of these flus stemmed from human interactions with other animals (Taubenberger et al. 2005; Belshe 2005), raising the question whether viral diseases that have emerged more recently in close connection with animal farming practices might trigger disease in large numbers of people. Box 3 provides some prominent examples of such viral diseases directly associated with the farmed animals' sector.

One example of a recently emerged zoonotic virus is the Nipah virus, a new paramyxovirus that emerged in Malaysia in 1998, affecting a number of pig farmers and slaughterhouse workers, causing encephalitis and death. This virus was proven to be caused by the presence of flying foxes (*Pteropus*, or fruit bats) on a large pig farm in Malaysia (Daszak et al. 2006). Forced by habitat loss, the bats in question arrived *en masse* to eat from the fruit trees that grew in an orchard near to the farm, passing on infection to the pigs by dropping half-eaten fruit that had been infected into the pigs' pens (Torres-Vélez and Brown 2004; Ka-Wai Hui 2006). The haemorrhagic virus outbreak of 1994–1995 in Queensland, Australia, is thought to have had similar origins, with horses rather than bats being the intermediate hosts (Ka-Wai Hui 2006).

Many animals are sold in live-animal markets (also called 'wet markets'), where they come into close contact with many other animals of various species. The capture and sale of bats in markets is thought to have caused the outbreak of severe acute respiratory syndrome (SARS) coronavirus in China in 2002, which infected people in Singapore, Vietnam, and Canada after some people from these countries had visited Hong Kong in March 2003 (Weiss and McMichael 2004; Ka-Wai Hui 2006). Another example of a disease that may have developed because of the crowded conditions in which animals are kept and sold is H5N1, an avian (bird) influenza that emerged in South East Asia in 2003 (Sims et al. 2005). By the end of December 2012, over 600 laboratory-confirmed human cases of H5N1, causing 360 deaths, had been reported to the World Health Organization (WHO 2012).

Pigs are considered to be good mixing vessels for the development of new zoonotic viruses as they are susceptible to both bird and human viruses, which is why pigs who enter into contact with both host species are particularly good virus creators (Ka-Wai Hui 2006). In 2009, a new influenza virus, the swine-origin influenza A H1N1 virus, started to infect human beings. Though there is much debate about the precise origins of this virus, there is a high level of agreement over a causal link with the farming of pigs (Escalera-Zamudio et al. 2012). By 1 August 2010, the virus had killed over 18,000 people (WHO 2010).

Box 3: Examples of zoonotic viral diseases directly associated with the farmed animals' sector

As high populations of farmed animals are maintained only because of human demand for their products, many consumers of animal products are more likely to impose diseases upon other human beings compared to those who refrain from such consumption: the probability that those who consume animal products will facilitate the emergence of a zoonotic disease that would cause illness and kill a large number of people is much higher than the probability that those who consume plant products will do so (B. Chen et al. 2009). An additional concern is that people who are relatively rich are more likely to consume animal products, whereas people who are relatively poor are more likely to suffer from zoonoses (Gunderson 2012; Karesh et al. 2012; Grace 2015).

1.3 Land use and degradation

Agriculture occupies about 38% of the earth's ice-free land, with 26% of ice-free land occupied by grazing and 12% by arable land (Foley et al. 2011). As the land that is used to farm animals includes both grazing and arable land, it has been estimated that the farmed animals' sector occupies about 70–75% of all agricultural land (Steinfeld et al. 2006; Foley et al. 2011). About one third of the earth's soil surface is unsuitable for arable production, though it either is or could be used for grazing or browsing (Penning de Vries et al. 1995). Provided that farmed animals eat plants that are not suitable for human consumption and do not rely (heavily) on feed, diets that include animal products need not necessarily use more land than could be used to feed the human population directly. In recognition of this fact, the opinion has been expressed that the ability of some farmed animals to turn plants that humans cannot eat into foods that people can eat 'may become increasingly important in terms of global food security' (Gill et al. 2010, 330). In reality, however, it is known that a lot of arable land is used to feed farmed animals; this is known principally by the fact that about 35% of the global harvest of cereals has been fed to farmed animals in recent years (Alexandratos and Bruinsma 2012, 71; Foley et al. 2011). In a study carried out in 2006, it was found that the area dedicated to this land use amounted to 400 million hectares (ha), or 4 million square kilometres, an area that is equivalent to the surface area of the 27 countries that then constituted the European Union (Aiking et al. 2006, 171).

The fact that a lot of arable land is used globally to feed farmed animals does not imply that this is the case right across the world. In many poorer countries most grain is consumed directly by people. Most nations in Africa and Asia allocate more than 80% of their arable land to the purpose of feeding people. Accordingly, it has been argued that in countries such as Kenya and Egypt, the current mixed agricultural system provides more human food compared to what a vegan system might provide, as the farmed animals in these countries rely mainly on resources that could not be used for direct human consumption

(CAST 1999). For a similar reason and because the significant unpredictability of rainfall limits arable farming, it has been argued that 'milking animals ... are crucial for maintaining human nutritional welfare in the drylands' of people living in Djibouti, Eritrea, Somalia, and Ethiopia, the countries that make up the Horn of Africa (Morton and Kerven 2013, 25).

In many more affluent countries, by contrast, large quantities of grain are fed to farmed animals. In North America and Europe, for example, only about 40% of all arable land is used to feed people. In addition, some affluent nations also use some of the land of less prosperous nations to feed their farmed animals: as land and labour costs are lower in poorer nations, the large agribusinesses that control a significant part of the farmed animals' sector benefit from sourcing some of their feed from poorer nations, in spite of the costs associated with transportation (Smil 2005). Some of this feed is grown on land that might have (had) more value by not being cultivated (for example, some rainforests) or by growing food crops. This is a growing concern as the amount of arable land that is being used to feed farmed animals is increasing rapidly. This is caused by the following factors: the explosion in the consumption of animal products; the fact that the greatest growth is not seen in the consumption of ruminants, but in the consumption of products from pigs and chickens ('monogastrics') who depend almost exclusively on feed in dominant farming systems; and the fact that a growing number of ruminants are being fed arable crops as substantial components of their diets (Weis 2013).

The use of arable land to feed farmed animals is very inefficient. This inefficiency varies between different areas and farming systems, depending on social and ecological conditions. In the context of farming in the USA at the dawn of this millennium, Smil (2002) calculated that 4.5 kg of feed is required to produce 1 kg of flesh from chickens, 9.4 kg of feed for 1 kg of flesh from pigs, and 25 kg of feed for 1 kg of flesh from feedlot-fed cows. Though chickens are the best converters of plant-to-animal-protein of all the main animals reared for their flesh, about 78% of all the plant protein that was fed to a chicken in the USA about a decade ago was not converted to protein that is eaten by human beings.

Accordingly, several studies (see box 4) have concluded that there are significant differences in the land requirements of different diets, depending on both the amount and the kinds of animal products that they include, with diets that include animal products generally requiring more land compared to diets that exclude them (Baroni et al. 2007; Reijnders and Soret 2003; Peters et al. 2007).

A study from the USA has claimed that 'an overwhelmingly vegetarian diet produced by modern high-intensity cropping' requires five times less arable land than 'the typical Western diet', which is calculated to use 'up to 4,000 m^2/capita' (Smil 2002, 619).

(Box continued on next page)

(Box continued from previous page)

A lower estimate is provided by a Dutch study, which concluded that the land used by an average Dutch household comprising 2.41 persons in 1990 to provide for a typical Dutch diet of 1990 equals 3,490 m² (Gerbens-Leenes et al. 2002). The authors add that this exceeds the land area of 444 m² calculated by another study (Penning de Vries et al. 1995) to feed a household at subsistence level by a factor of eight, largely because the former diet includes a much larger quantity of animal products.

A final example is a UK study which showed that a 50% reduction in the consumption of animal products in the UK, under a specific dietary scenario that provides other health-benefiting changes, including a reduction in the consumption of sugar, would—assuming that the proportion of food imports remained the same—reduce arable land usage by 265,000 ha in the UK and by 311,000 ha outside the UK, as well as release millions of hectares of grassland in the process (Audsley et al. 2011).

Box 4: Evidence that diets that include animal products generally use more land

In general, diets that include farmed animal products also contribute more to land degradation than diets that exclude them. The authors of the LEAD study claim that about 20% of the world's pastures and rangelands are degraded through overgrazing, compaction, and erosion caused by farmed animals (Steinfeld et al. 2006). What is ignored by the authors of this study is what may well turn into the most important issue associated with future strategies to counter land degradation: the loss of phosphorus obtained from mined rock phosphate, a key ingredient in most mineral fertilisers. Although the quality of reserves of rock phosphate is declining and mining costs are increasing, a recent study has estimated that the reserves that remain could be used up by the end of the century and that they could reach a peak (maximum rate) of use by 2033 (Cordell et al. 2009). The continent with the greatest food insecurities at the present time, Africa, exports more phosphate rock than any other continent, and a large and increasing percentage of phosphate rock is devoted to the farmed animals' sector, either through the cultivation of crops for feed or through feed supplementation. The production of fertilisers from phosphate rock yields large quantities of phosphogypsum, a toxic by-product that contains radionuclides of uranium and thorium. Some of these, as well as cadmium, end up in the soil when crushed rock phosphate is applied directly to it, as well as when processed phosphate fertilisers are applied that contain smaller quantities of these elements. Furthermore, although phosphorus can, unlike oil, be recovered and reused, large quantities of phosphorus leak from agricultural land. Long-term food security is therefore jeopardised both by soil pollution from phosphate rock and by the fact that remaining reserves are dwindling (Cordell et al. 2009; Wallis 2014).

Other than being undermined by the toxic components of mineral rock phosphates, soil fertility can also be compromised by other practices associated with the farming of animals. Apart from cadmium, some soils are polluted by other metals used in the farming of animals, for example by the zinc, copper, and arsenicals used as feed additives, as well as by veterinary medicines. The fertility of some soils is also jeopardised by nutrient loading—the accumulation of nutrients in the soil—caused by the application of excessive quantities of manure and fertilisers. Nutrient excesses have been documented to be particularly large in China, Northern India, the USA, and Western Europe (Foley et al. 2011). Over the long term, the soil is acidified by such excesses, resulting in reduced plant growth. Ammonia (NH_3) emissions also contribute to soil acidification, and about two thirds of anthropogenic ammonia emissions have been estimated to be produced by the farming of animals (Steinfeld et al. 2006). Ammonia acidifies the soil by combining with oxygen to form nitrogen oxide (NO_x) and nitrogen dioxide (NO_2), which can then combine with water and oxygen to produce nitric acid (HNO_3) and deposit as acid rain; as many ecosystems comprise organisms that cannot cope with the surplus nitrogen, this process also contributes to biodiversity losses. Nutrient loading, mentioned above, is a problem that is growing as more farmed animals are reared further away from their feed sources. An increasing number of animals are also reared in crowded facilities, which have been associated with relatively poor waste management practices due to their high concentrations of waste (Garnett 2009). Some soils are also waterlogged by a range of irrigation methods that are used by the farmed animals' sector to produce animal feed. Irrigation also contributes to salinisation, the mobilisation and accumulation of salts that are naturally occurring in soils. The salt scalds that are thus formed on top of the ground undermine soil productivity, restricting plant growth (Trout 2000).

A large amount of land also degrades through deforestation. Deforestation causes many land problems, including those associated with salinisation—the removal of trees allows ground water to rise, thus mobilising salt. Deforestation also leads to the erosion of fertile topsoil as most of the fertility of the soil that is found in rainforests is due to the soil being held together by trees. In 2000, Goodland and Pimentel (2000) estimated that about 60% of deforestation took place to make room for animal farming. Current expansion of agricultural farm land is mainly taking place in tropical areas. Tropical forests are very rich in biodiversity and provide many important ecosystem services. It has been estimated that about 80% of all new croplands in the tropics are situated in areas that used to be forests (Gibbs et al. 2010).

A large number of these are devoted to the production of animal feed, mainly in the shape of soybeans, the cultivation of which doubled to 22 million ha in the decade leading up to 2004 (Elferink et al. 2007) and then increased further, up to more than 111 million ha (yielding just over 276 million tonnes of beans) in 2013, a year in which more than 1 billion tonnes of maize was also grown, a large percentage of which, again, was used to feed animals (FAO 2015). Whereas the area that is devoted to growing maize has not increased as much as that used to grow soybeans, it has been estimated that it has grown by around 50% in the last 50 years (Weis 2013). The increases in yields of these two main animal feeds do not simply reflect increases in acreage—the former in fact surpass the latter increases, as global yield increases of soybeans and maize have, respectively, octupled and quadrupled over this same period of the last 50 years (Weis 2013). Most of the soybeans that are grown worldwide are crushed, producing 18.6% soy oil and 78.7% soy meal (as well as some waste), and—although the oil is used in a wide range of products (including biofuels)—almost all the meal is currently used to feed farmed animals (van Gelder et al. 2008). It has been estimated that only about 6% of all soybeans that are grown are directly consumed by people (Oliveira 2015). Though soybeans stimulate rapid growth of farmed animals because of their high protein content, by current yields they require more land relative to other crops that are grown to feed animals per unit of animal product (Elferink and Nonhebel 2007). In 2013, for example, about twice as much land was needed to produce soybeans as was needed to produce a similar mass of maize (FAO 2015). Brazil is a major producer of soybeans and a growing producer of animal flesh, and box 5 provides a good illustration of how the farmed animals' sector affects deforestation in a country with such large areas of remaining forests.

The country with the third largest production of body parts from land animals (with a production exceeding 20 million tonnes annually in recent years) and the second largest production of soybeans (with a production of 82 million tonnes in 2013), Brazil provides an interesting case study of the impact of the farmed animals' sector upon deforestation (Oliveira 2015; Weis 2013). The sector's expansion is the main cause of deforestation in the world's largest tropical rainforest, the Brazilian Amazon (Nepstad et al. 2006). Though the Amazon spreads out over eight countries in Latin America, the majority of it is located in Brazil. The LEAD study claims that the farmed animals' sector uses about 70% of the land in the Amazon that was previously forested as pastures, and most of the remainder of that land to produce animal feed (Steinfeld et al. 2006). To meet the high global demand for soybeans, some of the forest that had originally been cleared to expand grazing has been converted to soybean cultivation, leaving ranchers with large profits that some have invested in the acquisition of new forested land that either has been or is being deforested to increase grazing land. Increasingly, it is not only in the Amazon, but also in the *cerrado*—the Brazilian savannah, which equals the size of Mexico and occupies about 21% of Brazil's land—that soybean plantations spring up (MacDonald and Simon 2011, 10). The associated loss in biodiversity is huge, as both the Amazon and the *cerrado* used to be—and to some extent still are—very rich in biodiversity.

A lot of soybeans that are grown in Brazil are exported to distant places, particularly to China and the European Union. Most is exported to the former, and China is the country that has produced the largest annual share of flesh from land animals since 1990 (van Gelder et al. 2008; FAO 2015). The European Union, which banned the feeding of a range of animal products, including offal, to farmed animals (Regulation (EC) 999/2001), increased its importation of soybeans significantly after the BSE crisis. About 10 million ha of the soybeans that are grown in non-European countries are imported by the European Union annually, representing an area that corresponds to 10% of the arable land of the European Union (Elferink et al. 2007, 468). In the last decade, at least 20 million tonnes of soybean meal has been imported by the European Union annually, primarily from Brazil, to feed farmed animals (EC 2011; de Visser et al. 2014; van Gelder et al. 2008).

Box 5: The farmed animals' sector and deforestation in Brazil

To obtain a good picture of how much protein is used by the farmed animals' sector, I have calculated how many human beings could be nourished from the soybean meal that is fed to farmed animals if they consumed this meal directly, using the facts that roughly 20 kg of protein is recommended per human being annually and that 44% of the content of soybean meal is protein (Wallis 2014). In the European Union, 440 million people could satisfy all their annual protein requirements if we use a conservative estimate of the amount of soybean meal (20 million tonnes) that is imported annually by the European Union to feed farmed animals. This is almost 90% of the number of people living in the European Union. In the case of Australia, 11 million people could satisfy all their annual protein needs merely by the amount of soybean meal that it imports annually (at least half a million tonnes), which equates to about half of its human population.

In this survey I have shown that, on average, the farmed animals' sector uses more land to produce a unit of food than other agricultural sectors require to produce a similar quantity of food. In many situations, the sector also degrades more land than other agricultural sectors either are or would be degrading to produce a fixed unit of food. Finally, the case study of Brazil shows that a large proportion of the recent expansion of the farmed animals' sector has occurred in areas that are relatively rich in biodiversity.

1.4 Water use and pollution

The virtual water content of an entity is the amount of water that is required to produce it, which is captured by its water footprint (Hoekstra and Chapagain 2007). When talking about water, it is useful to distinguish between 'blue', 'grey', and 'green' water. The 'blue water' footprint of an entity refers to the volume of surface water and groundwater that is used—measured in terms of the surface water or groundwater that is lost—in its production; the 'green water' footprint stands for the rainwater that is consumed (excluding runoff) by the entity; and the 'grey water' footprint refers to the volume of freshwater that is required to assimilate the pollutants of the entity in question, based on existing ambient water quality standards (Mekonnen and Hoekstra 2012, 402). These distinctions are useful to highlight the fact that not all uses of water are equally problematic in terms of their negative GHIs.

Problems associated with water scarcity have particularly led to greater scrutiny of sectors that use large amounts of blue water. As many water sources are being emptied faster than the rate by which the hydrological cycle can refill them, a lot of blue water is used at unsustainable rates. Deforestation can also have a major impact upon the availability of water, as the loss of canopies reduces the soil's humus content and reduces local precipitation, resulting in reduced infiltration and water storage. Deforestation also makes the land more susceptible to fire, thereby increasing greenhouse gas emissions as well. It therefore contributes to climate change and its associated problems, including the loss of water from mountains that are losing snow and ice because of global warming.

The LEAD study estimates that the farmed animals' sector accounts for more than 8% of global human water use (Steinfeld et al. 2006). Not only does the sector use water to hydrate animals, to manage manure, and to clean animal housing, but—as soil compaction reduces infiltration rates—grazing animals and the use of heavy agricultural machinery also reduce the replenishment of freshwater sources by lowering water tables (Kirchmann and Thorvaldsson 2000). Though water usage in the sector varies between animals, their feed, the technologies that are used to obtain their products, and the ecosystems in which they live, are killed, and are prepared for human consumption, the production of farmed animal products generally requires more water compared to the production of other foods with similar nutritional content (Hoekstra and Chapagain 2007; Marlow et al. 2009; WWAP 2009). The sector accounts for 29% of the total water footprint from agriculture, which stems in large part (98%) from the water it uses to feed the animals: 1,463 Gm³/year for crops, and 913 Gm³/year for feed from grazing (Mekonnen and Hoekstra 2012). The total footprint for feed from crops amounts to 20% of the total water footprint of all crop production in the world, or 12% of the total blue water footprint of all crops (Mekonnen and Hoekstra 2012).

Mekonnen and Hoekstra (2012, 405) also reveal that the annual production of animal flesh, in tonnes, requires the following global averages of water: 4,300 m³/tonne for the flesh from chickens; 5,500 m³/tonne for the flesh from goats; 6,000 m³/tonne for the flesh from pigs; 10,400 m³/tonne for the flesh from sheep; and 15,400 m³/tonne for the flesh from cows, bulls, and steers. Per gram of protein, the water footprint of cows' milk, of eggs, and of chickens' bodies was estimated to be about 1.5 times larger than that of pulses, whereas for the flesh from cows, bulls, and steers, it was 6 times larger than the latter (Mekonnen and Hoekstra 2012, 410). The authors add that, with the exception of chickens, who rely heavily on feed regardless of whether they are kept in more extensive or more intensive systems, blue and green water usage increases hand in hand with intensification (in 'industrial systems'), as intensive systems rely more on the use of arable crops to feed animals. Where animals use grazing land that could not be used more efficiently for other purposes without substantial difficulties, the fact that they use a lot of water may not be such a problem, particularly if they rely mainly on green water. However, water scarcity is a growing concern, which is why the increasing usage of blue and grey water is particularly problematic.

Importantly, the global averages calculated by Mekonnen and Hoekstra (2012) exclude the grey water footprint associated with the treatment of a range of pollutants, including animal waste, pesticides, fertilisers other than nitrogen fertilisers, and other agrochemicals. One source of the farmed animals' sector's pollution is the soil that ends up in water through the erosion and sedimentation caused by farmed animals, either indirectly, through the deforestation that takes place for the expansion of the farmed animals' sector, or directly. Another problem is the creation of 'dead zones': the nitrogen compounds and the phosphorus excreted by animals, together with the application of excessive quantities of fertilisers to grow their feed, overfertilise rivers and seas and cause the algae that live in them to grow rapidly, a process known as eutrophication. When these short-lived algae die, they decompose; because any biological decomposition consumes oxygen, this causes oxygen depletion (hypoxia) of rivers and seas, leading to the suffocation of aquatic ecosystems (Eshel and Martin 2009). Eutrophication also causes human health concerns, for example by contributing to the development of *Pfiesteria piscicida*, an aquatic organism that not only kills fish but can also cause human health problems (Burkholder and Glasgow 2001). As an increasing number of animals are kept in confined systems that are far removed from nutrient-deficient fields that might benefit from the nutrients provided by their manure and urine, eutrophication is increasing (Smil 2002).

A further problem is the formation of nitrates from manure and artificial fertilisers. These nitrates can leach into drinking water supplies and filter through into the groundwater. The health effects of nitrate ingestion are the subject of considerable debate, as some studies have linked the human ingestion of nitrates with the occurrence of cancers and methaemoglobinaemia (Powlson et al. 2008; Katan 2009). Since many animals are fed from crops grown on arable land, of which large parts are devoted to monocultures, many methods used to farm animals increase the spread of pests and plant diseases, a well-documented problem associated with monocultures. This frequently leads farmers to use large quantities of pesticides—some of which are known to be harmful to human health—thus contributing to the development of pesticide resistance and to the presence of harmful pesticide residues in water and food (Koller et al. 2012; Matthews 2006).

Water is also polluted by the use of antibiotics and hormones, the latter of which are used to promote growth. Recombinant bovine somatotropin (rBST) is a hormone used in the USA, where it is administered to some dairy cows. It is unclear whether the use of these types of hormones might pose human health risks, but disruptions in the endocrine systems of several species of other animals have been associated with their use (Hotchkiss et al. 2008). Though its use is prohibited in the European Union and in many other countries, some other nations have allowed rBST. Other pollutants are the detergents, disinfectants, and antiparasitic agents that are used by the farmed animals' sector. Whereas some pathogens are undermined by some pollutants, others, for example *Cryptosporidium*, thrive in water polluted by the farmed animals' sector (Duffy and Moriarty 2003; Burkholder et al. 2007).

Though this is not intended to be a complete survey of all the water issues raised by the consumption of animal products, the negative water impacts associated with some forms of aquaculture must not be forgotten either, especially as about half of all fish who are currently consumed by human beings are produced in aquaculture systems (Bergqvist and Gunnarson 2013, 76). Some methods used to farm fish can be associated with relatively small negative water impacts; this is the case, for example, of the use of herbivorous species such as the common carp (*Cyprinus carpio*) or species of tilapia in small ponds (Bergqvist and Gunnarson 2013, 95). Others, however, have been associated with relatively large negative water impacts because of their use of algicides, fertilisers, pesticides, nutrients that cause eutrophication, (prophylactic) antibiotics, and other drugs that these methods use to raise fish (D. Cole et al. 2009; Bergqvist and Gunnarson 2013). The destruction of ecosystems associated with some forms of aquaculture also presents a growing concern. An example that has received some attention from academic scholars is the destruction of mangrove swamps in South East Asia that is taking place to meet the increasing demand—mainly from Western consumers—for shrimps, and its effects on coral reefs (Hendrickson et al. 2008, 320).

This survey shows that the farmed animals' sector uses a relatively large pro-portion of freshwater compared to other agricultural sectors and that it contrib-utes significantly to water pollution. Though diets that include products from pasture-fed animals may save water if they rely mainly on rainwater, dietary shifts towards vegan diets could also save large volumes of water and reduce water pollution in many situations.

1.5 The use of fossil fuels and atmospheric pollution

Diets that include animal products generally require more fossil fuels than diets that exclude them. The reason for this stems in part from the fact that a large proportion of the plants that are eaten by animals are not converted into food that people can or want to eat, but are merely used to keep the animals alive, as well as to produce manure and urine. Whereas the proportion of an animal that is actually consumed varies depending on the nature of the animal in question, one example of this inefficiency is provided by Loughnan (2012, 106), who esti-mates that 65% of the weight of a steer may not be consumed.

The explosion in the consumption of animal products that has occurred over the last century was facilitated to a large extent by the invention of the Haber–Bosch process, which is crucial in the production of artificial fertilis-ers. This process, which uses energy to capture nitrogen from the air, has been identified as the key factor in the exponential growth of the world population since its commercialisation in 1913 (Smil 2001). In addition, crop losses have been reduced significantly through the development and application of pes-ticides. What artificial fertilisers and most pesticides have in common is that their production uses large quantities of oil and gas (Hanlon and McCartney 2008).

Apart from relying on large quantities of fossil fuels, the farmed animals' sec-tor contributes significantly to a wide range of problems caused by atmospheric pollution, particularly because of the sector's rapidly increasing greenhouse gas emissions. The LEAD study calculated the relative share of emissions produced by the farmed animals' sector, claiming that the sector produced 18% of all anthropogenic greenhouse gas emissions in CO_2-equivalents (CO_2e) in 2002 (Steinfeld et al. 2006). The CO_2e of a substance measures its radiative forcing (or, less technically, its global warming) potential in units of carbon dioxide (CO_2). It stands for the amount of heat trapped by a quantity of gas as a factor of the heat trapped by one unit of a similar mass of CO_2.

Whereas a later, more detailed FAO study found that the total estimate provided by the LEAD study was 'in line with' the total estimate for the year 2005 (Gerber et al. 2013, 15), the former estimate has also been challenged: one study claims that the farmed animals' sector emitted 51% of all emis-sions in CO_2e in 2009 (Goodland and Anhang 2009). The main reasons for this significant difference from the LEAD study are attributed to the following issues: that the LEAD study did not include respiration as a source of emissions; that it undercounted the number of farmed animals (for example, by excluding farmed fish); that it overlooked some emissions produced by the production, distribution, and disposal of animal products, their by-products, and their packaging; that it ignored the emissions produced by the medical and pharmaceutical industries in their fight against diseases associated with the farmed animals' sector; and that an inappropriate CO_2e of 23, rather than the more appropriate figure of 72, was used for methane. With regard to this last reason, the authors justify their figure by pointing out that a 20-year timeframe (with CO_2e of 72) must be used for calculation rather than a 100-year timeframe, 'because of both the large effect that methane reductions can have within 20 years and the serious climate disruption expected within 20 years if no significant reduction of greenhouse gases is achieved' (Goodland and Anhang 2009, 13). The authors of the study also point out that the LEAD study ignored the opportunity costs associated with the fact that a lot of land (26% of grassland and 33% of arable land) that is used by the farmed animals' sector could regenerate as forest and capture much more carbon through photosynthesis (Goodland and Anhang 2009, 13).

The 51% figure provided by Goodland and Anhang (2009) has been contested. One study claims that respiration should not be included within the count as the CO_2 that farmed animals produce by respiring would have ended up in the atmosphere anyway by the decay of the plants that would not have been consumed by farmed animals anymore (Herrero et al. 2011). Goodland and Anhang (2012) have retorted by saying that this ignores that the earth's photosynthetic capacity cannot balance out all the carbon that is respired by farmed animals; the problem lies in the fact that the sector contributes to a loss in photosynthetic capacity through deforestation and forest burning, thus reducing the earth's ability to absorb carbon from the atmosphere. Goodland and Anhang (2012) do not explain, however, how they determined that respiration exceeds photosynthesis, resulting in a carbon loss. A second point made by the Herrero et al. (2011) study is that Goodland and Anhang (2009) factored in the opportunity costs of the farmed animals' sector, but not of other human activities that reduce carbon capture opportunities, for example urban development. This criticism is entirely justified. Goodland and Anhang (2012, 254) have also responded to this point, stating that they 'used a minimal figure for foregone carbon absorption in land set aside for livestock and feed production when the true figure would be much higher'. The problem with this is that they neither explain what this claim is based on nor how it would compare with the true figures for other domains of human activity.

In light of this lack of clarity, box 6 relies on data provided by the LEAD study and the later FAO study to provide a more detailed sketch of the most prominent contributing factors of the farmed animals' sector to climate change (Steinfeld et al. 2006; Gerber et al. 2013).

Firstly, the sector produces carbon dioxide. Animals respire, producing CO_2. Though some of the carbon that animals send up in the air when their lungs combine carbon with oxygen would also end up in the air through plants breaking down and through soils releasing gases had the animals not existed, some of the carbon released in the latter case would remain out of the atmosphere for longer by being locked either inside plants that live for a long time, such as trees, or inside soils that in the former case may not only release carbon, but also lose some of their potential to absorb carbon by being used to farm animals. In addition, fossil fuels are used to operate agricultural machinery, and most synthetic fertilisers and pesticides are derived from oil. This implies that carbon dioxide is released into the atmosphere through their production and use. About 25% of all synthetic fertilisers and pesticides are used to produce animal feeds (Steinfeld et al. 2006). Animal feeds are often grown far from where animals are kept and therefore require transportation. Animals are also often reared far from where they are killed, turned into products, and consumed. Energy is also required to house animals, as well as to transport and store the products that are derived from themovide room for animal farming are included, they have been estimated to ntributing to. Pimentel and Pimentel (2008) have calculated that, in the USA, the energy input from fossil fuels is more than 10 times greater for a unit of animal protein than for a unit of plant protein, although they add that the nutritional value of a unit of animal protein as human food is 1.4 times greater than that of a unit of plant protein. Though products derived from the bodies of animals are produced in different ways in the USA compared to how they are produced elsewhere, there is no doubt that the production of many animal products emits more carbon dioxide than the production of many other food products does. In total, the LEAD study estimates that the farmed animals' sector accounts for 9% of anthropogenic CO_2 emissions (Steinfeld et al. 2006), whilst the later FAO study estimates that it accounted for 5% of such emissions in 2005 (Gerber et al. 2013, 15).

The sector also produces methane (CH_4), mainly from enteric fermentation by ruminants and from stored manures, especially where these are stored in liquid form, as for example in lagoons. The full contribution of methane to climate change has been estimated to be more than half that of carbon dioxide (Shine and Sturges 2007). The LEAD study estimates that the farmed animals' sector accounted for about 37% of all anthropogenic methane emissions in 2002 (Steinfeld et al. 2006), whilst the later FAO study estimated that its share was 44% in 2005 (Gerber et al. 2013, 15). Though methane does not remain in the atmosphere

(Box continued on next page)

(Box continued from previous page)

for as long as CO_2, its CO_2e is 72 over 20 years, and 23 over 100 years (Forster et al. 2007). The fact that the farmed animals' sector produces a large amount of methane is primarily associated with the large number of ruminants that are used.

Chemical and organic nitrogen fertilisation also produces emissions of nitrogen oxide (NO_x), nitrous oxide (N_2O), and ammonia (NH_3). The creation of nitrous oxide in particular is a problem. The microbial production of nitrous oxide from soil nitrogen is promoted where the available nitrogen exceeds plant requirements. The LEAD study estimates that the farmed animals' sector is responsible for 65% of anthropogenic emissions of this gas, which has a CO_2e of 289 over 20 years (and a CO_2e of 298 over 100 years) and which also contributes to the hole in the ozone layer (Steinfeld et al. 2006; Forster et al. 2007); the figure given in the later FAO study is lower, at 53% for the year 2005 (Gerber et al. 2013, 15). In addition, the sector also accounts for almost two thirds of anthropogenic ammonia emissions (mainly from manure), which contribute not only to global climate change, but also to acid rain and the problems caused by soil acidification mentioned in section 1.3 (Steinfeld et al. 2006).

Box 6: How does the farmed animals' sector contribute to climate change?

Whereas my focus has been on the farmed animals' sector, we must not ignore the fact that many human diets also include products derived from animals who have not been farmed, particularly fish. Many diets that include fish who have been caught in the wild are associated with relatively high emissions compared to plant-based diets. Eshel and Martin (2006) estimate that typical Western diets, which include fish, are more inefficient compared to plant-based diets, especially since long-distance boat journeys are associated with the catching of fish preferred by Western customers. This long travelling distance is the reason for the high emissions of cod fishing calculated by Carlsson-Kanyama and González (2009, 1707S). A more general study was carried out by Reijnders and Soret (2003, 667S), who claim that, in Western Europe, trawler fishing—the prevailing fishing method in the area—uses 14 times more fossil fuels than would be used to produce an equal amount of plant protein. This figure excludes the high emissions that are frequently produced to process fish, for example the emissions produced by canning and refrigeration (Basurko et al. 2013).

The consumption of some fish, such as herbivorous fish kept in ponds that are situated close to consumers, can be associated with relatively small quantities of emissions. Many forms of aquaculture, however, are associated with serious concerns because of the emissions associated with their use of pesticides, prophylactic antibiotics, and nutrients that contribute to eutrophication, particularly their use of other fish as feed (D. Cole et al. 2009; Naylor et al. 2009). More generally, about one third of all the fish who are caught has been estimated to be used to feed farmed animals, which is why many diets that include the latter are associated with large emissions (Goldburg and Naylor 2005, 23).

Though figures on the magnitude of its contribution vary between different studies, it is clear that current human consumption of animal products contributes a great deal to climate change. The extent to which this might be mitigated will vary greatly with the alternatives that are envisaged.

One alternative that has been proposed is to reduce methane emissions by dietary or pharmaceutical interventions, but Webster (2013, 41–43) mentions that these interventions raise health concerns for the animals who might be affected. Rather than modify ruminant fermentation, a better strategy might be to reduce the number of ruminants. At the same time, however, it must be borne in mind that any reduction in the number of farmed animals is likely to trigger an increase in wild and feral animals who would occupy some of the freed-up space. However, though some of these would also produce methane, a reduction in the number of farmed animals is still likely to be accompanied by a decrease in methane emissions.

This is so for various reasons. Firstly, populations of wild and feral animals tend to be less dense compared to those of farmed animals. Secondly, the metabolic rates of these animals would be slower compared to those of many farmed animals—for example compared to cows (such as the Holstein-Friesian breed) who have been bred to produce large quantities of milk—thus reducing methane emissions. And thirdly, many ruminants would be replaced by animals who do not ruminate. In Australia, for example, reductions in the populations of sheep and cows would be likely to be accompanied by a growth in the number of kangaroos, who produce far fewer greenhouse gas emissions (Hoedt et al. 2015). Drastic reductions may not be achieved everywhere, however, depending on which animals might replace farmed animals. In the USA, for example, methane emissions might still be high if farmed animals are replaced by the animals who roamed across the land before the arrival of European colonisers. One study calculates that, if it is assumed that there were about 50 million bison before the arrival of European colonisers, methane emissions from bison, elk, and deer may have been about 86% of current methane emissions from farmed ruminants (Hristov 2012). This is in line with another study, which argues that current ruminant methane production in the USA is probably no more than 20% greater than what it was 300 years ago (when the author estimates there may have been 60 million bison), which is partly attributable to the fact that ruminants kept in feedlots—also known as feed yards—produce less methane (Webster 2013, 43).

Webster (2013, 43) adds the valid point that a focus on mere emissions of methane or of other gases is inadequate in light of the fact that the total impact of the animals concerned on the quantities of detrimental gases in the atmosphere must be considered. In this regard, Webster (2013, 195) points at recent research into the potentially positive role played by grazers, who ingest silica which is then excreted to end up in rivers and eventually in the sea to feed diatoms, a particular type of algae, which take up carbon dioxide by photosynthesis (Mike Packer 2009). The idea is that greater numbers of grazers lead to greater quantities of silica in the sea, which in turn triggers an increase in the number of diatoms and a greater capture of carbon dioxide (Carey and Fulweiler 2015; Vandevenne et al. 2013). Whereas Webster (2013, 43)'s claim that 'well-managed grasslands constitute a significant carbon sink' is contested as a necessary condition for this to be the case is that they must have been managed relatively badly beforehand (see e.g. P. Smith 2014), to assess the real potential of grasslands to reduce negative climate change impacts more research is needed to compare this type of management with how other ways in which the land could be managed might affect the concentration of different gases in the atmosphere.

Some have also suggested that the numbers of current populations of some farmed animals could be reduced by the replacement of some animal products that are associated with high emissions by other foods that have been derived from animals and production chains that produce fewer emissions, for example grasshoppers and other insects (Vogel 2010). Meyers (2013, 119), for example, has argued that 'we ought to engage in and encourage *entomophagy*, the practice of eating insects'. He arrives at this conclusion in light of the claim that 'ten kilograms of plant food yields only three kilograms of pork and only one kilogram of beef', but to 'about nine kilograms of insect meat', which is partly because 'insects are cold-blooded' and 'do not waste fuel keeping their bodies warm' (Meyers 2013, 124). To this he adds that many insects produce far fewer emissions and can eat things that human beings cannot eat. Before sharing in Meyers' excitement, however, we would need not only more precise ecological impact assessments of how different insect-rearing practices affect the environment, but also to address whether grasshoppers and other insects should be valued instrumentally for human consumption, a question that will be addressed in chapter two.

Many scholars have argued that radical changes in human diets are required in light of the significant contributions of the farmed animals' sector to problems caused by climate change (Macdiarmid et al. 2012; Scarborough et al. 2012b; McMichael et al. 2007). More generally, I shall argue in section 1.6 that such changes are required in light of all the negative GHIs that have been described. A range of websites now exist that provide people with the tools to calculate some of the environmental impacts associated with their food choices, such as the Agri-footprint website (http://agri-footprint.com) and the UNS website (http://www.ulme.ethz.ch, in German). Without wishing to endorse any of these, the usage of this type of websites may help readers to calculate the environmental impacts of their dietary choices, as well as guide dietary policy-making.

1.6 The moral imperative to reduce negative GHIs

The question of what counts as a good diet should be considered in light of the question of what counts as a diet that minimises negative GHIs (or maximises positive GHIs). In light of the dietary impacts that have been described previously, individuals and governments that take seriously the imperative to safeguard the right of all human beings to health care must encourage citizens to minimise dietary negative GHIs. Many negative GHIs should be allowed to be produced provided that positive GHIs are maximised. For example, in the case of the cultivation of rice, the fact that rice requires much more water than many other crops may be outweighed by the greater nutritional benefits of its consumption relative to other crops that could be grown, by local soil and climatic conditions, by the greater cultural meaning of rice, or by a combination of any of these factors. This example also shows that negative and positive GHIs that are difficult to quantify should not be excluded from our moral evaluations— for example the amount of pleasure that people derive from eating particular foods, the degrees of importance that they give to particular risks and uncertainties (for example those related to zoonotic diseases), the benefits that some people derive from the traction power or from the aesthetic values that some animals may provide, or any deontological constraints that should be accepted to safeguard moral agents' duties to strive for holistic health, for example those related to any duties that we may have towards other animals.

People may disagree about whether moral agents have a duty to prioritise more important over less important interests (or a duty to maximise positive GHIs) and about which impacts should count as positive or negative GHIs. However, in my view, there is overwhelming evidence to substantiate the view that many people, particularly those who live in relatively affluent countries, produce negative GHIs that ought to be avoided. In earlier work I suggested that those who contribute to the emergence and spread of zoonoses by consuming a wide range of animal products produce negative GHIs that ought to be avoided (Deckers 2011b). Elsewhere I provided a positive answer to the question whether the consumption of some animal products contributes to the existence of human hunger (Deckers 2011c). This is borne out at least partly by the fact that the consumption of many animal products contributes to the increase in human hunger that is triggered by one domain of human activity that is being taken increasingly seriously: anthropogenic climate change.

The evidence that can be provided to support the view that many people produce merely through their contributions to climate change negative GHIs that ought to be reduced is overwhelming. Climate change is expected to become more and more dangerous if the average global surface temperature increases by more than 2°C relative to pre-industrial times. According to a study by the Intergovernmental Panel on Climate Change (IPCC), the atmospheric concentration of greenhouse gases was about 375 ppm (parts per million) in CO_2e in 2005, and concentrations will have to stabilise at or below that level to avoid a more than 2°C warming relative to the pre-industrial age (IPCC 2007a, 20). If this is the case, global anthropogenic emissions must be cut by 50–85% relative to the 2000 level by 2050 (Shellnhuber et al. 2006; European Commission 2007). The IPCC claims with 'high confidence'—which is defined in terms of an 8 out of 10 chance—that, if we continue with a business-as-usual emissions policy, millions of people will suffer from negative health impacts associated with climate change (IPCC 2007b, 48). In Southern Asia, for example, the health status of millions of people has already been compromised through flooding, which has been reported to happen 'more frequently and more severely than before' (Douglas 2009, 127). The more the agricultural sector contributes to climate change, the more agriculture itself will be jeopardised by the adverse effects that have been associated with climate change, including increased droughts and floods. Several studies indicate that these problems will manifest themselves more in countries where people currently are relatively poor, thereby increasing the risks of their rights to health care being jeopardised (P. Smith et al. 2007; Lang and Heasman 2004; Parry et al. 2007; Stern 2006).

In light of these concerns, many governments have recognised the moral case for radical reductions in greenhouse gas emissions. By passing the Climate Change Act 2008, the UK Parliament, for example, has committed to reducing emissions by 80% by 2050, relative to emission levels in 1990 (Climate Change Act 2008). Similarly, the Australian Government has expressed the view that an 80% reduction in greenhouse gas emissions by 2050 relative to emission levels in 2000 would represent 'a fair contribution from Australia' (DCCEE 2011, xi).

Greenhouse gas emissions, however, are not the only things that matter morally. The development of a broader understanding of the negative GHIs associated with many human activities is facilitated by the notion of 'ecological footprint' (Wackernagel and Rees 1996). This concept was coined by Wackernagel and Rees (1996) to represent the 'amount of biologically productive land and water area an individual, a city, a country, a region, or all of humanity uses to produce the resources it consumes and to absorb the waste it generates under current technology and resource management practices' (Kitzes and Wackernagel 2009, 813; Rees 2003, 898). Though materials that are neither created nor absorbed by biological processes, such as plastics, are not represented, 'ecological footprinting' does include the effects that such materials have on biological systems (Kitzes and Wackernagel 2009, 814). Carbon dioxide emissions are included within ecological footprints by calculating the area of forest that would be required to assimilate those emissions, an approach that has been criticised not only because there are other ways in which these emissions could be sequestered, but also because the used conversion rates are debatable (Van den Bergh and Verbruggen 1999). A similar problem underlies the calculation of the ecological footprint associated with the use of nuclear energy, which has been equalised with the amount of forest that would be required to offset the CO_2-equivalent of nuclear energy (Moran et al. 2009, 1943).

In spite of these limitations, the ecological footprint provides useful information to assess the magnitudes of some of our negative GHIs because of its inclusion of a broad range of ecological parameters. Whereas the GHI concept measures the impact of human actions on the health of all biological organisms in one common unit, the concept of ecological footprint measures the impact of human activities on the nonhuman environment in one common unit: the use of 'bio-productive' (biologically productive) space, or the quantity of biological resources that is used to provide for any particular human activity. This is usually expressed in terms of 'global hectares' ('gha'), the amount of land that is needed to produce any particular thing that is consumed and to deal with its waste using currently available technologies at average global productivity. Whilst health is affected by much more than by the use of bio-productive space, it has nevertheless been claimed that the ecological footprint is 'the most comprehensive and most widely adopted overall measure of threats to environmental sustainability', and this indicator has been understood as one of the most important ways to measure the impact of 'environmental stressors' on human health (Dietz et al. 2009, 118; Dwyer 2009). As such stressors also affect the health of nonhuman organisms, the ecological footprint of humans is also concerning for those who question our impact on the nonhuman world.

The fact that our collective ecological footprint is large provides a very strong indication that our negative GHIs are substantial. In 2008, 2.7 gha was the ecological footprint of the average person, but the amount of biologically productive water and land that was available in that year per person was calculated to be no more than 1.8 gha (WWF 2012, 44, 48). On this basis, Rees (2006a) has used Catton (1980)'s concept of 'overshoot' to refer to the fact that resources derived from biological organisms are consumed faster than the rate by which they are replenished. Great differences between different people's ecological footprints can be observed. In 2008, the average Bangladeshi used less than 1 gha, whereas the average person from many more affluent countries, such as Denmark, the USA, the UK, or Australia, used more than 4 gha (WWF 2012, 43). In addition, the USA combines a very large national ecological footprint with a significant increase in population (Ehrlich and Ehrlich 1997, 1198).

Both our collective ecological footprint and the existence of large differences between people's individual footprints are morally questionable. The problem with the former is that future generations will have to try to secure their rights to health care whilst reducing their ecological footprints substantially. Future generations might well be able to find novel ways to safeguard their rights, even if their 'earth capacity' will be much reduced. However, the probability that the rights of many future people will be compromised is great as the odds are stacked against many of our future fellows. Take for example the people of Bangladesh: no clear answer has as yet been provided in relation to the question of how they will be protected from the likelihood of the large-scale flooding of coastal zones that is either caused or increased by anthropogenic climate change. Similarly, the health status of many Bangladeshis who are alive today has already been affected negatively by the November 2007 floods, which are likely to have been caused wholly or partially by anthropogenic climate change (Afjal Hossain et al. 2012). The fact that some people satisfy many desires that are not strictly necessary to enjoy a decent standard of health and thereby accumulate large ecological footprints causes severe problems for other people whose rights to health care are undermined.

We must therefore address not only what overshooting countries should do to reduce their ecological deficit, but also how many resources and how much waste each of us should be allowed to, respectively, consume and produce, and how many children we should have, without jeopardising the rights to health care of others unfairly. To help with this task, ecological footprint calculators that gauge individuals' footprints are useful. However, it must be recognised that the ecological footprint is no more than an aid, rather than the ultimate criterion to determine the morality of human actions. Clearly, some activities may be detrimental to the health of biological organisms, even if they use relatively few resources and produce little waste. An example would be killing someone, which might be considered positive if our sole aim was to reduce the ecological footprint of the entire human population. This example shows that a relatively large negative GHI (such as that of killing someone) need not be associated with a relatively large ecological footprint. The reverse also holds true. A relatively large ecological footprint need not be associated with a relatively large negative GHI. Compare, for example, the ecological footprint of a factory that produces shoes at a greater ecological footprint per shoe than a factory that produces shoes at a smaller ecological footprint. Should the former produce shoes that are significantly better for human health, for example by reducing bacterial infections, its average GHI per produced shoe might be more positive than the latter's. In spite of these considerations, the ecological footprint provides an important indicator of ecological stresses that may jeopardise human rights to health care.

In light of the magnitude of our ecological footprint, some ethicists have claimed that the occurrence of 'more hunger' is a certainty (Gjerris et al. 2011, 346). Rather than adopt such a pessimistic stance, I argue that negative GHIs that are not needed to fulfil our duties must be eliminated.

1.7 Reducing negative GHIs through dietary changes

A small but increasing number of studies have argued that dietary changes are required to reduce a wide range of negative GHIs associated with our dietary choices (Reijnders and Soret 2003; Carlsson-Kanyama and González 2009;

Baroni et al. 2007; Peters et al. 2007; Compassion 2007; Eshel and Martin 2009; Macdiarmid et al. 2012; Scarborough et al. 2012b). Some studies compare vegan with omnivorous diets (Eshel and Martin 2006; Carlsson-Kanyama and González 2009; J. Davis et al. 2010; Berners-Lee et al. 2012). Readers who wish to engage with these studies in detail are referred to box 7. A systematic analysis of peer-reviewed studies that report the land requirements and the emissions of 49 dietary options provides some indication that a transition to vegan diets in the European Union might reduce total greenhouse gas emissions by up to 20% and the demand for land needed to fulfil human dietary requirements by up to 60%, but the authors are rightly cautious about these claims as the review does not consider how non-diet related environmental impacts, for example those associated with leather replacements or the associated changes in health care costs, might be affected by such a transition (Hallström et al. 2015). A further reason why caution is needed is that most studies that compare different dietary scenarios consider vegan diets that are relatively unprocessed, where more emissions are likely to be produced by more processed vegan diets. A more general reason to be cautious is that there is a great deal of uncertainty associated with the impacts of a radically transformed agricultural system. In spite of this need for caution, it is clear that many people who consume animal products produce many more negative GHIs by doing so compared to those who abstain from doing so, and that dietary shifts towards vegan diets could reduce negative GHIs considerably.

A study from the USA revealed that the mean diet of a USA citizen, which includes 27.7% of calories from animal sources (comprising 41% from dairy, 5% from eggs, and 54% from a range of animal bodies), produces at least 1.5 tonnes more emissions in CO_2e per year than the emissions produced by a vegan USA citizen (Eshel and Martin 2006, 13). To obtain some idea of how this compares with the emissions produced by personal transportation, the authors point out that the average number of miles travelled by a USA citizen in 2003 was 8,332 miles, producing between 1.19 and 4.76 tonnes of CO_2 emissions, depending on which vehicle was used (Eshel and Martin 2006, 2–3). Drawing on their knowledge of the emissions produced by different car models, the authors make an interesting analogy. If we imagine that a person adopting the mean USA diet drove an averagely efficient car, the Toyota Camry, and that a vegan compatriot drove one of the most energy-efficient hybrid vehicles on the USA market in 2006, the Prius, the difference in diet-related emissions (for a given quantity of food with equal caloric intake) would amount to the difference in emissions produced by the former driving 143 miles in the less efficient car and the latter driving 100 miles in the more efficient car (Eshel and Martin 2006, 2–3). To understand

(Box continued on next page)

(Box continued from previous page)

the magnitude of this difference, a different analogy could also be used: the difference in emissions between the person adopting the mean USA diet and the person adopting the vegan diet corresponds to the difference in emissions between driving 8,332 miles in one of the most efficient cars and not driving at all.

A UK study measured the greenhouse gas emissions associated with 61 food categories that are sold in a mid-sized UK supermarket chain and used FAO 2010 statistical data to calculate the amount of food that is currently used in the UK (Berners-Lee et al. 2012). The calculation yielded a total of 3,458 kilocalories (kcal) per person per day, which is significantly more than what is actually consumed, revealing that a large amount of food is wasted. Subsequently, they described six dietary scenarios—each providing 3,458 kcal per day—and calculated the emissions that would be associated with each of them. Greenhouse gas emissions were reduced most significantly in the three vegan dietary scenarios. The vegan diet that produced the fewest emissions was not particularly healthy, and will not be discussed further. The two remaining vegan scenarios provide interesting food for thought. One of them embodied emissions that were 23% lower than the UK average diet. This scenario was based on scaling up the self-reported diets of vegans in the USA (Haddad et al. 1999) to the kilocalories associated with current UK usage levels, including both actual consumption and wastage. The other diet, described as the 'thoughtful' vegan diet, contained the highest level of carbohydrates, the lowest of added sugar, and the lowest of fat. It embodied 5.6 kg emissions in CO_2e per day, which is 25% less than the average UK diet's emissions per day. Interestingly, its annual cost was also found to be £380 cheaper than the average UK diet (Berners-Lee et al. 2012). In this study, it was assumed that an equal amount of food would be wasted for all 61 food categories. The problem with this is that it may well misrepresent vegan diets, for at least two reasons. Firstly, as foods derived from animal products are likely to go off more quickly and to be discarded more quickly because of their greater risks of causing food-borne illnesses, it is highly likely that omnivorous diets contribute more to food waste. There is some evidence for this in the literature, as research found that more than half of all the flesh that is available for consumption in the UK is wasted (Aston et al. 2012). Secondly, research has found that many people who adopt vegan diets do so at least in part for environmental reasons, which may indicate that they are more

(Box continued on next page)

averse to wasting food than people who adopt different diets (Fox and Ward 2008). Accordingly, it is likely that the reductions in emissions for the vegan dietary scenarios would be greater than those reported here.

Different dietary scenarios were also discussed in a Swedish study, which compared the greenhouse gas emissions of three Swedish meal options. Depending on which kinds of animal products were chosen, the difference between the hypothetical vegan meal and the two hypothetical meals that included animal products varied between a factor of three and a factor of eight, in spite of the fact that the former included soy imported from Brazil (Carlsson-Kanyama and González 2009, 1708S). A different study by the same authors, published with an additional co-author, compared the energy costs and greenhouse gas emissions from 84 common foods up to their point of import in a Swedish port, revealing that the importation of vegan protein used much less energy and emitted far fewer emissions than protein derived from animal products (González et al. 2011). The same study found that animal products produced more emissions when they contained more protein, whereas the reverse applied for plant products and protein levels.

A wider range of impacts was explored in a study that estimated the environmental impacts of four different meals with roughly similar nutritional content by means of the life cycle assessment methodology, which aims to measure the 'cradle-to-grave' impacts of products (J. Davis et al. 2010). The four meals that were compared for hypothetical consumption in both Spain and Sweden were the following: 1/ a meal consisting of chopped pieces of pigs who had been fed with cereals and with soy meal imported to Europe from American countries, with potatoes, raw tomatoes, wheat bread, and water; 2/ a meal consisting of chopped pieces of pigs who had been fed with a feed based on peas, rapeseed, mostly European-grown cereals, and some imported soy meal from American countries, with potatoes, raw tomatoes, wheat bread, and water; 3/ a meal consisting of chopped pieces of pigs who had been fed in the same way as in the second scenario that were turned into a sausage that also contained 10% of peas, with potatoes, raw tomatoes, wheat bread, and water; 4/ a meal consisting of a burger made from peas grown in Europe, with potatoes, raw tomatoes, wheat bread, and water. In the Swedish scenario, it was assumed that all foods would be produced in Germany, except for the potatoes, which would be produced in Sweden, and the tomatoes, which would be produced in Spain. In the Spanish scenario, it was assumed that all foods consumed by people were produced in Spain.

(Box continued on next page)

(Box continued from previous page)

It was found that the energy use of the fourth option would be almost as high as the energy required for the other options as the assumption was made that these burgers would be sold and stored as frozen and that slightly more frying would be required because of the higher volume of the burgers compared to the fried items in the other meal options. The authors point out, however, that the study assumed that the pieces of pigs had been bought fresh, but that energy use would be much different had the assumption been made that these had been frozen. It was also found that the global warming contribution of the fourth option would be about half that of each of the other three options—which all had similar global warming contribution levels—in Sweden, but about two thirds of that of the meals that contained animal products for Spain, largely because the pea burger requires significant amounts of energy at the pea burger factory, the retailer, and the household level. The discrepancy between Spain and Sweden for the global warming contribution of the fourth scenario is attributed to the fact that the latter nation generates much more energy from nuclear power plants and water. Regarding the contribution to eutrophication, it would be less than half for the fourth option than the high levels associated with the other options, which is due primarily to the high quantities of nitrates and ammonia that are produced by pig farms. The contribution of the fourth option to acidification would be even lower compared to the other options. The authors did not calculate differences in land use, but point out that the fourth option would use considerably less land. Finally, rather than rely on processed pea burgers, many people in Sweden and Spain might actually prefer to eat raw or cooked peas, which can reasonably be expected to reduce energy costs quite considerably.

Other studies at European and global levels also report significant differences between diets that include and diets that exclude animal products, in favour of the latter (Tukker et al. 2006; Tukker et al. 2011; Stehfest et al. 2009; Foley et al. 2011). One study revealed that the farmed animals' sector contributes no more than 6% of all economic value in the European Union, but that it produces about 24% of all monetarised environmental impacts from the consumption of all goods (Weidema et al. 2008, 6). This finding suggests that the sector produces relatively large quantities of negative GHIs, even if the exact quantification of this will vary depending on which and how environmental impacts are measured.

Box 7: Comparing the negative GHIs associated with omnivorous and vegan diets

1.8 The case for a radical transformation of agriculture

Though some vegan diets produce fewer negative GHIs than other diets, two obstacles manifest themselves when the results of the studies that I have discussed in the previous section are used to stimulate dietary change towards veganism. The first is that they measure a limited number of negative GHIs that are associated with current production systems, rather than the negative GHIs that might be produced by very different agricultural systems. Future vegan diets would be very different from those that are adopted by vegans living today if they were accompanied by a shift—whether more or less radical—from our current mixed agricultural farming system towards a vegan system. Such a system would, for example, require very different methods to maintain or improve soil fertility, including a much greater reliance on the use of green manures (plants that are grown to provide manure for other plants) and human manure and urine, the latter of which are now frequently wasted, causing losses of nitrogen and—more importantly—phosphorus. The use of green manure could also be accompanied by the use of plant-based anaerobic digestion, which would produce digestate that is rich in nitrogen to stimulate plant growth and methane that could be used for energy purposes. It has also been remarked that such a system would need to rely more on chemical fertilisers (Korthals 2012); whereas this need not be the case if both green and human manures are used, there is no doubt that a radical shift to a vegan-organic system would pose a significant challenge in relation to the goal of maintaining and boosting soil fertility (Darlington 2010).

Reliable studies of how shifts to vegan diets might reduce negative GHIs must therefore incorporate estimates of the negative GHIs that might be produced by very different agricultural systems, where relatively little may as yet be known about how such systems might perform. Such estimates, however, would be highly relevant. For example, to determine whether sufficient fruits and vegetables would be available to provide for healthy diets in a particular location, it is important to know what kinds of foods could be grown in that area and how much they might yield. This does not imply that locally sourced diets will always produce the least negative GHIs, particularly as it has been shown that current transportation of foods accounts for a relatively small percentage of their greenhouse gas emissions (Weber and Matthews 2008; González et al. 2011).

The second problem is that we should not ignore the possibility that a reduction of negative GHIs in one domain of human activity might increase negative GHIs in another domain, or even overall. What we eat affects many other things. Accordingly, the negative GHIs of human diets should not be isolated from the negative GHIs of other human activities, for example the production of footwear. Should the adoption of a predominantly vegan agricultural system be associated with a decline in the supply of leather, for example, people would need to increase their production of non-leather shoes. Any uncertainties related to what kinds of shoes might be produced and how this might be done result in difficulties to estimate these shoes' potential negative GHIs.

The existence of these uncertainties might persuade some to favour conservative strategies that support (the development of) production systems that reduce the negative GHIs associated with the consumption of animal products, rather than to support strategies that aim to reduce their consumption as such. Many strategies could be adopted to reduce the negative GHIs associated with the consumption of animal products, including better manure management, changing from warm-blooded to more efficient cold-blooded animals, reducing negative GHIs associated with the slaughtering of animals and the distribution of their products, improving breeds of farmed animals and of plants used for their feed (for example through the genetic engineering of animals and plants), and developing lab-grown (also known as cultured, synthetic, or in-vitro) flesh. In a study funded by New Harvest, an organisation that supports this last technology, it is claimed that in-vitro flesh that is assumed to be able to be cultivated by using cyanobacteria as a growth medium might lower energy use, greenhouse gas emissions, and land and water usage very substantially compared to conventionally produced flesh in Europe, but the authors also point out that its public acceptance may be marred by public concerns over its unnaturalness (Tuomisto and de Mattos 2011), a theme that will be explored in section 2.12. Empirical research, however, has found that this is not the only thing that people are concerned about regarding in-vitro flesh, and that their concerns include issues of safety and taste (Hocquette et al. 2015; Laestadius and Caldwell 2015).

Whereas some of these technologies may reduce some negative GHIs considerably, the LEAD study has claimed that 'the environmental impact of livestock production will worsen dramatically … in the absence of major corrective features' (Steinfeld et al. 2006, 275). If this is so, it must be doubted whether approaches that merely aim at changing production will be sufficient, particularly since many studies estimate that reducing the sector's environmental impacts may turn out to be rather difficult (Weidema et al. 2008; Wirsenius and Hedenus 2010; McMichael et al. 2007). With regard to the sector's greenhouse gas emissions, for example, it has been claimed that a 20–25% reduction per unit of product derived from the bodies of animals might be possible (Weidema et al. 2008; DeAngelo et al. 2006). However, it must be doubted whether even modest reductions could be achieved, at least in the short term. A working group on agriculture for the IPCC concluded that 'little progress has been made in the implementation of mitigation measures at the global scale' (P. Smith et al. 2007, 500). Though the past may not be an accurate basis from which to predict the future, reducing the negative GHIs associated with the consumption of animal products significantly per unit of product may be difficult. Any technological progress that may be achieved must be situated within the context of future agriculture, which will be compromised by the negative impacts that have been produced in the past, including the decline in reserves of rock phosphate and fossil fuels, loss of soil fertility, land degradation, and water scarcity and pollution, as well as the negative impacts associated with atmospheric pollution. Any technological advances that might be made also rely on investments in science and its infrastructure, thus increasing emissions in the short term.

Even if significant reductions per unit of product might be achievable, the rapid adoption of diets that include (a greater quantity of) animal products is problematic in light of the fact that the human population is growing at an unprecedented rate, resulting in an increased demand for food (World Bank 2008; Royal Society 2009). On the basis of recent demographic and consumption trends, the LEAD study predicts that global demand for farmed animals' products will double by 2050 relative to the production level in 2000 (Steinfeld et al. 2006, 275). If this demand materialises, significant reductions in negative GHIs per unit of product may fail to bring about an overall reduction of negative GHIs. The argument has been made, however, that there is limited potential for further expansion of agricultural land, and that food increases will therefore have to come mainly from land that is in production already (Lal 2009). This may be difficult, especially because the gap between actual yields and maximum yields under ideal growing conditions is rather small in many countries (J. Huang et al. 2002). Whilst crop yields increased by 56% between 1965 and 1985, Foley et al. (2011) found that they only increased by 20% between 1985 and 2005. Indeed, serious questions have been raised over whether higher yields could be obtained without compromising long-term sustainability, particularly because these even higher yields are likely to be associated with large losses of phosphates and nitrogen (Smil 2011).

A further reason why merely reducing negative GHIs per unit of animal product does not go far enough relates to the fact that human beings need other things apart from food, for example energy. To replace fossil fuels, it is likely that an increasing amount of land will be required to provide energy in the future. The World Bank (2009) predicts that by 2030 even as much as 40% of our global grain production could be used as biofuels. Though this prediction may be wrong, the increase in pressure on agricultural resources from the energy sector provides further evidence to suggest that many diets that include relatively large quantities of animal products are highly problematic.

Clearly, conservative attempts to reduce dietary negative GHIs merely by altering production methods are grossly insufficient. I mentioned before that the UK Parliament, for example, has committed to reducing greenhouse gas emissions by 80% relative to its emissions in 1990 (Climate Change Act 2008). To obtain a better understanding of how drastic this reduction is, it must be borne in mind that it has been calculated that current dietary emissions in the UK are as high as 2.7 tonnes CO_2e per person per year, and that those who adopt a vegan diet sourced from within the current food production system have been estimated to reduce their emissions by no more than about 25% (Berners-Lee et al. 2012, 190). Given that total consumption-related emissions have been estimated to exceed a UK average of 14 tonnes CO_2e per year per person (Aston et al. 2012) and that they should total around 2.8 tonnes CO_2e to reach the 2050 target of an 80% reduction, it is extremely unlikely that this target could be reached if the average person's allocated quota was to be filled almost entirely by their dietary emissions alone.

Unless dietary changes are made, it would leave the average UK citizen with no more than an allowance of 0.1 tonnes CO_2e annually for non-diet related sources. The same applies to other citizens who live in countries with similar levels of emissions that may be committed to similar reductions. As such drastic reductions in non-diet related emissions seem totally unrealistic I would like to imagine what the world might look like if everyone who could adopt a diet that did not include animal products without compromising the right to health care of any human being would adopt such a diet. Though the answer to this question will vary between different areas, depending on social and ecological factors, I have selected the example of the United Kingdom, partly because Simon Fairlie (2010) has envisaged what 'a vegan permaculture' system might look like if it were adopted in the UK. This system would not only avoid synthetic fertilisers and pesticides, but also produce some biofuels, as well as some flax and hemp to produce 7.25 kg in textiles per person per year (replacing the wool and leather that is used for these purposes under the current system).

Fairlie (2010) estimates that such a system would be able to feed about eight people from one hectare of land. As there are currently about 61 million people in the country, approximately 7.7 million ha of the approximately 22 million ha of non-urban land that is available in the UK would be required to feed this population. Each person would be provided with 2,767 kcal of food per day, which is more than the recommended daily intake values (FAO/WHO/UNU 2001), thus allowing for some food waste. However, it can be expected that bodily energy needs would be higher than what they are today, as more people would carry out harder physical work under such a scenario than within the current agricultural system, which relies heavily on fossil fuels through the use of machinery, pesticides, and synthetic fertilisers, thus saving on human labour. More than 14 million ha of non-urban land would be left for non-arable purposes. Though there is no doubt that some of this land would need to be used for human purposes unrelated to food production, including the production of timber and firewood (Heaton et al. 1999), some land that would not be used for arable purposes could nevertheless still be used to produce food, for example by being cropped with fruit trees.

Fairlie's proposal is modelled largely on the kinds of foods that are currently produced in the UK, that is, cereals, potatoes, sugar, rapeseed oil, dried peas, vegetables, fruit, and nuts, where he envisages that over half of all the arable land would be occupied by cereals, potatoes, and rapeseed (for oil). These crops are currently frequently grown in large monocrops, which are notoriously poor in biodiversity. It is therefore likely that any vegan agricultural system that is more sustainable might look very different from the scenario depicted by Fairlie

(2010). Out of a concern for biodiversity, even if it were valued only to sustain a rather narrow conception of human health, we must move away from the large monocrops that now dominate world food markets, and seek new ways to increase variety through a renewed emphasis on growing (a broader range of) fruits and vegetables. Our current agricultural system jeopardises food security by focusing on a very narrow range of plant foods. The FAO has estimated that 75% of the plant varieties that were cultivated on farms in the beginning of the 20th century were no longer cultivated by its end; that human beings obtain about 60% of their calories from only three plants (rice, maize, and wheat); and that only about 200 of the 250,000 to 300,000 known edible plant species are consumed by us (FAO 2004). Whatever the precise form might be of a UK vegan agricultural system, such a system should increase the range of plants that are consumed and be accompanied by a move away from the few food crops that now dominate the UK, as well as the global, food market.

The negative GHIs that would be associated with such a system would be much smaller than those that are associated with the current UK agricultural system. Some of the benefits of a modified version of the system envisaged by Fairlie (2010) include: the avoidance of pesticides and synthetic fertilisers and a reduction in the use of fossil fuels; a greater diversity of plants grown for food, resulting in more varied diets and greater long-term food security; a reduction in the loss of phosphates and nitrogen and in the eutrophication process associated with such a loss; a reduction in acidification; and greater availability of land that can be reforested to produce timber and firewood. Fairlie's scenario would also eliminate food imports and must therefore also be amended where a good case exists for the importation of some vegetables and fruits with relatively small negative GHIs.

As omnivorous diets are associated with more negative GHIs than vegan diets in many locations, similar benefits can be expected if the global agricultural system was transformed into a predominantly vegan agricultural system. However, in light of what has been described in the introduction to this chapter, namely that the lives of some people currently depend on using animals, an exclusively vegan agricultural system would not be optimal to minimise negative GHIs unless it could be shown that removing their dependency would decrease negative GHIs. To assess this issue fully, as well as to assess comprehensively whether my case for a radical transformation of agriculture survives further scrutiny, the GHIs associated with any duties we may have towards the nonhuman world must be explored, an issue that will be addressed in chapter two.

1.9 Conclusion

Many human moral agents produce negative GHIs that ought to be avoided, jeopardising the rights to health care that are possessed by all human beings. Although not all diets that include animal products result in relatively large negative GHIs, I have shown that, in many eco-social settings, diets that include animal products produce more negative GHIs than vegan diets. Using the UK as an example, I argued that a wide range of diet-related negative GHIs could be reduced significantly if current agriculture was transformed into a predominantly vegan agricultural system. As I have ignored the GHIs of different human diets on the entities that make up the nonhuman world, it might be possible that the greater negative GHIs associated with many omnivorous diets are outweighed by the greater positive GHIs that such diets produce on the nonhuman world. The chapter that follows aims to document the GHIs that have so far been ignored to provide a holistic picture of the GHIs associated with human diets. Without this picture, it is not possible to assess which diets compromise each moral agent's duty to safeguard their holistic health. The conclusions that have been drawn here, however, stand firm in light of an assessment of all the interests that must be tended to in order to fulfil one's holistic health care duty.

CHAPTER TWO

The Ethics of Qualified Moral Veganism

2.1 Introduction

Whereas the first chapter abstracted any GHIs that may be associated with how other organisms ought or ought not to be treated by us from the argument, no assessment of the GHIs associated with the consumption of animal products can be complete without considering the impacts of such a consumption upon the nonhuman world and how these impacts affect moral agents. The consideration of these two last points is the objective of this chapter. Much of the literature in animal ethics has focused mainly on the concern that the consumption of animal products is frequently associated with the infliction of pain or suffering on animals (Singer 1975; Marcus 2001; Hills 2005; Safran Foer 2009; Cochrane 2012). Pain can be defined as an 'aversive sensation' associated with nociception, the latter of which in turn has been defined as 'the ability to perceive a noxious stimulus and react in a reflexive manner' (Barr et al. 2008, 745). Much debate has been held over the question of which animals might be capable of experiencing pain, which can be distinguished from nociception as the latter perception of a noxious stimulus can be unconscious. An example of nociception that does not trigger pain sensations is provided by Palmer (2010, 13), who discusses a study reported by McPhail (1998) that showed that nociception continues in human beings with severed spines who report not to be in pain.

The capacity to feel pain must also be distinguished from the capacity to suffer. A very small number of people are born with congenital insensitivity to pain as they lack functional nociceptors, which Varner (2012, 110–111) defines as 'specialised elements of the peripheral nervous system whose function is to respond to damaging or potentially damaging stimuli'. People who lack functional nociceptors may nevertheless still be able to suffer, for example from the emotional impact of not being able to register tissue damage. This might occur, for example, when they fail to withdraw from a hot surface and consequently

How to cite this book chapter:
Deckers, J 2016 *Animal (De)liberation: Should the Consumption of Animal Products Be Banned?* Pp. 51–105. London: Ubiquity Press. DOI: http://dx.doi.org/10.5334/ bay.c. License: CC-BY 4.0

sustain burns. The reverse is also possible. Masochists are able to feel pain, but they do not appear to suffer from feeling some kinds of pain. If individuals are capable of experiencing either pain or suffering, it is appropriate to say that they are sentient. More precisely, sentience is associated with the capacity to experience pain or suffering, as well as its reverse, the capacity to experience pleasure or joy.

In this chapter I shall recount some personal experiences that I have had with some of the main groups of animals who are used for human food purposes, complemented by the experiences of others. The aim of this exercise is to provide a reasonably good picture of how animals fare in the food industry. It will thus become clear that the human consumption of animal products supports practices that inflict pain and suffering on numerous animals. This will be followed by a discussion of the moral relevance of sentience in section 2.6 and by other sections where I shall identify and discuss the moral relevance of a number of other concerns associated with how human beings regard and treat other animals. A new moral theory will be developed to address these concerns: 'qualified moral veganism'. Those who are familiar already with how animals are treated in the food industry may wish to skip the ensuing sections (2.2–2.5) to continue reading from section 2.6.

2.2 The lives of chickens

On one of the farms where I used to help out, the chickens were kept in tiny cages that each held four birds. There were long rows of these battery cages, and a big lagoon of droppings underneath them collected the excrement that fell through the wired mesh of each cage. Hens were placed in the cages when they arrived from chicken breeders, just before they started laying. At this stage, they had already been debeaked to avoid injuries from pecking at each other. Whereas pecking is a normal activity for chickens, excessive pecking at each other is an example of redirected behaviour, which Webster (2013, 76) defines as normal behaviour that is directed at the wrong object and which he identifies, together with stereotypic (aimlessly repetitive) behaviour, as signs of frustration and deprivation. Debeaking is a process whereby about one fourth of the beak of the chick is removed by means of an electrically heated blade that cauterises the chick's blood vessels as part of the animal's beak is snipped off.

After they had arrived to live on the farm, chickens left their cages either after they had died or when they were transported to the slaughterhouse. They experienced little daylight during their lives, could hardly move, and spent their entire lives on metal wires. Profit margins were tight, so that all chickens would be sent off to the slaughterhouse when the costs of keeping them outweighed their yield in eggs. They were then replaced by new chickens and the whole process would start again. The male chicks who were bred by the people who bred these hens were killed as soon as they had hatched. I am not sure how this occurred, but a common method that is still used today to dispatch of these useless birds is to gas them. Marcus (2001, 102–103) also claims that the practice of throwing them into plastic bags where they are slowly smothered under the weight of other chicks is applied widely, as is the practice of killing them by means of a grinder.

Chickens would actually lay more eggs if they were looked after better, for example by reducing the number of birds placed in each cage, but the reason why this tends not to happen is that it would reduce the number of eggs that would be produced per cage. Financially, it pays more to stack a larger number of chickens into each cage than to reduce the number of birds who live in each one of them. According to Marcus (2001, 106), stocking densities have now increased to a density of five birds per surface area no bigger than 30.5 by 50.8 cm for the vast majority of 'layers'—the name given to hens who are kept to lay eggs—who are kept in the USA today. Even more restrictive space allowances have been reported for India, Brazil, and Ukraine (Hawthorne 2013, 18). In the European Union, however, conventional battery cages have recently been phased out, as Council Directive 1999/74/EC was fully implemented in 2012. The directive allows enriched or 'furnished' cages to be used, which must contain litter, roosts, and 'claw-shortening devices' (scratch mats), and which must be at least 45 cm high and provide each bird with at least 750 cm² of space, including 150 cm² for a nest-box (Council Directive 1999/74/EC). Webster (2013, 215) claims that evidence supports the view that these enriched cages cater for the welfare of chickens as well as many free-range systems (see e.g. M. Appleby et al. 2002). Whereas it is unclear why this is concluded, it may relate to the fact that mortality in furnished cage systems has been documented to be lower than in any other systems, and foot health tends to be better—as the incidence of footpad dermatitis and bumblefoot tends to be lower (Sherwin et al. 2010). At the same time, parasitic diseases tend to be more common, and the range of behaviours displayed has been observed to be more limited (Lay et al. 2011). In addition, some furnished systems have also been associated with an increased risk of cloacal cannibalism (Moinard et al. 1998).

When birds are kept in tiny cages and become aggressive with each other, they cannot escape from each other's company, resulting in injury and death. When ventilation systems fail or are inappropriate, many birds can die from overheating, a problem that may aggravate with climate change. Marcus (2001, 107) and Loughnan (2012, 60) also describe the practice of forced moulting, whereby birds are kept in the dark for a long period of time and their food intake is withdrawn for up to two weeks or altered to a very-low-nutrient diet in the hope that this will stimulate moulting and boost egg production afterwards. This practice may trigger stress, greater morbidity—caused, for example, by *Salmonella* Enteritidis—and death for a large number of chickens. After about one and a half to two years of laying, all chickens are replaced by new chickens who lay more eggs. I remember participating in a process that was called 'the catching of chickens', a process whereby birds are pulled out of their cages and transferred to crates that are loaded on trucks to transport them to the slaughterhouse: I used to pull all the chickens out of each cage, hold each chicken by one of their feet, walk down the corridor, and put them inside the crates used to transport them. This appears to be common practice, and many hens sustain leg injuries as a result of being carried in this way (Broom 1990).

Chickens are by far the land animals the most frequently consumed by humans in the world, accounting for more than 80% of all flesh consumption (Weis 2013). In Australia, for example, the per capita consumption of chickens increased from half a bird per year in 1950 to 27 birds per year in 2010 (Wallis 2014). Broiler chickens—who are named after the way in which they are cooked—are different varieties of chickens who put on weight faster compared to hens who are kept because they lay eggs. This is why male chicks of breeds kept for laying are considered to be useless, resulting in their being killed at the hatchery. Unlike chickens who are kept because of the fact that they lay eggs, chickens who are kept for their flesh are housed on concrete floors. Stocking densities have been reported to average between 10 and 20 birds per square metre in the USA and in Australia (Marcus 2001, 110; Loughnan 2012, 56). In the European Union, the law makes their individual lives abstract by expressing stocking densities in terms of kilograms per square metre. Stocking densities should not normally exceed 33 kg/m^2, even though they could be allowed to reach up to 42 kg/m^2 under specific conditions (Council Directive 2007/43/EC, art. 3). If we add the fact that chickens currently weigh about 2.4 kg at slaughter (Tuyttens et al. 2014), it can be concluded that the European Union allows the co-existence of up to 17 mature birds per square metre.

Breeds that are used today put on seven times more flesh around their breast by the time they are eight-weeks-old than did nine-week-old chickens around their breastbones in 1976 (Marcus 2001, 109). As the chickens used today grow older, their movement becomes more and more restricted. As they are fed high-protein diets, they grow so fast that their bones find it hard to support this rapid increase in weight, leading to a wide range of problems, including lameness. Other problems include leg deformities, dislocated joints, fractures, and various metabolic disorders, including convulsions and ascites, a disease of the liver related to fluid build-up in the abdominal cavity. Blisters, hock burns, and footpad deformities are also common as birds spend a lot of time lying down (Turner 2010). Many of these problems are particularly present in those animals who are kept for reproductive purposes: as they live longer than their offspring, their particularly large size poses significant health problems (Webster 2013, 31).

Most chickens who are kept for their eggs or their flesh are kept in vast barns where many processes that are used to look after them are automated, so that the amount of attention that each bird receives from farmers is reduced to a minimum. By consequence, farmers are unlikely to identify birds who are in poor health. Incidentally, most turkeys are kept in a very similar fashion. Because genetic selection has been so successful in increasing the size of turkeys, they can no longer mate—which Webster (2013, 180) claims does not present any welfare issues; this is why turkey farmers use artificial insemination to breed turkeys.

The vast majority of chickens do not die naturally. Most are killed in slaughterhouses. For most chickens who are kept for their flesh, this happens within 40 days after hatching; for most hens kept for their laying qualities, this happens about a year and a half after birth. Chickens are hung upside down on a conveyor belt with their feet in overhead shackles before they are killed. Chickens may suffer from inversion (being hung upside down) and suspension as they do not experience this posture at any other stage during their lives. In a research project funded by the UK's Department for Environment, Food and Rural Affairs, it was shown that the 'welfare' of chickens might be slightly improved when their breasts are supported before they enter the water bath used to kill them, yet breast support conveyors appear to increase the risk of birds disengaging their legs from the shackles (Lines et al. 2011). Some birds have wide legs that do not fit easily into these shackles, so that their legs may be pulled hard to make them fit into the shackles, resulting in compression. Birds tend to become agitated, which causes bruising, and wing flapping causes haemorrhaging of the wing tips. Shackling is known to cause pain, particularly for birds with joint problems and bone fractures, some of which they may sustain through being handled.

After being shackled, chickens move towards electrified water baths where their heads touch water that is charged electrically in order to stun them, which aims to cause loss of consciousness and to induce cardiac arrest. Some birds touch this water with their wings first, which results in their sustaining small electric shocks before being stunned. Research has shown that many birds are not stunned effectively and that they therefore either recover consciousness or do not lose consciousness before the next stage (Shields et al. 2010). It has also been found that some birds are stunned inappropriately by the process taking place too slowly. Some birds who appear to be unconscious may actually not be, but merely be undergoing muscular paralysis. The food quality of the corpse that is used for human consumption is influenced by the frequency of the electric shock that passes through the animal, which is why many birds are not stunned in such a way that they lose consciousness. Stunning efficacy is also influenced by many other factors, including the presence of other birds, the quality and resulting conductivity of the water in the water bath, the depth and duration of immersion, the size of the water bath, the size and nature of the birds, and the nature and tightness of the shackles (Hindle et al. 2010).

After being stunned, chickens are pulled through a tunnel and meet a rotating blade that makes a ventral neck cut that may sever either one or both of the chicken's carotid arteries in the neck. Cutting both arteries has been found to be most effective at bringing about a quick death. Chickens are known to regain consciousness if this takes place too long after stunning, or if the cut is inadequate, which has been shown to occur due to differences in bird size; some slaughterhouses decapitate birds immediately after stunning, but this does not lead to immediate loss of consciousness in the severed head. The chickens then move through a scald tank of boiling water and their feathers are plucked out. Those animals who had not yet been killed now drown and burn in the boiling water. Their feet and heads are then cut off, and they are eviscerated. Finally, they are packed for sale (Shields et al. 2010). As many of these processes inflict pain on these animals, some have suggested that alternative systems should be developed; one of these alternative systems could be 'controlled atmosphere killing', a method that uses gas to render birds unconscious, but it has been remarked that many slaughterhouses may find this system 'too expensive to implement' (Lines et al. 2011, 129).

2.3 The lives of pigs

I used to help out on pig farms too. The numerous health risks associated with intensive pig farming have been well-documented and are summarised by Webster (2013, 142). I shall not list them here as I prefer to focus on the systemic problems that underlie these more specific health issues.

The vast majority of pigs who are kept for their flesh are kept inside barns where they are crowded together and experience no or little daylight until they are herded into trucks to be transported to the slaughterhouse. They are kept on concrete slats, which reduce labour requirements as excrement falls in between the slats to be stored in lagoons inside concrete pits under the pigs' living spaces. The farms where I worked were no exceptions: sows were kept in sow stalls and farrowing crates, which are known to increase the risk of lameness, for long periods of time. Sow stalls are metal-barred crates that measure no more than a few metres long and less than a metre wide. The sows could stand in them but not turn around. The sows were confined even more when they were moved, just before giving birth, into farrowing crates, where they lacked opportunities to engage in nesting behaviour. The main purpose of these latter crates is to keep the sows as immobile as possible during the early days of nursing, to avoid piglets being crushed between the sow's weight and the concrete floor on which she stands.

Whereas the European Union has now banned the use of sow stalls during the early stages of pregnancy (Council Directive 2008/120/EC), it is worth pointing out that the problems associated with spatial confinement have been aggravated by a change in consumer preference, developed over the last 50 years, for less fatty flesh (Webster 2013, 31): this triggered a trend to kill pigs at earlier stages of their lives, when they were significantly smaller and leaner than their mature-sized mothers, who have been selectively bred to reach a very large size when they reach maturity.

On the farms where I worked, piglets were kept with their mothers until they were big enough to be weaned off, when they were about three weeks old.

Webster (2013, 143) comments on this practice as being 'profoundly unphys-iological' as their intestines are not well-adapted to this dietary change and they struggle to keep warm, necessitating the purchase of expensive feed and machinery to keep them warm inside buildings that are kept as sterile as pos-sible, as well as vaccines and antibiotics. In the earliest stages after weaning, the piglets would be most susceptible to enteritis and post-weaning multi-systemic wasting syndrome (PMWS). By that time, males had been castrated, their needle teeth had been clipped, and their tails had been docked, all without anaesthetic. Tail-biting is an example of redirected and stereotypic behaviour for which the main risk factors appear to be a lack of space and a lack in oppor-tunities to forage (Taylor et al. 2010); tail-docking results in the creation of amputation neuromas, which increases the sensitivity of the docked tail, thus acting as an incentive for the pig to avoid being bitten. Both tail-docking and the reduction of corner teeth are now illegal in the European Union unless 'there is evidence that injuries to sows' teats or to other pigs' ears or tails have occurred' (Council Directive 2008/120/EC, annex 1, chapter 1, par. 8), but research has found that this law is flouted routinely (Lerner and Algers 2013). All of these practices are measures that aim to reduce aggression or the conse-quences thereof. Castration is also supposed to improve the taste of pigs, and to speed up the rate of growth. Aggression increases with high stocking densities, which are maintained in many systems so that pigs gain weight rapidly, rather than expend energy on moving. Hormonal growth promoters—synthetic hor-mones that were created about 30 years ago, such as porcine somatotropin—are also used in some countries to the same effect of rapid weight gain (Marcus 2001, 121–122; Wolfson and Sullivan 2004, 218).

Because many pigs were in such poor shape at the farms where I helped, sev-eral pigs died from heart attacks or had to be given drugs whilst they showed signs of breathlessness when I helped to transfer them between buildings or to herd them on to the trucks that moved them to the slaughterhouse when they were about half a year old. Pigs do not always move easily in the direc-tion in which farmers want them to move. Shouting and slapping were some of the methods used to make pigs move in the desired direction. The mixing of pigs who are not familiar with each other has also been reported to increase stress, as well as has the fact that pigs are not provided with opportunities to forage, a lack of opportunity which encourages bar-chewing and tail-biting. Webster (2013, 144) interprets that these behaviours are not primarily aggres-sive acts, but acts that stem from the animals' frustration at being kept in thor-oughly uninteresting surroundings, a situation that cannot easily be remedied by the provision of enriched environments—now mandatory in the European Union—as pigs become bored quite easily with things like tennis balls as they do not offer rewards, whereas 'ethologists will recognise similarities in the behaviour of sows foraging for worms in the mud and punters working the slot machines in Vegas'. One farm that I worked for also used plastic tubs suspended on cables from barn ceilings to try to reduce boredom, which presumably also would have done little to help the cause. Marcus (2001, 116) documents that in typical farms in the USA each pig may not receive more than 12 minutes of human care during his or her lifetime.

When pigs are taken to the slaughterhouse, they are often moved to where the workers want them to be by means of electric prodders. Pigs are slaughtered after being stunned, which aims to make them unconscious. This can happen by various means: an electric current can be applied to the head to cause a grand mal seizure; a bolt can be fired through the skull by means of a captive bolt pistol; or they can be gassed using CO_2. The use of this last method appears to be increasing, as other methods are deemed to pose greater welfare concerns (Atkinson et al. 2012). The pigs are then shackled and hoisted up before being stuck in the neck with a sharp knife that aims to cause the pigs to bleed to death. Sometimes, this takes a considerable amount of time, so that some pigs regain consciousness before dying (Anil et al. 2000). The pig's body is then submerged in hot water where a pig scalder removes the pig's hair. Big scissors and a blow-torch may also be used in this process. The pig is then eviscerated, and the head is usually removed, as well as the body cut into two halves. The body is subsequently fragmented and processed further before being consumed.

2.4 The lives of cows

I worked on three dairy farms too. In the 1970s cows were tethered continuously during the winter months and milked in the places where they stood. In the summer months they would spend a lot of time in the field and come into the stable twice a day to be tethered while they were being milked and provided with additional feed. Each cow had their own place in the stable, and the name of each cow was written on the rafters that stretched out across the stable to support the roof underneath which the cows lived. I remember some of their names, including Nora, a cow whom I held in admiration, as she had defied the odds merely by still being alive whilst she was already about 12-years-old. Most cows had long gone by then as the cost of replacing them by a younger cow who produced more milk and had fewer health problems was smaller than the cost of keeping the older cow. By the 1980s this system had changed: cows were no longer tethered in their stables, so that they could move around more in what is known as a 'loose house'. Milking took place by cows learning to queue up outside the milking parlour, which they would enter in order to be milked whilst being fed concentrated feed pellets. Automated systems now read the computerised information held on a chip around each cow's neck to provide them with the correct quantity of pellets that they need for optimal production.

These systems are now used very widely. The fact that cows have been able to move around in stables since the 1980s means that the farmer has less of an incentive to send their cows out into the field. Many farms now operate systems whereby dairy cows spend their whole productive lives inside stables while all their food is brought to them. Even if this suppresses natural grazing behaviour and increases the risks of disease triggered by inadequate bedding, cubicles, and nutrition (Webster 2013, 127), farmers may still lose money by sending their cows out into the field as any energy that is spent walking around by the cow is energy that is not spent on producing milk. Cows now produce about twice as much milk as they did 40 years ago. It is almost impossible to find cows who are allowed to live as long as Nora lived for. By the time they are about four- to six-years-old, most cows are killed to be replaced by younger cows who produce more milk (Whitaker et al. 2004). In order to produce as much milk as possible, dairy cows are inseminated about three months after they have delivered their first calf. This process is repeated after every new calf they deliver to maintain high milk yields. Cows are also routinely de-horned, a process whereby cows' horns are removed to reduce risk of injury to the farmer.

As dairy herds are not as suitable for the production of flesh as other breeds—such as the Belgian Blue with their 'double-muscling' traits, who are bred specifically because their muscles develop much more quickly—in dairy herds many male calves and a smaller number of females who are surplus to requirements are shot as soon as they are born. Calves who are not killed are frequently taken away from their mothers immediately after birth, and one of the farmers I used to help out uses 'the bag' (an oesophagal feeder) for calves who do not learn to suck from a rubber teat shortly after they are born: a plastic tube that is connected to a bag filled with colostrum (the milk that is produced just after the birth) is inserted into the mouth of the calf and a valve is opened once the farmer thinks the tube sits deep enough in the calf's throat. Sometimes the tube is inserted in the wrong place, in the windpipe rather than in the oesophagus, resulting in the milk being released inside the calf's lungs, with lethal consequences.

The same farmer has also used recombinant bovine somatotropin (rBST), also known as recombinant bovine growth hormone, which is produced by genetically engineered bacteria. Its use is banned in the 27 countries of the European Union as well as in some other countries, but is legal in more than 40 countries (Fredeen 2006). When I asked him why he used this, he answered that it increased milk profits as the cost of each injection of rBST was smaller than the price of the additional milk the cow would consequently produce. Any other concerns that he may have had were side-lined. I am unsure whether the farmer in question still uses rBST, but its use has declined in the USA in recent years, which Webster (2013, 71) attributes to the fact that its use was demanding so much from cows who were already stretched to the limits of productivity that it was unsustainable.

Research has found that cows who receive rBST have increased risks of mastitis and lameness, but that these concerns may not be significant enough for farmers to avoid its use because of cows' increased productivity (Dohoo et al. 2003; Fredeen 2006). Together with a perceived lack of fertility and unacceptable yield, the two conditions of mastitis and lameness are, however, the most common reasons given by UK dairy farmers in relation to why they send their animals away to be slaughtered (Whitaker et al. 2004). Mastitis is a very common inflammation of the udder that has increased in frequency as bacteria have more opportunities to enter the udder due to selective breeding for greater milk production (Turner 2010). Cows nowadays spend more time on milking machines, unless these machines pull harder to get the milk out—where malfunctioning machines that pull too hard are a significant concern related to mastitis. Lameness, which can manifest itself in various forms, including infections of the horn of the cloven hoof or of the surrounding skin, is also very common. Webster (2013, 72, 131) estimates that it features in about a quarter of dairy cows, resulting in 'more or less severe pain', and he identifies inadequate foot hygiene and the use of wet silage (instead of dry hay) as major concerns.

Veal is the name given to the flesh taken from calves. Most veal is produced from dairy breeds, as almost all bull and about three quarters of heifer calves are not needed by the dairy industry. There are at least three different kinds of veal. 'Bob veal' is produced from slaughtered calves when they are no more than a few days old. Formula-fed or 'milk-fed' veal is produced from calves who are fed a diet that contains milk as well as other things, and that is deliberately low in iron, making the calf anaemic. This produces flesh that is light in colour. These calves are slaughtered when they are about 16 to 20 weeks old. Veal that is darker in colour is produced from calves who are killed when they are slightly older and who have been fed a more varied diet. The rennet that is found within calves' stomachs is also used to produce cheese. Some calves are tethered and kept in crates wherein they can hardly move, which results in their flesh being tender. To this effect, they are also fed very restrictive diets, increasing their chances of contracting pneumonia, diarrhoea, and abomasal ulceration (which is associated with high milk diets). They are also kept in the dark, as well as in isolation from other animals. Several jurisdictions have now banned the use of crates, including Australia and the European Union, but the practice continues in many other countries (Webster 2013, 139).

Beef is the name given to the flesh that is taken from cows and bulls who are usually from non-dairy breeds. Many of these bulls are turned into steers by being castrated, usually without anaesthetic. To identify the animals, some are branded, a process whereby a mark is burned on their bodies. Tags that may be pierced through the animals' ears may also be used for this purpose. Some breeds, for example the Belgian Blue, are so big—partly because of careful selection for a natural genetic mutation in the myostatin gene—that they struggle to give birth naturally. Many animals are delivered by caesarean section, causing injury and pain to the cow. As many cows are out in the field, farmers may not notice for a long time that their cows are in distress, particularly if they possess large numbers of them. Many cows who are kept primarily for their flesh enjoy outdoor lives, but this necessitates a lot of chasing by farmers. I remember an incident when a cow was chased for several hours after she had escaped from the field.

Whilst many cows, bulls, and steers who are raised primarily for the nutritional value of their bodies spend parts of their lives in fields, many are moved to feedlots during the last few months before they are slaughtered. Here, the animals are locked up into outdoor pens and their diet is changed from one that consists mainly of grass to one that is very high in grain. The extra calories and protein fatten them up, but the animals' digestive systems are not able to cope very well with this new diet. Feedlot illnesses are mainly caused by these inappropriate diets. They include acidosis (a digestive condition), laminitis (a condition affecting the horny laminae of the hoof), ergot poisoning (through grain contaminated with ergot fungus), polioencephalomalacia (PEM, caused by vitamin B1 deficiency), vitamin A deficiency, bladder stones (caused by the overconsumption of phosphorus, which is fed as a supplement to some animals), and urea poisoning (Webster 2013, 136; Loughnan 2012, 51–52). Bovine respiratory disease is also common amongst feedlot cows and stems from cows having been subjected to a range of stresses (Engler et al. 2014). Ionophore poisoning also occurs where cows are given synthetic growth promoters, which are allowed in many countries (Kart and Bilgili 2008). Apart from these diseases, foot lameness, diarrhoea, and pneumonia are also common (Webster 2013, 137).

The 'shackle and hoist' method used to be the dominant mode in which cows, bulls, and steers were slaughtered: animals were shackled on one of their legs and lifted into the air before their throats were cut. They would often suffer broken bones and torn ligaments before being slaughtered. Whereas many Jews and Muslims still prefer slaughter to occur in this way (Farouk et al. 2014), motivated by their respectively kosher and halal traditions, most animals are now hoisted into the air after being stunned in a box that restrains them: a captive bolt stunner or pistol is used to drive a bolt, made out of an alloy such as stainless steel, through the skull of the animal, in the hope that this will render the animal unconscious soon after. Exsanguination is then attempted by cutting the main veins or arteries in the throat or by a stab in the chest close to the heart. I am unaware of the extent to which concerns about the spread of mad cow disease via brain tissue may have altered stunning practices in slaughterhouses, but Grandin (2014) has written that 'effective stunning and reducing skull fracturing are two opposite goals', where the latter goal serves to reduce the risk of people contracting nvCJD.

2.5 The lives of fish

I used to engage in recreational fishing too. Fish include animals from several taxonomic groups. The more than 32,000 species that have been identified make up more than half of all vertebrate species (C. Allen 2013). In relation to this diversity, C. Allen (2013) mentions the interesting anecdote that the coelacanth is more closely related to us than to tuna, who themselves are more closely related to us than to sharks.

Even if I used to fish as a child, there has never been any doubt in my mind that fish are capable of suffering and that fishing inflicts suffering. Whilst some scholars deny that fish are sentient (e.g. Rose et al. 2014), some animal welfare scientists have conjured up sophisticated experiments to determine whether fish might suffer, and many provide a positive answer when they interpret the findings resulting from these experiments (Chandroo et al. 2004; Braithwaite 2010).

Many fish may live far better lives than farmed animals as they are allowed to live relatively free from human intervention until they are caught. This freedom allows them to behave in the self-directed ways for which there is much less scope in factory farms. However, the number of fish who are used for human consumption is much greater than the number of other animals who are consumed. Modern boats benefit from ever more sophisticated methods to catch fish, including bottom trawling, which has already damaged more than 50 million km^2 of seafloor, which is partly why a recent review states that 'humans have had profoundly deleterious impacts on marine animal populations', even if this has been 'less severe than defaunation on land' (McCauley et al. 2015, 1255641–5). Whilst fish from approximately 1,500 species are caught, about half of all fish who are now consumed have lived in aquaculture systems, a number that has increased rapidly in recent decades (Anthony et al. 2013). The farming of some fish, such as salmon, also results in significant impacts upon their wild relatives, as large quantities of wild fish are caught, killed, and used to feed farmed fish (Naylor et al. 2009).

Aquaculture is sometimes called the 'Blue Revolution', comparably with the 'Green Revolution' that greatly increased agricultural production in less affluent countries. This rise in productivity has been associated with significant animal welfare concerns. Mason and Finelli (2006, 110) refer to aquaculture as 'the factory farming of aquatic species'. Various health concerns have been reported (Bergqvist and Gunnarson 2013). These include malformations of the spine resulting from the lack of genetic diversity in many species who are bred for maximal productivity and fast growth, as well as from environmental factors, for example the keeping of fish at water temperatures that are unhealthy for them and their being provided with inadequate nutrition. Other concerns include injuries and stress caused by handling and by hormonal injections and vaccinations that are administered to control, respectively, spawning and exposure to diseases. Female fish may also experience stress whilst being subjected to a process called 'strip-spawning', whereby they are taken from the water and squeezed to extract their eggs (Hawthorne 2013, 32). Bergqvist and Gunnarson (2013, 78–83) also report increases in aggression, stress, and injury in some species, increases that are associated with inadequacies in water quality, housing systems, stocking densities, feeding methods, and transfer systems such as the pumps and pipes that are used to transport farmed fish. Finally, aquaculture also traps migratory fish, for example salmon, preventing them from engaging in natural behaviour.

Further concerns include the effects of fish farms that are situated in oceans or rivers on wild fish who come into close contact with their farmed relatives and who may contract their diseases without having the benefits of all the drugs that the farmed species are given. Fish are frequently crammed together in small cages that provide good environments for the spread of disease, for example infection by sea lice (Mason and Finelli 2006, 111). Fish farms use a wide range of pharmaceuticals to keep these diseases at bay, and this also results in negative health impacts on other species. Some anti-parasitic drugs that have been used to treat sea lice infestation in Atlantic salmon, for example, have been found to be toxic to lobsters and shrimps when they were exposed to these drugs in high concentrations (Haya et al. 2001). Another concern is that many farmed fish escape from fish farms and interbreed with wild relatives, which may reduce the genetic variety and resilience of the latter. A related concern is that wild species may be transformed radically now that the commercial use of one genetically engineered species, a type of salmon, has been legally approved in the USA (Issatt 2013; Waltz 2016).

A range of concerns have been raised in relation to the methods that are used to kill fish. In the days when I engaged in recreational fishing, we used hooked fly maggots or worms to lure fish, and sometimes we impaled other fish on hooks in our attempts to catch pike. These methods are also used by many others in the fishing industry. Most fish, however, are caught in nets, which can injure other animals and cause severe damage to underwater ecosystems. Fish who are caught by deep-sea trawlers are dragged from the bottom of the sea. The presence of large numbers of fish stresses the animals, and many fish die before they are hauled on board by being crushed under the weight of other fish, resulting in death by injury and suffocation. Those who are still alive when they are on board either die from being cut open when they are being 'cleaned' or are left to die whilst being stored in ice water, which results in anoxia. Some species lose consciousness only after several hours of being immersed in ice. Other stunning and slaughtering methods include clubbing, spiking, gassing (leading to narcosis), bleeding, and electrocution. In the Netherlands, eels are also killed by immersion in salt baths followed by evisceration, during which they can remain conscious for several hours (Bergqvist and Gunnarson 2013, 85–87).

2.6 The moral imperative to take sentience seriously

From the account presented in the preceding sections—which has focused on the main categories of animals who are used for human food, but could be complemented by other reports and personal experiences with other animals who are also used for human consumption—it should be clear that the consumption of animal products inflicts a lot of pain and suffering (see also Brambell 1965; FAWC 2009). Whilst the infliction of pain can sometimes be positive, for example when people undergo painful operations in order to remedy health problems, most people, apart from some masochists, generally seek to avoid pain and suffering. Therefore, human beings have an interest in avoiding pain and suffering, and anyone who proposes to subject other people to pain or suffering ought to either have their consent or make a convincing case for wishing to do so.

Similarly, there is no reason to suspect that other animals lack an interest in the avoidance of pain or suffering. Though many animals may not be aware of the fact that they have such an interest, the question whether they are seems irrelevant: human infants are not aware of the fact that they have an interest in the avoidance of pain either, but nobody seems to doubt that they have such an interest. More importantly, barring exceptional circumstances, of which I mentioned one in the preceding paragraph, I have not been able to identify a good argument that it would be acceptable to inflict pain on human infants. It is generally recognised that they, as well as older human beings, possess a right not to be harmed through the human infliction of pain or suffering that should be respected in most circumstances. By analogy, it could be argued that we ought to grant such a right also to all sentient organisms where the infliction of pain or suffering does not serve their interests.

Before we decide on granting such a right, however, we must consider a complicating issue. The question must be asked whether there is such a thing as an insentient organism. If there is no such thing, we might have a problem. If we assume that it is acceptable for us to eat other organisms, any moral theory that adopts a duty to avoid inflicting pain or suffering would stipulate a duty that would be violated routinely if all organisms were able to experience pain or suffering, which would perhaps call into question the relevance of such a moral theory. A lot has been written on this topic. Although I shall engage with a number of studies, I must emphasise that I do not endorse some methods that have been used to explore the matter as some of the experiments in these studies have inflicted a lot of pain and suffering or death upon animals.

In earlier work, I grappled with this insentient-organism problem by discussing what Whiteheadian scholars—scholars who are influenced by the work of Alfred Whitehead—have written on the theme (Deckers 2011d; Deckers 2011e). One such scholar whose view on this matter I did not engage with previously is Palmer (2010, 14, 18), who thinks that many organisms may only be capable of 'unconscious responses to pain', by which she may mean that they are only capable of nociception (given that pain is, by definition, a conscious experience), and who takes the 'relatively conservative view' that only mammals and birds are capable of feeling pain. Whereas Palmer (2010, 12) thinks that 'many organisms, including some plants and amoeba[e], move away from noxious stimuli', she adds that 'it seems extremely unlikely that they feel pain'. The evidence that she provides for this conclusion is that 'research on human fetuses indicates withdrawal reflexes before the development of the thalamo-cortical circuits associated with pain perception' (Palmer 2010, 12). One of the problems with this claim is that the fact that foetuses can experience pain once they have obtained 'thalamocortical circuits' does not imply that they are unable to feel pain before the emergence of these circuits; another is that neither plants nor amoebae are human foetuses, which calls their comparability with the latter into question.

A different Whiteheadian scholar, whose work I engaged with before, is Dombrowski (2006, 225), who claims that clams (also known as bivalves; a group of animals that includes mussels, scallops, and oysters) may not be sentient as they 'only have a cluster of ganglia' and lack 'a central nervous system'. This is in line with Singer (1975, 188)'s early position, where Singer draws the 'prudential' line between sentient and insentient organisms 'somewhere between a shrimp and an oyster'. In the second edition of *Animal Liberation*, however, Singer (1990, 174) expressed doubt about this position, which is perhaps not surprising as the study of pain and suffering in other animals is complicated. This may be related partly to the fact that most, if not all, nonhuman animals are unable to communicate to us that they are in pain, as all lack the power of speech. However, the significance of language should not be overstated, at least if we accept that talking about pain and feeling it are two very different things. Though clams are not able to tell us whether they are sentient, animal welfare approaches typically focus on anatomical, physiological, and behavioural data to explore whether an organism might be sentient.

If we focus on clams, starting with anatomical evidence, we may agree with Dombrowski's claim that they lack central nervous systems, but whether we do depends on our understanding of what counts as a central nervous system. If the possession of a brain or a brain-like organ that both receives information from and exercises a great deal of control over all parts of the body is assumed to be a necessary condition for the possession of such a system, then a clam may not have a central nervous system. If, however, all that is required for the possession of such a system is the ability to act as an integrated individual where the organism as a whole can respond to and direct its parts, then clams would possess central nervous systems (as the clam as a whole would be brain-like). Whereas I shall not engage with the question of which definition we should adopt, the main point in this discussion is not whether clams have central nervous systems, but whether they are sentient. Crucially, the possibility that they may be sentient cannot be ruled out by the potential absence of a central nervous system. Nervous tissues are clearly present in clams as they generally have three pairs of ganglia: the cerebropleural ganglia that control the sensory organs and the mantle cavity, the pedal ganglia that control the foot, and the visceral ganglia. These are connected with each other and with other body parts by means of various connections, allowing clams to act in integrated ways. Physiological support for the possibility that some clams may be able to experience pain comes from the observation that the common mussel (*Mytilus edulis*) releases substances that are similar to the dopamine that mammals release, when they are thought to experience pain, to produce analgesic effects (Stefano et al. 2008).

In spite of these observations, the existence of significant physiological and anatomical differences between human beings and clams may have tempted Dombrowski (2006) and Singer (1975) into thinking that clams lack sentience. The cognitive ethologists Bekoff and Sherman (2004, 179), however, question the 'view that only big-brained creatures' have developed modes of awareness— a view which they claim stems from anthropocentrism. Apart from focusing on anatomical and physiological similarities and dissimilarities between different animals, we may also learn something about an organism's mental capacities by studying their behaviour. Common mussels, for example, close their shells rapidly when they identify toxic chemicals, whilst scallops start swimming when they detect starfish as they try to escape from these predators (Crook and Walters 2011, 188). These observations do not imply that these organisms are capable of feeling pain. However, the same could be said about any other animal who exhibits an evasive response in the presence of a negative stimulus, prompting the question of why some animal welfare scientists accept this kind of behaviour as an indicator for sentience in some species, but not in others (J. Smith and Boyd 1991). More generally, as similar physiological and behavioural features have been associated with sentience in other species, it might therefore be inferred from these features that the common mussel may be capable of experiencing aversive sensations, and the same applies to any other clams who possess features that can be interpreted similarly.

Accordingly, what Varner (2012, 105, 112) calls the standard response in relation to the question of which animals are sentient, namely that vertebrates probably are, and that invertebrates are not, with the possible exception of the group of cephalopods (octopuses and squid), is doubtful. This standard picture results from the standard approach that has been used to conduct research on sentience, which has focused almost exclusively on whether the following features are either present or absent: particular neuro-anatomical structures that might be associated with affective states, for example the lateral pallium in fish; structures that might be interpreted as nociceptors; substances that can be interpreted as endogenous opioids (substances that are produced by the body to reduce pain); and a narrow range of behavioural features, including whether organisms respond to damaging stimuli in ways that are analogous to how human beings normally respond and whether they can vary such responses after being exposed to substances that are known to be analgesics (Anthony et al. 2013; J. Smith and Boyd 1991). In light of this approach, the view that mussels may not be sentient seems surprising, but I guess that the answer that will be given would depend a great deal on how much weight is given to the presence or absence of particular features. Those who consider mussels to be insentient arguably bestow great weight on the absence of neuro-anatomical structures that are sufficiently similar to the neuro-anatomical structures of animals who are believed to be sentient, but this need not be the only solution to this puzzle.

The more general problem with those who rely exclusively on the standard approach is that it ignores the possibility that organisms who lack what we perceive to be (central) nervous systems may have developed radically different ways to detect pain, as well as other endogenous and behavioural responses. The existence of these difficulties does not imply that we should abandon the standard approach. Some have argued that an anthropocentric bias—which results in a tendency to anthropomorphise—is inevitable: the possibility of ascribing sentience to other organisms would necessarily depend on our capacity to detect similarities between human beings and organisms who belong to other species (Proctor 2012). I do not think that this interpretation is accurate. We should rather speak of an individualistic bias: it is from my own experiences of pain or suffering that I am able to ascribe similar capacities to others, where the concept of 'others' includes other human beings. Accordingly, someone who is not capable of experiencing either pain or suffering would not be able to identify pain or suffering in others. The idea that there is such a thing as an anthropocentric bias merely results from the belief that there is a strong consensus that all human beings experience pain and suffering in similar ways. If we bear in mind that absence of evidence is not tantamount to evidence of absence, we must remain open to the possibility that organisms who are radically different from us may have capacities to experience pain and suffering that are hard or even impossible for us to understand much about. Crucially, any evidence that might be presented one way or the other will always be constrained by our individualistic bias, 'a single point of view', which prevents us from feeling what it is like to be another (Nagel 1979, 167).

Accordingly, the view that is held by Varner (2012, 123) and by J. Smith and Boyd (1991, 63) that earthworms do not respond to damaging stimuli in ways analogous to how human beings normally respond need not be taken to indicate that earthworms lack sentience. The fact that they behave differently should hardly be surprising. These organisms are so different from us that it may be hard for us to imagine what might constitute a response from them that would indicate pain sensitivity. This lack of understanding is compounded by the fact that invertebrates in general have received relatively little scientific attention and constitute a more difficult study group because of their biological differences (Proctor 2012). However, anyone who has ever tried to pull an earthworm out of the ground may think that they resist, and anyone who has ever injured an earthworm may also think that their movements can be—to use the words that Naess (1995, 15) once used when he saw the death struggle of a flea through a microscope—'dreadfully expressive'. One person who studied worms more than just about anyone else is Darwin (1881, 98), who thought of them as possessing 'some degree of intelligence' whilst also recognising the widespread bias against this possibility: 'This will strike every one as very improbable; but it may be doubted whether we know enough about the nervous system of the lower animals to justify our natural distrust of such a conclusion.' A similar bias surrounds the question whether earthworms might be sentient.

To return to the class of crustaceans, research found that not only mussels but many other crustaceans release hormones when they are exposed to situations that might be stressful (Elwood et al. 2009). Not only have *Chasmagnathus* crabs been shown to be able to learn to avoid electric shocks (Fernandez-Duque et al. 1992), but shore crabs (*Carcinus maenas*) have also been observed to vary their avoidance behaviour depending on whether several aversive stimuli are present, showing that their avoidance behaviour is not an uncontrollable reflex that might have indicated no more than unconscious nociception (Elwood et al. 2009). Also, crayfish (*Procambarus clarkii*) can learn to move to a safe spot by associating the turning on of a light with a shock that is given 10 seconds later (Kawai et al. 2004), and glass prawns (*Palaemon elegans*) have been observed to groom and to rub one of their antennae against the flank of a tank after noxious stimuli had been applied to the antenna in question (Barr et al. 2008). Several species of crustaceans have also been shown to respond in ways similar to how vertebrates respond when they are given analgesics (Elwood et al. 2009). The grooming and rubbing observed in glass prawns, for example, stopped when the animals in question had been treated with benzocaine, a local anaesthetic in humans (Barr et al. 2008).

Regan (1983, 30) has expressed the view that he is inclined to think that a snail cannot feel pain, but this is doubtful too. In an experiment with snails (*Helix* sp.) carried out by Balaban and Maksimova (1993), snails had to displace the end of a rod in order to receive electrical stimulation. Compared to a control group, snails who received stimulation to the parietal ganglion decreased the frequency with which they touched the rod, whilst snails who received stimulation to the mesocerebrum—which is known to fulfil a role in sexual activity—increased the frequency with which they did so. Sherwin (2001, 111S) provides a thought-provoking comment on this research: 'if this experiment had been conducted with a vertebrate species, we would almost certainly ascribe these responses as being due to the animal experiencing sensations of pain or discomfort when self-stimulating the parietal ganglion, and pleasure when self-stimulating the mesocerebrum'. In arthropods, some spiders (*Argiope aurantia*) have been observed to autotomise (to cast off from their bodies) a leg when ambush bugs (*Phymata fasciata*) sting the leg in question in an attempt to escape from being caught by the spiders, while autotomy was avoided when the leg was merely being grasped (Eisner and Camazine 1983). These spiders also cast off legs when they are injected with various venomous substances, some of which are known to cause pain in humans. These findings suggest that autotomy may be triggered by pain rather than by an unconscious reflex triggered by nociception, with the effect of saving life in the presence of a noxious stimulus. Several examples of other invertebrates who have shown similar behaviour are provided by Elwood et al. (2009).

The possibility that some invertebrates might be sentient is also supported by recent research that explored whether honeybees might, like human beings, develop negative cognitive biases when they experience negative feelings, where negative cognitive biases, also known as the 'glass-half-empty syndrome', are expectations of negative outcomes (Bateson et al. 2011). Bateson et al. (2011, 1070) explored whether honeybees show negative cognitive bias 'when they are subjected to an anxiety-like state induced by vigorous shaking designed to simulate a predatory attack'. They found that shaken bees had a greater propensity for interpreting later ambiguous stimuli 'as predicting punishment' and that honeybees are therefore likely to be able to experience emotions (Bateson et al. 2011, 1070). After bees were conditioned to extend their mouthparts (probosces) in the presence of a positive odour and to withhold their mouthparts in the presence of a more negative odour, it was found that shaken bees showed similar behaviour to the control group in the presence of the more positive odour, but that they showed a greater propensity to withhold their mouthparts from the less positive odour and from a selection of odours that were similar to the less positive odour that they had been exposed to before being shaken. The experimental group and the control group therefore differed in their perceptions of either the impact or the probability of what is referred to as 'being punished': the former were more likely to interpret ambiguous stimuli as threats. Bateson et al. (2011) also found that shaking reduces the presence of particular hormones (dopamine, octopamine, and serotonin) that might affect the olfactory memories of the bees, resulting in the observed cognitive bias.

But why stop at honeybees? Animals who may appear to be much simpler than honeybees may also be sentient. Even unicellular eukaryotic organisms, such as *Physarum polycephalum*, have been observed to exhibit remarkable behaviour, including: solving mazes and geometrical puzzles; controlling robots; and adjusting their behaviour in response to their anticipation of unfavourable conditions (such as cold temperature and humidity) that they had already been exposed to at regular intervals in the past (Pershin et al. 2009; Saigusa et al. 2008). If no nervous system is required for these actions, the capacity of sentience may not require what is commonly understood to be a necessary prerequisite for its existence.

Even plants are described as 'sensitive organisms' in a recent review of research into 'plant neurobiology', a discipline which the authors claim has had a 'difficult start' because of the existence of a 'deeply-rooted, almost "dogmatic", view of plants as passive creatures not in a need of any neuronal processes and capabilities' (Baluška and Mancuso 2009, 61), a view that the authors trace back to Aristotle, but that they think might have been partially overcome by Darwin and Darwin (1880, 573), who thought that plants have sensitive zones at the tips of their radicles that act like the brains of animals (Baluška et al. 2009). Accordingly, Darwin and Darwin (1880, 199–200) compared the behaviour of plant roots with the behaviour of moles who carefully feel around to detect where the ground is most fit for burrowing. Baluška and Mancuso (2009) also argue that the neurosciences associate complex neural systems primarily with animals who move, but that recent research on animals who are sessile, for example on corals such as the purple sea urchin (*Strongylocentrotus purpuratus*), or on animals who move slowly, for example *Trichoplax adhaerens*, a marine animal that is only about 1 mm long, has revealed their 'surprising neuronal complexity', in spite of their great similarity to plants (Baluška and Mancuso 2009, 61; with references to Pennisi 2008 and to Materna and Cameron 2008). Perhaps the most interesting thing about plants in relation to the topic of whether they might be sentient is that some have been observed to rapidly increase their production of ethylene when they are exposed to stressful situations (Baluška and Mancuso 2009, 62). Until recently, ethylene was used as an analgesic in human medicine. Could it be that some plants increase their endogenous production of ethylene when they are in pain? It has been argued that 'plants lack central nervous systems, nociceptors ... and other morphological features associated with the capacity for sentience' (Steiner 2013, 221), but I think it is a mistake to interpret the absence of traits that we confidently associate with sentience as evidence of the absence of sentience.

And why stop at plants? Even bacteria can communicate with other bacteria by means of quorum sensing, a chemical way to communicate that leads to coordinated behaviour; they can also anticipate events that are about to occur in their environments (Waters and Bassler 2005; Shapiro 2007). Could it be that they vary their behaviour to avoid painful experiences? Nagel (1979, 168) may have been right sociologically that 'if one travels too far down the phylogenetic tree, people gradually shed their faith that there is experience', but this should hardly be surprising in a culture that is dominated by dualistic and reductionist-materialistic ontologies, where both ontologies share the view that there are things that are wholly devoid of subjective experience, but where only the former allows for some exceptions. Where the latter is unable to account for mental phenomena, the former faces the problem of how they could emerge in a world that would supposedly once have been totally devoid of them. Elsewhere, I expressed my support for the theory that all simple and what Hartshorne (1972) called 'compound' individuals (as opposed to aggregates such as stones) possess mental or experiential capacities, but that the degrees to which they have such capacities may vary with entities' relative material complexities (Deckers 2011d).

The most elaborate defence of this Whiteheadian ontology against the rival ontologies of reductionist materialism and of dualism is by Griffin (1998), who coined the label of '*panexperientialism*' to describe it. Whereas my position differs from Griffin's as I consider the universe as a whole to be an aggregate rather than a compound individual (God) and as I consider plants to be compound individuals (rather than aggregates of cells), I think that my position might also be called '*pan-sentientism*'. Whilst Dombrowski (1988) has made a distinction between individuals whom he considers to be 'proto-sentient' and others whom he considers to be sentient, I do not think that we can infer the existence of an experiential capacity in any individual unless we think of that individual as possessing the capacity to experience things either positively or negatively. Whitehead (1978, 211–212) did not think that a neutral experience was possible, speculating instead that reality was the stuff of emotions or feelings. In this light, sentience can be understood as a capacity, held by all individuals, to distinguish between what is positive (or pleasurable) and what is negative (or painful), which can then be used to make emotional decisions on how to act that either may or may not be mediated by thoughts about one's emotions.

This Whiteheadian ontology clashes with the views of most ethicists, who adopt the view that sentience features only in a select number of biological organisms. For organisms that have an interest in staying alive, it seems plausible to hold the view that the evolutionary function of pain may lie in warning the organism so that it can avoid that which may undermine its health or result in death. When it comes to thinking what the function of pain might be for, for example, a water molecule, it is much more difficult to envisage any purpose. However, it might perhaps be said that a similar function operates here: could it be that a water molecule uses its feelings to try to maintain its structure? Whereas I provide an affirmative answer to this question, it must also be emphasised that Whiteheadians do not adopt the view that the feelings of entities at different levels of reality have the same intensities. In order for a complex individual such as a human being to exist as a unity, the billions of feelings that constitute the individual must be integrated, which is thought to generate a greater depth of experience than the level of experience that might feature in, for example, a single cell or a water molecule. In this ontology, the concept of nociception still refers to an unconscious perception of damage, but only to refer to the individual as a whole being unaware of this damage; at a more localised level, for example in the leg of someone with a severed spine, the conscious feeling of pain after injury still exists.

I shall now address the relevance of these considerations for the question whether all sentient organisms should be granted a right to be free from the human infliction of pain or suffering. If we accept that human beings should be allowed to consume other organisms, it might be argued that it will be problematic to grant other organisms such a right on the basis of the view that it would justifiably be violated as a matter of routine practice. If we accept that we must eat living beings and that all organisms may be able to experience pain, it may not be possible to feed ourselves without inflicting pain or suffering. However, the fact that we may inflict pain and suffering through eating does not imply that we should refrain from granting all sentient organisms a *prima facie* right to be spared from the human infliction of pain. As mentioned in the introduction, the words '*prima facie*' are important: in the absence of other morally relevant considerations, it would seem to be highly appropriate to give other organisms such a right, given that sentient organisms generally seek to avoid painful experiences. Indeed, it would seem to be odd to hold the view that we ought to be concerned about inflicting pain on other human beings, but not about inflicting it on our more distant relatives. Accordingly, it makes sense to say that someone who steps deliberately on an earthworm, for example in an attempt to release their frustration, violates unjustifiably the earthworm's right to be spared from pain. Similarly, it is meaningful to say that someone who tramples on a plant for a similar reason wrongs the plant in question. As a general rule, we should, all other moral considerations being equal, inflict as little pain and suffering on other organisms as possible when we make dietary choices. Where we fail to do so, we act immorally as we fail to minimise negative GHIs.

When it comes to deciding which organisms we should use to feed ourselves, it is appropriate to allow ourselves to be guided by evidence about the differences in the capacities of different organisms to experience pain and suffering, without losing sight of the fact that what it means to be another individual will always be a matter of speculation. Consequently, moral agents are not accountable for any errors that they may make in assessing differences in organisms' capacities to feel pain and to suffer, provided that they have not been negligent in their attempts to assess such differences. Any differences that might plausibly be held to exist in the psychological complexities or in what Birch and Cobb (1984) term the capacities for 'richness of experience' of different organisms would seem to be relevant, as it would, *ceteris paribus*, be more problematic to consume organisms who might endure more pain or suffering than others in the process of being turned into food.

This is illustrated by the following example. If we are correct to assume that a lettuce does not feel much pain by being confined in its growing space, but that a pig may undergo much more pain and suffering by being confined—which may prompt her, for example, to start biting bars out of frustration when she is kept in gestation or farrowing crates—we are right to be more concerned about confining pigs. Accordingly, I would argue that a pig's interest in not being confined to a small space ordinarily outweighs any human interest in confining a pig, but that any interest in not being confined that a lettuce may possess does not trump the human interest in confining the lettuce. The desire to confine a lettuce, for example, could be motivated by the desire to reduce weeds, which would seem to be an appropriate desire to act on. The desire to minimise the human infliction of pain and suffering on other animals is precisely what motivated Singer (1975; 1990) to write his *Animal Liberation*, which shows limited support for the project of 'ceasing to rear and kill animals for food', even if the goal of 'stopping the suffering' and the infliction of pain on animals cannot be reached (Singer 1990, vii, xii).

It is time to take stock. Many ethicists have argued that it is more problematic to use (particular) animals than to use plants for food, arguing that this is merely related to only the former being sentient. This picture has been questioned. Nonetheless, I have endorsed the view—adopted by many animal ethicists—that sentience matters and that, *ceteris paribus*, we ought to make dietary choices that minimise pain and suffering. An animal ethic that rests only on Singer (1990, 228)'s main concern, namely the 'wrongness of inflicting suffering' and pain, however, is unsatisfactory.

2.7 Is the minimisation of pain and suffering all that matters?

The *prima facie* duty to minimise inflicting pain and suffering does not *ipso facto* provide grounds for an obligation to abstain from eating animals. Many animals die naturally or accidentally, for example; in a moral theory that focuses only on the avoidance of inflicting pain and suffering, these would be legitimate candidates for consumption. Even the consumption of animals who are killed deliberately would be allowed, provided that they are killed painlessly. This issue was brought up for discussion by Singer at the second Minding Animals conference, which took place at Utrecht University in the Netherlands in July 2012. Specifically, Singer questioned whether it would be wrong to kill a cow by going up to her in the field and shooting her in the head with a well-aimed shot, an example of a general issue which has presented a 'real difficulty' (Singer 1990, 228) for him for quite a long time.

Whereas I have questioned, in the preceding section, whether it is ever possible to kill painlessly, there is nevertheless sufficient evidence, for example from surgical operations on anaesthetised people, to suggest that people can be anaesthetised to such an extent that it may be possible to kill while inflicting hardly any or no pain at all on the individual as a whole. This is why I adopt the view that it is possible to kill individuals painlessly, even if the cells, molecules, atoms, and sub-atomic particles that compose an individual may continue to experience pain after death.

If the painless killing of an individual is possible, a theory that values only the minimisation of pain and suffering could not object to the painless killing of a cow. Indeed, a theory that valued only this goal would find it difficult to object to the killing of a human being if death could occur painlessly. Such a theory clashes with our moral intuition that it would, in many situations, be very wrong to kill a human being. The reason why killing may be wrong, therefore, cannot lie simply in the fact that killing might cause pain or suffering.

In attempting to solve this problem, many philosophers have argued that a distinction should be drawn between those organisms who merely seek to avoid pain and suffering and those who also value a continued life. For Singer (2006, 6), an organism who is able to value a continued life would be able to have 'a clear conception of the ... (possible) future', in the sense of being able to form clear 'hopes and plans' of what the future may hold in store for them. Accordingly, the painless killing of many human beings would be problematic in view of the fact that many human beings value continued life. Though Singer (1990, 20) does not answer the question of which 'capacities are relevant to the question of taking life', he proceeds by stating that 'the life of a self-aware being, capable of abstract thought, of planning for the future, of complex acts of communication, and so on, is more valuable than the life of a being without these capacities'. Elsewhere, he comments on the moral relevance of this difference: 'Since neither a newborn human infant nor a fish is a person, the wrongness of killing such beings is not as great as the wrongness of killing a person' (Singer 1995, 220).

In a similar vein, Varner (2012, 219) has argued that special significance should be given to those human beings who possess a biographical sense of self, a sense that would not be possessed by any other animals. Yet, unlike Singer, who merely distinguishes between animals who are persons and animals who are not, Varner (2012, 219) claims that special significance should also be given to what he calls 'near-persons': animals who possess the capacities to 'remember pleasant and unpleasant events', as well as to form 'more complicated, longer-term desires than merely sentient animals are capable of'. Accordingly, he uses scientific evidence to claim that great apes, cetaceans, elephants, and corvids (ravens, crows, jays, magpies, and nutcrackers) should be included within the category of near-persons, and he proceeds by stating that 'contemporary societies' are not justified in killing near-persons for food (Varner 2012, 249).

But while persons and near-persons should not normally be killed for food, it would be acceptable, according to these theories, to kill the vast majority of animals—the 'merely sentient'—in many situations, provided that this could be done without inflicting pain or suffering on them. A scholar who is very clear in this regard is Scruton (2000, 126, 141–142), who argues that cows and bulls can justifiably be killed as a matter of routine farming practice, 'provided they are killed humanely', in light of his view that 'to be killed at one year is not intrinsically more tragic than to be killed at two or three ... for that they must be killed is evident, this being the reason why they live'. Whereas Scruton (2000, 142) would probably exempt human infants from this moral imperative on the basis of the putative 'affections' of others and the positive value of allowing them to achieve things in their lives—a subject that he does not deal with clearly—Singer (2006, 6) has claimed that, provided that 'parents agree that it is better that their child should die ... perhaps it is *not* wrong to take the life of a severely brain-damaged human infant' [emphasis in original]. However, it is unclear why he picks this particular example, given that he writes elsewhere that 'we value the protection given by a right to life only when we want to go on living', where personhood, a category from which he excludes all infants, rather than just those who are severely disabled, is held to be a necessary condition for the existence of this want (Singer 1995, 218–219).

Whereas I am at one with Singer that there may be situations where continued life is a curse and death a blessing, I do not adopt the view that human beings who lack a biographical sense of self and 'merely sentient' animals should not be granted *prima facie* rights to life. In reflecting on these issues, Cochrane (2012, 65) has argued that 'ordinarily [vertebrate] animals have an interest in continued life' because it would give them opportunities for 'well-being' or 'pleasant experiences'. The ability to value continued life is here distinguished from the ability to value other things, for which being alive is a prerequisite. Even if many animals may not be able to value continued life in the sense that they would be able to pursue 'self-chosen life goals', which may presuppose the ability to attribute negative value to one's death, Cochrane (2012, 66) appears to argue that a vertebrate animal's interest in continued life relates to their ability to value many things that keep them alive, such as water and food. We might thus be able to derive the fact that such animals have an interest in the continuation of their lives from the fact that they act in ways that serve the preservation of their lives. Even if many animals may not be able to develop ideas about the projects that they wish to pursue in the future, the mere fact that they strive to avoid things that could jeopardise their existence in the future would be sufficient to recognise that they have an interest in continued life.

In this regard, Cochrane's view about killing animals appears to be similar to Regan's, even if the latter is much less clear on the issue. In his early work, Regan (1983, 243) claims that we should ascribe a right to life to those animals who are what he calls 'subjects-of-a-life', where 'individuals are subjects-of-a-life if they have beliefs and desires; perception, memory, and a sense of the future, including their own future; an emotional life together with feelings of pleasure and pain; preference- and welfare-interests; the ability to initiate action in pursuit of their desires and goals; a psychophysical identity over time; and an individual welfare in the sense that their experiential life fares well or ill for them'. Such subjects would include 'normal mammalian animals, aged one or more' (Regan 1983, 78, 247). However, it is unclear why these animals would stand out from others. An animal who is capable of having 'a sense of ... their own future' would seem to possess the ability to imagine themselves to exist in the future, a necessary condition for an animal to have the capacity to value a continued life. Evidence is lacking to suggest that this capacity, which may depend on the ability to have thoughts about thoughts, is possessed by most mammals (Carruthers 1992; Bermúdez 2003).

What is even more questionable is that, in a later edition of *The Case for Animal Rights*, Regan (2004, xvi, xl) widens the category of animals whom he considers to be 'subjects-of-a-life', writing that birds are also included, and that fish 'may be' as well, but that 'plants and insects' are excluded. In this respect, Cochrane's account is similar, as he draws a distinctive line between vertebrates and invertebrates. Though Regan does not—at least to my knowledge—question his 'subject-of-a-life' criterion and definition explicitly anywhere, in his later work he first appears to shift his focus to 'noncognitive criteria ... such as sentience' (Regan 1997, 110), and then appears to identify those who are not and those who are subjects-of-a-life with, respectively, those who are 'in the world but not aware of it' and those who are both in the world and aware of it (Regan 2004, xvi). Regan appears to broaden his category of animals who are subjects-of-a-life here and, like Cochrane, adopt the view that animals need not be able to value a continued life in order to possess an interest in continued life.

Though I accept the view that animals may possess a *prima facie* right to life in spite of the possibility that they may not be able to attribute value to a continued life, the claim that this right is grounded in the fact that animals take an interest in things that keep them alive has devastating consequences for the theories defended by both Regan and Cochrane, as well as for the theories espoused by many other ethicists. The reason for this is that evolution has selected for all living beings possessing an interest in seeking out things that serve the continuation of either their own or some of their species' members' lives and in avoiding things that might undermine life. Regan (2004, xvi) claims that 'amoebae ... are in the world but not aware of it' and Cochrane (2012, 24) claims that 'we can be reasonably sure that creatures such as amoebas and oysters lack the capacity for consciousness', but I reject these claims. Consequently, any theory that distinguishes between the painless killing of (some) animals who are not able to ruminate on their future lives and the painless killing of plants based on the assumption that these animals, unlike plants, have interests in continued life adopts a moral distinction on the basis of what I take to be a false assumption. If the possession of interests in things that serve the continuation of their own or their species' members' lives is sufficient for it to be meaningful to say that an animal has an interest in continued life, it is impossible to distinguish between the painless killing of animals who are unable to value continued life and the painless killing of plants. If the making of such a distinction makes any sense, the reason for it must lie elsewhere.

2.8 Is the killing of anaesthetised animals for food acceptable? Weaknesses of existing theories

Cochrane (2012, 65)'s answer to the question whether animals whom he considers to be sentient should ordinarily be allowed to be killed for food is negative, as he finds that it would deprive them of 'pleasant experiences', where it would not be too demanding of us to allow these experiences to occur. Someone who is inspired by his account but accepts that invertebrates and plants also possess interests in pleasant experiences would be faced with a tricky dilemma: should any moral distinction be made between killing anaesthetised animals and killing anaesthetised plants for food?

Whereas Cochrane (2012, 205) does not deal with this particular question as he dismisses that plants may be sentient, there is no doubt that a Cochranean interest-based theory would resolve the issue by weighing up the different interests 'in not being made to suffer and in continued life' of 'moral patients'—which I define in this book as any others who might be affected by the actions of human moral agents—and choose the action that would inflict the least harm on them, where harmful actions are defined as those that harm the above interests the most. This approach is associated with some problems.

One issue is the problem whether to prioritise the interest in not being made to feel pain or suffer or the interest in continued life. If the former deserves priority, it does not necessarily imply that plants would lose out, given that we lack knowledge about how they might be anaesthetised. If the latter deserves priority, we must address the epistemological problem of how we might be able to know which organisms have greater capacities to enjoy pleasant experiences compared to others. As mentioned before, relatively little research has been done on the mental capacities of invertebrates and plants. Even if more research had been done, the questions would remain of how we might be able to infer from our external observations what might take place inside the bodies of other organisms and how we might rank the values of different experiences (Nagel 1979). Whereas I am prepared to assume that animals are normally capable of having richer experiences, this assumption does not answer the question why we should value the lives of those who may be able to enjoy richer experiences over those who may only be capable of enjoying less intense experiences. Whilst I am also willing to adopt the view that we should grant more weight to the former, my main concern with Cochrane's approach is that he ignores some relevant, important interests that human moral agents may have, but more importantly ought to have, which should complement his focus on weighing up the competing interests of moral patients. My unease is illustrated by the consistent way in which Cochrane ought to deal with the question of what to do with the bodies of animals who either are killed justifiably or die naturally, as well as with the inconsistent way in which he deals with the question whether the act of killing animals for food might, in some situations, be preferable to its alternatives.

In relation to the first question, Cochrane (2012, 132) appears to agree with my view that it is acceptable to kill some animals for their own good in some situations. For example, if a nonhuman animal has been hit by a car and experiences severe pain and suffering associated with irreparable damage to her body, both Cochrane and I agree that euthanising the animal in question would be justifiable. Incidentally, this is in line with the recently implemented European Union Directive 2010/63/EU on the protection of animals used for scientific purposes, which accepts that it may be appropriate to kill other animals who are 'likely to remain in moderate or severe pain, suffering, distress or lasting harm' (Council Directive 2010/63/EU, art. 17, par. 2). I am not satisfied, however, with what Cochrane should conclude in relation to the question of what to do with animals who are killed mercifully (to save them from agonising deaths where imminent death is inevitable through injury or disease), which—incidentally—should also apply for animals who die accidentally or naturally. If animals could be euthanised without the use of drugs that may be harmful to human beings, or if it were (made) safe to eat animals who had been killed mercifully or those who had died naturally, this theory would oblige us to eat them to avoid harming the interests of others either intentionally or accidentally, given that Cochrane (2012, 88–89, 206) cannot see anything wrong with eating the corpses of nonhuman animals *per se*. I shall reject this theory in section 2.10.

If Cochrane had been consistent, he should also have granted that diets that avoid the deliberate killing of animals in order to procure their body parts for human consumption are not necessarily better than other diets. However, Cochrane (2012, 101) claims that they are, at least where the killing concerns animals whom he considers to be sentient, as diets that refrain from killing such animals in order to use their bodies for food would result in 'the fewest animal deaths overall'. Steven Davis (2003; 2008) has mounted a powerful objection to this claim, arguing that some vegan diets inflict much more harm on moral patients than other diets. This is so because numerous animals are killed by agricultural practices that are used in arable farming—for example ploughing. Several authors have engaged with Steven Davis's challenge (see e.g. Matheny 2003; Lamey 2007). The most recent challenge comes from Cochrane himself (2012, 98–102), who argues that Davis does not get his numbers right. If Davis had calculated the number of deaths per consumer (rather than assumed that an equal amount of land would feed the same number of human beings, regardless of which diet they adopted), Cochrane argues that he would have come to the conclusion that diets that refrain from killing the farmed animals that he is concerned with cause fewer animal deaths.

This last claim is extremely implausible. Cochrane and Davis base their estimates on the assumption that crop cultivation kills about twice as many animals as ruminant grazing. Cochrane admits that the accuracy of these figures is compromised by a lack of research data on how different farming practices affect other organisms but, if invertebrates were included in this calculation, I estimate that the real figures would reveal a much greater difference, this time in favour of grassland, with the number of animals killed there much lesser. In the South of England, for example, it has been recorded that managed pasture contains about 354 earthworms per square metre (D. Knight et al. 1992), and it has also been estimated that ploughing may halve this number (Darlington 2010, 275). Cochrane might retort that this is not a problem for his theory, given its lack of interest in invertebrates, but Schedler (2005) has reported rightly that arable farming kills many vertebrates too, for example voles and mice.

The questionable nature of Cochrane's conclusion becomes even clearer when we take note of the fact that his calculations simply take for granted that the current practice of feeding large quantities of feed from arable crops to farmed animals constitutes a necessary practice of diets that include products taken from grazing animals. Though it is correct to assume that, in reality, many diets that rely on the consumption of animal products use more arable land than vegan diets as the farmed animals in question are fed large quantities of feed—a concern that I mentioned in the previous chapter—it is very unlikely that vegan diets necessarily result in fewer animal deaths. A large amount of land is unsuitable for arable cropping. If farmed animals graze on this land and if they are allowed to eat nothing other than grass, particularly when they are kept in low densities and when browsing animals are kept (rather than animals who graze closer to the roots of plants), it is highly likely that an omnivore who uses some of these animals for food will be responsible for fewer animal deaths than someone who adopts a vegan diet. In light of his preference to choose the diet that causes 'the fewest animal deaths overall', Cochrane (2012, 101) is therefore not justified in claiming 'that livestock animals have a right not to be killed by us in agriculture, but that field animals do not', where 'field animals' are understood to be the wild and feral animals whom Cochrane considers to be sentient. The necessity to adopt a diet that includes the consumption of sentient animals would be even greater if Cochrane (2012, 205) had not ignored his other main concern in this context: 'animals' interests in not being made to suffer'. Indeed, the balance would shift even further in favour of some omnivorous diets if we consider the fact that the killing of animals who are used for food occurs relatively quickly, in sharp contrast to the killing of many animals who die by the cultivation of arable land, who do not benefit from quick deaths as they are cut into pieces by agricultural machinery.

The fact that omnivores may, in some situations, inflict less pain, suffering, and death upon animals than vegans is also a problem for the theories espoused by many other scholars in animal ethics, for example Francione (2010a). Though I agree with Francione (2010a, 72) that 'the fact that animals are accidentally ... killed in the cultivation of crops is different morally from intentionally killing individual animals', it must nevertheless be pointed out that there are situations where the foreseeable but accidental killing of animals is worse than their being killed deliberately. Francione (2010a, 72) draws an analogy between the accidental killing of animals in arable farming and the accidental killing of human beings in road accidents, where the practices that result in these deaths are nonetheless acceptable. Though the analogy works in showing that there is a moral difference between accidental and deliberate killing, as well as that some activities that may result in accidental killing, for example driving a bus, should not necessarily be banned, it ignores an important distinction between the two scenarios: some carnists might argue that road casualties should be tolerated because of the high value that many people attribute to some forms of modern transport, but that the extra deaths that are caused by some vegan diets do not serve any purpose, for example where vegans refuse either to consume animals who were killed intentionally out of compassion—to relieve the animals' suffering—or to eat those who die naturally or accidentally. In such situations, the vegans in question could avoid the extra deaths that their diets inflict on any animals who are killed accidentally but foreseeably through arable farming. They might add, contrary to Francione's suggestion, that many animals who are killed in arable farming are killed intentionally, for example through the use of pesticides, and that even vegan-organic (or veganic) farming systems that do not rely on chemical pesticides might need to resort to intentional killing in some situations, as I shall document in sections 3.5.2 and 3.5.3.

2.9 Recognising that speciesist and animalist interests are morally relevant

Like interests should be treated alike, regardless of which species the individual with interests happens to belong to. In this respect I do not disagree with the positions developed by many animal ethics scholars (e.g. Singer 1975; Cochrane 2012). What I do take issue with, however, is the view that any interest that a human moral agent may have to attribute special moral significance to those moral patients who happen to be or to have been human beings, regardless of whether they possess particular capacities, should be dismissed as irrelevant. We might call this interest a '*speciesist*' interest: an interest to attribute special moral significance to human beings merely on the basis of the fact that they either belong or, in case they had died, once belonged to our species. Whereas it would be more accurate to refer to this as a human speciesist interest, given that the term '*speciesism*' could be used to refer to a tendency to privilege any species, human or otherwise, I shall in this book simply speak of a speciesist interest whilst assuming that the interest privileges a human interest. If speciesism, conceived of in this way, is a fundamental, morally relevant human interest, which is required to maintain good human health, I believe that good human health also demands that we recognise that we have interests in attributing moral significance that is less than the moral significance of human beings, but nevertheless greater than that of other nonhuman organisms, to: other animals, whether they be dead or alive, because they are biologically more closely related to our species than other (non-animal) organisms are; and those animals who are biologically closer to us than other animals are. I shall refer to the former interest as an 'animalist' interest and to the latter interest as an 'evolutionist' interest.

The reason why these interests should be morally relevant is informed by my reflection upon three considerations. Firstly, as all biological organisms are related to each other, there is no boundary between species in the sense that they would be distinct kinds. Though in organisms that reproduce sexually a species could be defined—if we accept what is known as the 'biological species concept'—as a group of organisms who are able to breed with each other (Lewens 2012), so that members of one species are separated from members of another by the fact that they are not able to interbreed, accepting this definition does not imply that there is no biological continuity between species. The Darwinian view, which I support, is that all species have descended from a common ancestor (Darwin 1859). All living organisms are our kin. Secondly, though we are all related, we are more closely related to other animals than to plants. Animals are closer kin than plants. Thirdly, human beings have been endowed with the ability to recognise, using phenotypic information, that there are various degrees of proximity in how different organisms are related to them, similarly to how other animals—even if their capacities may be more limited—recognise animals who are and who are not closely related. Recently, some genotypic knowledge has also been gained, which may correct phenotypic understandings. Even then, we may not always be right in our judgements, but people who are sceptical of this capacity to differentiate closer kin from further kin biologically might be persuaded that we possess it if they ponder whether we are more closely related to chimpanzees than to mussels. Some animals are closer kin than others. In my view, these biological facts matter morally, which is why my account differs from that developed by Diamond (1978, 474): whereas I agree with her that the notion of an animal as a 'fellow creature'— which she claims to be relevant for animal ethics—'is not a biological concept', biological facts are nevertheless relevant to determine how much of a fellow any other is, bearing in mind that what ought to count as a 'biological fact' will always be determined by normative assumptions.

Before explaining why I believe that the biological perception that there are varying degrees to which other organisms are related to the human species matters in relation to the question of how we should make dietary choices, I would like to argue for the moral relevance of a speciesist interest. Cochrane (2013, 671) imagines a situation where the right to life of a human being would clash with that of a rat, arguing that—all other interests being equal—the right of the human being in question would win out given that 'the human interest in continued life is ordinarily much stronger than that of rats'. The problem with this claim is that the devil is in the detail. Whilst this interest may 'ordinarily' be stronger, it may not apply to those human beings who are largely dependent on others for their lives to continue, such as severely disabled or demented people. In such situations, Cochrane would be obliged to prioritise the life of the healthy rat, given that healthy rats are able to experience things that are beyond the sorts of things that can be enjoyed by a severely disabled human being. Even if, for the sake of the argument, we adopt the unlikely view that there might not be much of a qualitative difference between their experiences, Cochrane would at least be obliged to toss a coin to resolve the conflict.

Those who adopt a relational approach to ethics might aver that it would still be possible to prioritise the human being in question on the basis of their relationship with other human beings, but the problem with this is that the rat in question might be a companion animal, in which case an approach that points at the moral relevance of relationships only might again settle the matter by means of a coin toss, which is precisely what May (2014) has argued. Whereas I do not adopt the view that contingent relationships—any relationships that are based on a subjectively felt closeness to the entity that one relates to—are irrelevant to morality, the relational approach clashes with the views of many scholars, including myself, who would adopt a moral duty to prioritise the lives of human beings, however badly disabled they may be, at least as long as it cannot be deemed to be in their own interests for their lives to be ended, in which case our care should still be directed primarily towards them (Crary 2011; Deckers 2005a; Diamond 1991).

It is also impossible to make sense of why many people feel that they have particular duties towards human beings who have died without adopting the view that we ought to have a speciesist interest. Cochrane (2012, 88) tries to deal with this issue when he ponders the acceptability or otherwise of human cannibalism. In his view, the thought that one might consume dead human beings or be consumed by human beings after one's own death is unpleasant. This is why he adopts the view that people ought not to eat the corpses of other human beings. The problem with this is that he cannot accommodate this conclusion within his own theory, which appears to demand merely that we ensure 'that our use of animals does not cause them to suffer or be killed' (Cochrane 2012, 206). As Cochrane himself recognises, those who are dead do not have any interests, and therefore are not in any way disadvantaged by being consumed.

In this light, one would expect Cochrane to approve of their consumption, given that doing so would safeguard the interests of any others who might be consumed otherwise. A fairly rational human being who accepts Cochrane's theory might admit that they have emotional concerns with the thought of being eaten by or of eating someone else, but they would be expected to reject these ethically irrelevant perceptions to safeguard the morally important interests of those who might be eaten instead, which they can be expected to find even more upsetting to ignore. If we should not ignore these interests in other situations, it is unclear why a mere dislike of cannibalism should be sufficient to override these interests. Cochrane (2012, 88) tries to resolve the problem by arguing that what is required to spare the consumption of those who have died is 'a significant set of individuals who are happier in the knowledge' that particular organisms are spared from being eaten. It is unclear why the question whether one is a legitimate candidate for consumption or not should be settled by the arbitrary matter of whether it happens to make some group happy. The logical outcome of this view would be that we should also honour the view of an imaginary group of people with a great love for particular plants who may argue that they would be really upset by the thought of their being eaten.

If we adopt the view that human moral agents ought to have a speciesist interest, on the other hand, and that this interest ought to outweigh the interests of other organisms, which we may decide to consume instead of a human corpse, a coherent justification is offered why we should not normally engage in human cannibalism. The gustatory or nutritional benefits that we might derive from eating a dead human body should normally not stand in the way of our greater, morally significant interest in showing proper recognition to other human beings by not eating them. Some people may well have an interest in eating other human beings or in being eaten by them, but any such interests should normally be overridden by our speciesist interest. Giving adequate consideration to the special moral significance of human beings demands that we refrain from consuming dead human beings.

One objection to speciesism is that adopting it or—perhaps more accurately—recognising its existence would imply that we should also adopt racism, given that we are more closely related to people from our own race than to people from a different race. I am not convinced by this objection. I know that a moral agent from a different race would object to me giving less moral significance to them, and I also know that I would object to being granted less moral significance by them. In spite of our biological distance, which should not be overstated, it would therefore seem wise if we both agreed to grant each other (as well as members of both races who may not possess moral agency, but are nevertheless held dearly by the imaginary parties) equal moral significance, at least if it is agreed that no party should be allowed to occupy the moral high ground. A world in which I experience discrimination on racial grounds and discriminate against others on racial grounds would seem to be worse than a world in which there is no such discrimination. Our interest in human equality therefore trumps any interest that we may have to attribute marginally more moral significance to someone who belongs to one's own race.

When it comes to the question of what a nonhuman animal might think about being granted less moral significance than a human animal is, by contrast, we have no answer. The fact that nonhuman animals have no concept of what it means to be granted less moral significance would seem to be relevant here. I might wrong a nonhuman animal by not giving them their due, but the resentment that such an animal may feel towards me for being wronged is of a different—in a morally relevant way—order to the resentment that a human moral agent from a different race might feel. The perception that another human being is one of us, in spite of our differences—racial or otherwise—seems unquestionable, as well as its moral relevance. I am therefore unpersuaded by the charge that speciesism would be as questionable as racism (see also e.g. Brennan 2003).

2.10 Animalism's distinctive answers in relation to the morality of killing and consuming animals

In a similar way to how tending to our speciesist interest stands in the way of killing human beings and consuming dead human beings other than in exceptional circumstances, animalism sheds new light on the questions whether the killing of anaesthetised animals for food is acceptable and whether it is acceptable to refrain from consuming animals who die naturally or accidentally.

I have argued that we should not normally (i.e. in situations where human beings can consume other things without great difficulties) kill human beings or use their corpses for food, even in situations where refraining from doing so may result in the killing of other animals and in their associated loss of pleasurable experiences, for example those associated with the loss of animals killed accidentally in arable farming. In an animalist perspective, in similar circumstances other animals should not be killed for food either, and neither should animals who die naturally or accidentally be consumed. Their consumption should normally be taboo, a word that Milner (2011, 105) documents to have been introduced into European languages by the explorer Captain Cook and his successor, Captain King, who described how the concept was used in Polynesia—for example to refer to tabooed women who were forbidden to touch the flesh of animals after they had touched human corpses, as well as on some other occasions.

Research has revealed that the consumption of some animal products has been tabooed in many cultures and that taboos on the consumption of animals are far more common than any other consumption taboos (Fessler and Navarrete 2003). Many people accept taboos in relation to the consumption of some animal products. The kosher and halal practices of, respectively, many Jews and Muslims are well-known, yet one need not be religious to adopt a taboo in this domain. Think for example of some people who would not wish to eat certain body parts, for example an animal's eyes, in spite of their nutritional benefits, or of people who have companion animals and who refrain from eating their animals after the latter's natural or accidental deaths. Many people who object to the thought of eating their companion animals when the latter are, for example, rabbits nonetheless eat their companion animals' species members, so the question remains why a taboo should be accepted, and, if it is, where to draw the line.

In earlier work I argued for a taboo on the basis of the possibility that consuming the bodies of animals might whet people's appetite for turning living animals into corpses (Deckers 2009). This position also appears to be endorsed by Gruen (2011, 102–103). According to this line of reasoning, the displeasure that ought to be associated with killing animals may be weakened by the pleasure derived from eating animals. Whereas the latter would not be problematic *per se*, it would be problematic if those who eat animals were more likely to support the killing of animals for food. Whilst many people who consume animal products did not kill the animals from whom their products derive and the idea of doing so may never cross their minds—indeed they might even abhor the thought of doing so—one's gustatory pleasure at eating animals might still motivate one to be more supportive of practices that kill animals unjustifiably.

The problem with this (slippery slope) mode of reasoning is that the sheer fact that a practice that is in itself good might motivate one to be more supportive of a similar practice that is bad may not be sufficient to justify a ban on the former. By using a plane for a justifiable cause, I might develop an appetite for the morally questionable practice of travelling by plane for pointless reasons, but the fact that I may do so does not seem sufficient to justify a ban on the former practice. However, the difference between this example and the problem discussed in this section is that banning the justifiable use of plane travel would seem to undermine a very important interest, whereas it might be argued that the same cannot be said about banning the consumption of animals where doing so does not rely on a violation of their interests—as any interest in eating them could, at least in many situations, also be fulfilled by eating plants. Some might argue that the relative absence of important interests that might be harmed in the latter case and the fact that human beings may be prone to

slippery slope reasoning, particularly when they are influenced by their gustatory pleasures, must be taken into consideration in the development of a moral
theory—perhaps a more general ban could be justified on this basis?

I am no longer persuaded by this mode of reasoning. As I have mentioned
already, refraining from consuming animals in situations where doing so does
not violate their interests does not imply that no morally significant interests
are sacrificed. Any choices that we make to eat other foods also harm, both
intentionally and accidentally, the interests of many nonhuman organisms. In
many situations, this harm includes harm to animals, even if they are not actually eaten. This is a real problem for the theories in animal ethics that I have
encountered so far: if—once any nutritional, zoonotic, and human resource
concerns have been given adequate consideration—a human moral agent's
main concern should be to safeguard the interests of any moral patients who
may be affected by their food choices, it would be their duty to consume animals where doing so minimises harm on any moral patients who might be
affected. If a general taboo on the consumption of animals can be justified, its
justification must therefore lie elsewhere.

It might be objected that a mere interest in healthy food is sufficient to
ground such a taboo given that foods derived from animals may be more likely
to affect physiological human health negatively than plant foods because of the
fact that many pathogens thrive in the tissues of both nonhuman and human
animals, particularly shortly after death (Fessler and Navarrete 2003). Whereas
this might account for the fact that we have good reason to avoid unsafe animal products, it does not explain why a taboo should be adopted where safety
concerns can be minimised. Rather, I do not think that the moral relevance of
the perception of various degrees of commonality between different animals
and human beings can be ignored. If this perception is not neutral, but morally
laden, our psychological health may be undermined if we consume animals,
perhaps because our emotions should stand in the way of objectifying those
whom we should have related to as subjects before they died.

Those who struggle to accept either the existence or the moral nature and
claimed relevance of this emotion might wish to consider whether a fairly general taboo on the consumption of animal products ought to be adopted in light
of the question whether they would consume their companion animals after
they had died. Whereas some people who refrain from consuming their companion animals and their companion animals' species members might claim
that there is something special about the nature of the species of the animals in
question that sets them apart from other animals, my view is that a necessary
condition for this claim to be satisfactory is that it fits with our evolutionist
interest. In other words, for this claim to be valid, these people ought not to
consume animals who are more closely related to us either. Whilst recognising
the significance of this interest implies that some species—i.e. those who are
more closely related to us than others—are better candidates for a taboo than
others, it does not imply that there are no grounds for a general taboo.

If people have an interest in the consumption of animals—an interest that appears to have been selected for in the evolution of our species—it would seem strange for taboos to emerge and to be maintained unless there is also something that human moral agents across the world find objectionable about eating animals. Anthropological research reveals that many cultures adopt taboos on the consumption of particular animals, for example of animals kept for companionship, in spite of the fact that they may kill their species members for food. Whereas this does not rule out that the development of one's gustatory pleasure might make one more likely to approve of killing animals for food, it shows at least that it does not prevent the adoption of a taboo. Indigenous populations of the Caribbean and of lowland South America, for example, reserve a taboo only for those individuals within particular species who are kept as 'iegue'—a Carib term that can denote both an adopted child and a tamed animal, the latter of which meaning is thought to have influenced the meaning of the word 'pet' when it was first defined in an English dictionary in the early 18th century (Norton 2015).

Some might argue that what is doing the moral work here is the 'pet bond'. Whereas I do not wish to question the view of those who claim that eating one's pet poses a greater moral problem than eating a member of one's pet's species, a theory that is based on animalism generalises the feeling of moral revulsion that one ought to have towards eating one's pet to a moral interest in the avoidance of consuming all animals. It supports the view that speciesists might adopt, namely that it is normally inappropriate to consume the bodies of dead human beings because of the conflict of such a consumption with honouring our interest in a 'species bond', but it expands this principle to a concern with consuming the bodies of all animals based on an 'animal bond'. Our evolutionist interest explains why it might be particularly troublesome not to adopt such a taboo when it concerns the consumption of animals who are relatively close to us in evolutionary terms.

To the extent that 'perceived intelligence' acts as a proxy for the perception of relative evolutionary similarity, empirical research supports the view that people experience more disgust when they contemplate eating animals who are more similar to them than other animals (Ruby and Heine 2012, 49). In addition, sociological evidence supports the view that greater empathy for companion animals is causally related to greater feelings of discomfort not only with eating them, but also with eating animals who are farmed for food and who are, presumably, empathised with as well based on the perception that they bear an evolutionary similarity to one's companion animals and to oneself (Rothgerber and Mican 2014). Indeed, it is perhaps only through having developed some empathy with some animals, who need not necessarily be pets, that we can develop the kind of empathy that is required to embrace the idea of 'universal benevolence' that Mancilla (2009, 15) recognises in the work of Adam Smith (1982, 235), who writes that 'we cannot form the idea of any ... sensible being, whose happiness we should not desire, or to whose misery, when distinctly brought home to the imagination, we should not have some degree of aversion'. Similarly, Scruton (2000, 36) writes: 'Two of our sympathetic feelings are of great moral importance: pity towards those who suffer and pleasure in another's joy'. What I have argued here is that this empathy can survive the animal's death and that we ought to foster such a culture of empathy to protect and promote holistic human health.

In spite of the fact that we have capacities to empathise with all sentient beings, I have argued that we are bound to empathise more with some than with others. Some might accept that our capacities to empathise with plants are more limited, but nevertheless argue that we should extend our evolutionist interest further. Accordingly, they might argue that plants that have died naturally ought not to be eaten by us either, and *a fortiori* that they should not be killed for food in situations where we can consume other things. To avoid killing plants, we could consume parts of plants without killing them, or use only fruits and berries to feed ourselves, being careful not to damage seeds in the process. As only a small percentage of many plants would be used whilst others (for example plants of which only the roots are edible) would not be used at all, adopting this proposal would lead to: a much greater demand for agricultural land, aggravating its associated problems; a significant increase in demand for agricultural labour, with the potential to jeopardise other important human endeavours; and, finally, more restrictive diets and greater food insecurity that may undermine human health. In light of these considerations, I consider that plants are sufficiently remote from us in evolutionary distance to justify the view that their consumption by us is the lesser evil. In addition, the view that living plants have more limited capacities to experience harm than living animals seems plausible, as well as morally relevant.

It might be objected that human beings also have health interests in eating animals, and that their interests in eating the body parts of pigs, for example, would be thwarted unjustifiably if they had to refrain from doing so. I disagree with this perspective in situations where human beings can safeguard human health without eating animals. Compared with the human interest in relating appropriately to pigs and with pigs' interests in, for example, wallowing in the mud, which they cannot fulfil by being killed, the putative human desire to eat pigs' body parts seems to pale into insignificance, at least in situations where human beings can eat nutritious foods that are not derived from the bodies of animals or products from animals who are more distantly related without increasing negative GHIs. Accordingly, for all people who take animalism seriously, the human interest in relating appropriately to pigs and the pigs' interests in doing things that keep them alive should be sufficiently weighty to impose a strong *prima facie* obligation to refrain from eating pigs, where the former interest alone should be sufficiently weighty to impose a strong *prima facie* obligation to refrain from eating pigs who have died naturally or accidentally.

To make the central claim defended in this section more concrete and show how it differs from the claim made by those who argue against the implications of animalism, let us imagine a group of vegans on their way to their allotments, where they have planned to harvest some fruit and vegetables in order to have a garden party. One vegan individual drives the car and accidentally runs into a deer who is crossing the road; the individual laments the fact that the deer has been killed by the collision, as well as the error of not seeing the deer in time to avoid the animal. Rather than risk harming further sentient animals in their garden in the process of harvesting, scholars such as Singer (1975), Regan (1983), Varner (2012), and Cochrane (2012) should argue—if they are consistent with their own theories—that the group ought to eat the deer instead, at least if we assume that it would not make the group more likely to support killing animals for food and that it would not increase nutritional or food safety concerns relative to the alternatives. Admittedly, to enjoy a balanced meal the group might need to supplement the flesh from the deer with some fruits and vegetables, but this does not detract from the point.

This is precisely what our imaginary car driver suggests. Remembering the days when eating the bodies of animals was a habit, the driver decides not to waste an opportunity and tells everyone: 'Vegan party is off, barbecue is on.' Anyone who thinks that there is something odd, something surreal, about this fellow may understand that qualified moral veganism cannot be based on the desire to minimise the infliction of pain, suffering, and death upon other animals. Rather, it is motivated by the feeling, rooted in animalism, that we should not eat animals. A theory that takes our animalist interest seriously adopts the view that we have a moral duty to avoid eating the deer, at least in the vast majority of situations. Giving proper recognition to the deer demands that the deer's body be not regarded as a consumable object by human beings, even after the deer has died, at least in situations where people are able to feed themselves adequately by other means without increasing negative GHIs.

2.11 Human health, the genetic engineering of animals, and animals' interests in living independently

A human moral agent undermines their health not only by rejecting speciesism and animalism, but also by ignoring or downplaying our interest in protecting the integrity of nature. A major threat to this interest is the genetic engineering of animals, which has been carried out for various purposes, including the provision of human food. In thinking of the scenarios of 'decerebrated' animals envisaged by Rollin (1995, 193) and the 'living egg machines' imagined by Comstock (2000, 152), Varner (2012, 276–278) has welcomed the conventional breeding and the genetic engineering of animals that aim to make them insentient. One scenario that he finds particularly attractive is no longer in the realm of science fiction, but concerns a strain that was created by the selective breeding of chickens who suffered from a natural mutation that caused them to be blind; this strain was found to be useful to overcome the problems posed by feather-pecking, comb-pecking, and cannibalism amongst confined chickens, as the blind chickens did not engage in these behaviours (Ali and Cheng 1985). Whereas I am not aware that any farmers have started using blind chickens since their creation over 30 years ago, in light of a positive assessment of these blind chickens' welfare (Sandøe et al. 1999, 321–322), which has been thought to be better than the welfare of other strains within the systems that dominate the farmed animals' sector, Varner (2012, 277–278) would welcome the replacement of sighted chickens with blind strains, although he recognises that the existence of a 'yuck factor' might imply that 'consumer preferences cannot be changed by the waving of a philosophical wand'.

I am less pessimistic about philosophers' abilities to change people's preferences. The problem might actually lie in the kind of wand that the philosopher waves, rather than in the possibility that others may resist change. What is being approved of here appears to be analogous to an employer who gives his employees pills so that they are better able to cope with the miserable conditions that they are working in, for example by forgetting about them. It might be objected that the right way to address these miserable conditions is not to give pills to one's employees, but to improve their working conditions. Some might say that giving pills to one's employees under these circumstances would violate human dignity. Though the concept of human dignity is difficult to define, its meaning could be clarified—in true Wittgensteinian fashion—from how the concept is used. Diamond (1978, 475) invokes the concept in discussing the moral issues related to animals performing circus tricks, which she calls an 'indignity'. Whereas I am unsure about the precise meaning of the term for Diamond, I would relate this concept back to my fundamental interest in health, conceived holistically. Unless there is no other way to improve one's employees' health, it might be unhealthy for an employer to provide these pills, even if they might improve the employees' welfare. Whereas it is hard to imagine how they could, as employees may feel that swallowing such pills would be degrading, it is nevertheless possible to imagine that they might, for example if employees lacked awareness of swallowing them because the employer gave them covertly, for instance by adding them to the employees' drinks. The employer should tend not only to the welfare of others, however, but also to his own welfare, which might not be compatible with the pill-giving practice: merely entertaining the thought of addressing the problem in this way may indicate that one has the wrong attitude towards one's employees.

Similarly, if the sighted strains of chickens engage in fighting and cannibalism, it would seem to be appropriate to question whether the conditions under which these animals are kept could be altered so that chickens may be able to display more normal behaviours. As fewer chickens engage in fighting and cannibalism when they are kept in slightly better conditions, for example when they are allowed to live outdoors for some of the time, another solution than the breeding of blind chickens ought to be preferred to the problems caused by chicken aggression.

Some might object that this is an ideal-world solution that fails to consider the real world in which we live, where farmers may be forced by the competitive market to keep chickens in conditions that are far from ideal. Consequently, these farmers might favour out of economic necessity the technological solution proffered by the creation of blind chickens. Barring exceptional circumstances, for example where the farmer's own survival would depend on adopting this solution, I am not persuaded by this line of thinking. One might argue that farmers should explore and adopt better alternatives to the problem posed by the human infliction of pain and suffering upon chickens.

The problem remains, however, that, given that many farmers and consumers are currently unwilling to refrain from using chickens for food, focusing merely on the ideal scenario fails to do something right now about the conditions in which many animals are kept. Consequently, it might be argued that a dual strategy should be adopted where one part of the strategy advocates the adoption of vegan diets where appropriate, whilst another part advocates the genetic engineering or the selective breeding of farmed animals as a temporary measure, in the hope that the latter part of the strategy will at least reduce animal welfare concerns in the short term. To add force to this objection, one might even consider that the welfare of blind chickens or of any genetically engineered or selectively bred animals might be better than the welfare of, respectively, sighted chickens and non-selectively bred animals, even if the last two groups were kept in the best possible conditions. This also shows why the project of what Thompson (2008) refers to as the 'disenhancement' of animals, where the concept of 'disenhancement' suggests that animals gain something (for example reduced exposure to violent behaviour) whilst losing something else (for example sight), presents a significant moral challenge.

One way to tackle this objection is to deny the empirical claim on which it rests by arguing that whenever animals are bred to lose some function their welfare actually deteriorates as well, regardless of whether there may be improvements in specific areas of their lives. In this vein, Sandøe et al. (2014, 735) have recently questioned Ali and Cheng (1985)'s contentions in light of new research into the welfare of blind chickens, concluding that 'blind laying-hens do, after all, have poor welfare compared with similar sighted birds'. The authors proceed to state, however, that this does not yield a principled objection against animal 'disenhancement' as there may be cases where such projects do increase the welfare of other animals overall. Whereas the authors may be right in this regard, it is important to recognise that this issue must not be considered in light of the question of what may or may not increase different entities' purely subjective experiences of welfare, but in light of a normative account of what ought to be deemed to be constitutive of good welfare for all affected parties, regardless of any differences in subjective perceptions.

In this light, the authors point out rightly, albeit cautiously, that the welfare of nonhuman animals might be improved by these projects, but they conclude wrongly that 'arguments that disenhancement is "disrespectful of telos" do not seem to stand up to critical scrutiny' (Sandøe et al. 2014, 740). More specifically, this conclusion is wrong because, when we consider the question whether to alter the *telos* or nature of an animal, we must consider not only how the genetic engineering or the selective breeding of animals might affect the health of the nonhuman animals concerned, but also how it might affect human health.

Regardless of any differences in subjective assessments of our health or welfare, I claim that human health *is* undermined by the selective breeding of blind chickens and, more generally and *a fortiori*, by the genetic engineering of animals. Whereas I do not adopt a 'nature knows best' philosophy, I nevertheless adopt the view that we must adopt a *prima facie* duty to safeguard the integrity of nature in order to protect good human health. Looking after our own health interest demands that we cultivate the right attitude towards nature. When I use the word 'nature' in connection with the concept of the 'integrity of nature', the word refers in the first place to everything that is not affected by conscious human design (rather than to the extended sense of 'nature' which encompasses everything, including human beings). A paradigm case of the 'natural' in this sense is a dinosaur, whose existence was not in any way influenced by human beings, given that we were not around at the time that the dinosaurs existed. However, now that we do exist, few natural things exist that have not been affected by human beings. Still, even a wild animal who lives today is more natural than a farmed animal. Classifying things in terms of whether they are natural is therefore not a simple 'yes' or 'no' matter, but a matter of degree. To explore how natural or unnatural something is, it is therefore important to question not only whether human beings affected it, but also how they did so.

In the Whiteheadian ontology that I adopt, all natural individuals have autonomous teleological (or goal-directed) centres that drive their development. In this light, a computer is not a natural individual. Even if its programme works to accomplish particular goals, these goals have been designed not by the computer itself, but by an external designer. Whereas a computer is composed of billions of natural individuals, such as molecules, atoms, and sub-atomic particles, that do possess autonomous teleological centres, the ways in which these individuals function may not be changed much by their being assembled into a computer. Or, to provide another example, when driftwood is used to develop a sculpture, the teleological centres of the molecules inside the wood are also unlikely to be altered much by the human design: they do what they do regardless of the shape that is imposed upon the wood.

This differs from the processes that used artificial selection to bring about modern breeds of cows and bulls. It is unimaginable to think, for example, that nature might have selected for the creation of cows with very high metabolic demands that facilitate the production of milk at the rates that modern dairy cows produce it, or to think that it would have selected, as for example in the case of the Belgian Blue breed, for the creation of cows who are so muscular (through selection for a 'double-muscling' trait) that they can hardly or no longer give birth naturally. The integrity of nature has been undermined by these projects as the internal teleologies of these cows have undergone significant changes compared to the internal teleologies of their distant ancestors, so that they are now programmed to do very different things. These cows have been designed by the external teleologies of human beings who aimed at increasing the production of milk and flesh, in similar ways in which the natural creation of blindness in some chickens might be selected for by chicken breeders. In some situations, this external design has been so successful in modifying the internal teleologies of the cows who are used to produce dairy products and flesh that their survival depends on human beings, rather than on their internal teleologies. The Holstein-Friesian cows who dominate the dairy industry, for example, rely on the human provision of high protein concentrates to satisfy their high metabolic demands, whereas the Belgian Blue cows rely on caesarean section to reproduce.

The genetic engineering of animals differs from these conventional selective breeding methods in that the animals' teleological centres are altered from the inside, rather than from the outside. To produce change, conventional selective breeding methods rely on indirectly manipulating the internal capacities of organisms or gametes (by selecting males and females for sexual reproduction, which introduces change through the creation of offspring with given traits) whereas genetic engineering frequently alters the internal capacities of organisms or gametes directly. I write 'frequently' as there are exceptions. Some genetic engineering techniques used on bacteria, for example, rely on the internal capacities of bacteria to alter themselves through a process that is known as horizontal or lateral gene transfer, a process whereby bacteria spontaneously adopt genetic material from their surroundings. Some genetic engineering techniques exploit this intrinsic capacity, for example by heating bacteria, which triggers the desired adoption behaviour. The genetic engineering of multi-cellular animals, by contrast, does not rely on coaxing the natural capacity of an organism to incorporate foreign DNA.

Even if the changes that occur either through conventional breeding or through genetic engineering might favour the welfare of the animals thus created, I question whether they are desirable in light of my claim that we should adopt a *prima facie* duty to safeguard nature's integrity to protect human health or welfare. In a world that is manipulated to a great extent by human design, which has conferred significant benefits to humans, I believe that we must also give some moral weight to the autonomous, internal capacities of all individuals to direct their own developments. Consequently, any proposal to modify other organisms, particularly if the method involves genetic engineering technologies that force genetic changes on organisms that—whilst they may be able to respond well to those changes—lack the natural capacities to bring about those changes themselves, must provide a positive answer to the question why forcing external (or 'unnatural') changes on these organisms would outweigh my *prima facie* concern. I am not arguing that nature always promotes the health of organisms better than human beings may be able to do, but that giving due consideration to our own health demands that we ascribe some positive value to maintaining the autonomous capacities of all biological organisms.

In this light, the human creation of blind strains of chickens, for example, is not a positive thing. The dual strategy objection, however, remains. If the (unlikely) assumption is made that blind chickens do actually fare better within some current farming systems and that we are unable to move away from these systems by campaigning for the adoption of vegan diets, it might be argued that approving of the creation of blind chickens may be the lesser evil, even if it is granted that doing so undermines human health by allowing human beings to be relatively unrestrained in controlling nature. Advocates may concede that care must be taken to avoid the possibility that alleviating some animal welfare issues in this and similar ways might undermine broader human health and animal welfare objectives. The underlying concern could be articulated as a worry that people might habituate to these new methods and, consequently, become less likely to adopt vegan diets because of the fact that they have accepted the objectification of animals, which might be more readily accepted because of the associated improvements in the welfare of other animals. Whilst acknowledging this concern, advocates might argue that it nevertheless would be insufficiently strong to justify a prohibition.

The rationale underlying this way of reasoning might be illustrated by returning to the analogy mentioned above. Imagine an employer with many employees who are treated badly and a moralist who talks to the employer about improving conditions on the factory floor. The employer does not want to listen to the moral argument and the employees cannot escape from the fact that they are treated badly. The moralist might either continue to argue with the employer or invest their energy in supporting a change in the law on drugs so that the employees could be provided with new pills that they could take so that they would become less aware of their predicaments, and consequently suffer less. I would argue that the moralist should be allowed to support the lat-ter option, provided that they maintain their primary focus on their long-term goal and that there are very good grounds to believe that supporting the latter option does not undermine this long-term goal.

I am not persuaded, however, that this case provides a good analogy to sup-port projects that undermine the integrity of animals in radical ways. A better analogy for these projects is the sale of human kidneys. Some who support a dual strategy might point out that we should also allow the sale of human kidneys as long as human poverty continues to exist. Given that there are poor people in spite of efforts to eradicate poverty, the argument might be made that we should allow poor people to sell one of their kidneys, provided that we have reasonable grounds to believe that the greater good of reducing their poverty in this way outweighs any health concerns for those who might decide to sell a kidney and that it will not undermine the goal of reducing poverty overall. Should we deny them this option by prohibiting the sale, even if doing so may impose greater health risks upon them than permitting the sale of kidneys?

I believe that we should, as the negative GHI associated with allowing people to compromise their bodily integrity in exchange for money outweighs the negative GHI associated with denying some people this opportunity to escape from poverty.

Whereas the 'disenhancement' of animals is dissimilar from the sale of kidneys in that the lure of a financial incentive is irrelevant to the former *per se*, what the suggested solutions to the dilemmas posed by these two scenarios have in common is that it is not necessarily wrong to allow pain and suffering even where something could be done about it as safeguarding the integrity of nature, of which safeguarding the integrity of the human body is one particular instantiation, ought to be the overriding interest. Incidentally, this does not imply that we should also prohibit people from donating kidneys voluntarily; allowing this voluntary practice does not remove the morally relevant fact that kidney donation relies on altering the natural functioning of a human body, but the risk of coercing someone else into using their body for this purpose through the offer of money is more problematic than the negative value associated with appropriating part of one's own body, where I believe that only the latter can be justified as a voluntary contribution to the greater good.

None of the above implies that anyone who makes the dual strategy objection fails to make a valid point, which is why I believe that minor compromises on the value of maintaining the integrity of nature are justifiable if they reduce the human infliction of pain, suffering, and death upon farmed animals. If it was found that a particular strain of chickens coped much better with current farming conditions than another strain where the reason for this did not stem from the removal of a basic physiological trait such as the capacity to see, for example, greater human intervention in the breeding of chickens (through artificial selection for the desirable trait, for instance) might be justified in order to replace the latter by the former. Great care must be taken, however, that any support that is given to this strategy does not undermine the objective of promoting vegan diets.

Attributing sufficient value to the integrity of nature demands not only that we question the breeding of animals through artificial selection and genetic engineering, but also that, where appropriate, we allow animals to live independently. In relation to the possible interest that some nonhuman animals may have in living independently, my position is different from that of Cochrane (2012, 13), who denies that most nonhuman animals have such an interest, for example where he argues that dogs 'are not rational autonomous agents with an interest in leading their own freely chosen lives', and that they therefore should not be provided with a 'fundamental right to be free'. If freeing dogs or any other animals caused them more harm, Cochrane (2009) also suggests that their liberation may not be appropriate. I disagree with this view for two reasons.

Firstly, a nonhuman animal's right to freedom need not necessarily hinge on the question whether the animal in question has the capacity—which Cochrane rightly appears to consider necessary for the dog to be a rational agent—to compare reflectively the options of a free life with that of a life under human domestication or, more generally—in Cochrane (2009, 660)'s words—to 'frame, revise and pursue their own conception of the good'. Though I share Cochrane's assumption that dogs (as well as most other animals) are not rational agents, and accept that some breeds of dogs seek out the company of human beings in some situations and that many would struggle or even be unable to live independently from human beings, the dingo provides a good example of a domesticated animal who turned to a feral existence upon being introduced into Australia (Savolainen et al. 2004). The dingo may well have a serious interest in living independently from human beings that might be undermined by a domesticated life. Given the right environmental context, for example the presence of sufficient prey animals, some other breeds of dogs may well have a serious interest in living independently too. Whilst this need not imply that we should always grant them a right to be free—given that feral dogs might attack human beings, for example—those animals who may thrive better whilst living independently must at least be given a *prima facie* right to be free. The same applies to animals who are being farmed. For this reason, I am puzzled that the release of domesticated animals does not appear to be considered by Francione (2010b, 36), even if I agree that it would not be a good idea to release 'domesticated nonhumans to run wild in the street'. Even if there might be good reasons why human beings should not allow animals who used to be farmed to roam wherever they like (as feral pigs might, for example, destroy arable crops), nonhuman animals need not be rational agents in order to be granted *prima facie* rights to roam freely.

Secondly, the question whether to release an animal from human domestication need not depend on the animal being better off by being liberated from human interference. Whereas the nonhuman animal's welfare is relevant, any decision to liberate an animal should ultimately be decided by whether it is best for us to relinquish our control over a particular animal. Where animals have at least some interest in living independently, it may be appropriate for us to liberate them as our health interest demands that we value nature's integrity, which in turn may demand that we relinquish some of the great control that we exercise over our fellow earth inhabitants.

2.12 Human health and in-vitro flesh

The virtue of maintaining a focus on one's holistic health can be undermined in many ways. Mark Packer (1996, 58) considers that, one day, flesh for human consumption may be grown from cultured human somatic cells, extracted painlessly from consenting humans, and comments that 'consumers might be willing to pay more in order to enjoy the naughty thrill of cannibalism without any pangs of conscience' as 'nobody would suffer any pain, and no one would be killed'. The consumption of in-vitro flesh that has been developed from a tiny skin cell previously removed from the body of just one consenting human being might well be healthy in a narrow sense that it could provide people with adequate nourishment, but if health is understood more holistically, the development of such flesh is not normally healthy, neither for those who consume it nor for those who might develop it. Human body parts are not the sorts of things that people should normally perceive to be good candidates for human consumption. Apart from the fact that human cells do not grow naturally outside human bodies, the value that is relevant here, additionally to this interest in 'naturalness', is our speciesist interest.

This raises the question whether we should be equally concerned about the creation of synthetic flesh from nonhuman animals. Laestadius (2015) has reported that discussions over in-vitro flesh started at least from 2000 when a NASA-funded project cultured goldfish cells into tissue with the aim to explore its potential as a possible food source for astronauts—even if the actual tissue was not consumed. The first time that in-vitro flesh was actually consumed was in 2003, when cells were taken from frogs and grown outside their bodies to be consumed in an art installation called 'Disembodied Cuisine', which was part of the L'Art Biotech exhibition in Nantes, France (Catts and Zurr 2013).

The controversy over lab-grown flesh has grown significantly, however, since August 2013, when a team from Maastricht University created the first lab-grown burger, which was consumed publicly in a media event held in London (Post 2012; Jha 2013). The burger was created by extracting satellite cells (skeletal muscle-specific stem cells) from a cow through a needle biopsy. The cells were then cultured on a scaffold in a lab. Whereas the development of the burger in question relied on the use of foetal bovine serum as a growth medium, efforts are being made to steer away from using animal products as a growth medium, and Post (2014, 30) has expressed the view that this seems 'attainable' in light of the fact that many other cells can already be cultured in media that do not include any animal products, for example in those containing amino acids obtained through bacterial fermentation.

If we assume that these efforts will pay off so that the technology would rely only on the usage of animals to extract the cells from which the flesh is cultivated, the question must be asked whether this technology should be embraced. Arguably, such cells might be able to be obtained from animals without inflicting any pain on them as it might even be possible to obtain them immediately after the animal has died. Whilst the cells in question, as well as their descendants, would—in accordance with a Whiteheadian ontology—still be sentient, it seems plausible to assume that the sentience of these cells would pose much less of a question in terms of whether pain or suffering should be allowed to be inflicted on them than using a whole animal for human consumption would.

Whilst proponents of this technology may concede that the technology may not eliminate pain, they might argue that the production of food in this way, particularly when it is done in a carefully controlled laboratory environment, may inflict less pain and death upon sentient life than other modes of producing food. Some vegans might even warm to the prospect of eating lab-grown flesh as their decision to refrain from consuming flesh need no longer rest on a choice between killing animals or killing plants for food. Rather, the choice would now be between killing the latter or killing animal cells, where the question of which might impose more harm on moral patients may be much less certain. Even if answering this question also depended on the processes involved with the development, use, and transportation of any growth media that were used, the view that consuming animal cells might be associated with a reduction of the pain, suffering, and death that is imposed on moral patients seems plausible.

Whereas many concerns that have been expressed over in-vitro flesh might be allayed by these considerations, an animalist perspective also considers this topic by starting from my speciesist unease with the consumption of human flesh. Both Cochrane (2012, 116) and Varner (2012, 276–277) argue that the concerns of those who object to the development and the consumption of in-vitro flesh from nonhuman animals should not really be taken seriously as they would be based on nothing more than aesthetic feelings or matters of taste, rather than on considerations related to 'well-being', but neither rule out the possibility that the health of those human moral agents who consider this technology to be—in the words used by Rollin (1995, 193)—'aesthetically abhorrent', as well as the health of others (who might be affected negatively without being conscious of it), might be undermined by the realisation of the in-vitro flesh project. As for lab-grown human flesh, I believe that the production and the consumption of in-vitro flesh derived from other animals presents a holistic health care problem.

I have argued already that holistic health may be jeopardised by projects that undermine the integrity of nature. Even if my concern with safeguarding the integrity of nature is less pronounced with in-vitro flesh than with the genetic engineering of animals, it is not allayed altogether. Research has already found that many invoke the concept of the 'unnatural' when they comment on this former technology (Laestadius and Caldwell 2015). I think that people are right to invoke this concept in this context: cultured flesh is more unnatural than conventional methods to produce flesh as stem cells do not grow into flesh outside living bodies without human intervention. However, the technology is likely to be more natural than genetically engineered flesh, depending on the extent to which the attempt to merely coax or trick these cells into doing what they might have done had they still been inside living organisms is successful. Whereas the teleological centres of the cells that are extracted from the animals who are used in the process may not be altered as much as the teleological centres of any animals who are engineered through anthropogenic genetic alterations, it is not because the latter present a greater concern in relation to safeguarding nature's integrity that the former should be acceptable.

However, as I argued in relation to the creation of blind chickens, the concern that I have with the ideology, which is perpetuated by in-vitro flesh, that conceives of animals' body parts in terms of flesh that can justifiably be eaten by human beings in many situations and the concern that I have with the jeopardising of nature's integrity are only two concerns that I have in relation to the consumption of animal products. If, in order to avoid malnutrition, I had to choose between consuming lab-grown flesh, developed in the fashion envisaged here, or consuming flesh taken from animals who had been killed for food, I would choose to consume the former on the basis of the fact that, in the circumstances described, only the former would avoid the killing of animals for food. Accordingly, I would support the development and use of in-vitro flesh if it could be argued convincingly that a serious concern, such as human malnutrition, could be minimised by its development without increasing overall negative GHIs compared to other options that might be available.

More realistically, it might be argued by those who support the dual strategy outlined in the previous section that there is a moral imperative to develop in-vitro flesh given that there is no sign that large numbers of people are willing to switch to vegan diets and that, in most if not all jurisdictions, legitimate procedures to prevent people from consuming animal products are lacking. As the human use of cells poses fewer moral concerns than the human use of whole animals since mere parts rather than whole individuals are manipulated, and as the processes involved with the development of in-vitro flesh appear to be more natural than those involved with the genetic engineering of animals as these cells appear to be merely coaxed to do what they naturally do in a different environment, I agree. I am cautious, however, as our resources could also be used to support other projects that reduce the human infliction of pain, suffering, and death upon other animals, where careful consideration must be given to which option maximises positive GHIs and to how any short-term gains should be balanced with the aim to maximise positive GHIs in the long term.

However, the environmentally responsible production of in-vitro flesh ought to be welcomed at least for one other reason, which has nothing to do with the human consumption of animal flesh, but has to do with the consumption of animal flesh by companion cats. If we assume that it is not justified to euthanise these cats—an assumption that I cautiously support—and that they cannot be weaned off either partially or wholly from human domestication without unacceptably large welfare concerns, it will be necessary for human beings to continue feeding them. If cats cannot thrive without consuming animal flesh—a subject that is not without controversy (see e.g. Gray et al. 2004)—and if they cannot be fed from animals who die naturally or accidentally or from those who are killed justifiably, the production of in-vitro flesh would seem to be preferable to the alternative of killing animals in order to feed them. My stance on this, however, is also one of caution. Whilst the promotion of research into the adequacy or otherwise of vegan cat diets must be encouraged, other options—discussed by Milburn (forthcoming)—may be preferable at the present time, including the feeding of eggs from rescued hens, the feeding of flesh that would otherwise be disposed of and that is obtained without giving out any financial or other compensation, or the feeding of flesh obtained through skip diving. As these products would become very scarce if large numbers of people converted to vegan diets, however, the development of in-vitro flesh in order to feed cats would seem to be a positive development.

2.13 The duty to adopt qualified moral veganism

In my opinion, the ethical concerns that I have described in this and the preceding chapters can only be given the consideration that they deserve by the adoption of qualified moral veganism. My commitment to veganism is qualified as my theory does not demand that human beings abstain from eating animal products in all situations. It is a moral, rather than a dietary, position that can be adopted by everyone, even by those who ought not to adopt vegan diets for justifiable personal, social, or ecological reasons: in a similar way to how even those who might justifiably resort to consuming human bodies in emergency situations may agree with the view that it would not be appropriate to do so in more ideal situations, my claim is that even those who might justifiably eat animal products in some situations ought nevertheless to refrain from doing so (with the exception of consuming human milk and—in very specific circumstances—honey) in more ideal situations. It is a vegan theory in the sense that vegan diets ought to be the default diets for the majority of the human population. Recall that I defined a vegan diet as a diet that does not include animal products, apart from human milk and honey.

In the first chapter I argued that many people's diets fail to minimise negative GHIs. This conclusion has been bolstered in this chapter as I have argued that, in many situations, omnivorous and vegetarian diets increase negative GHIs by neglecting our duties towards the nonhuman world. Though we must give moral consideration to how our actions affect both animals and plants, I argued that animals, and particularly those who are most closely related to human beings, should be granted greater moral significance. In this light, I recognised that some vegan diets can, in some situations, impose greater negative GHIs upon other animals than other diets. However, I also argued that, in many situations, this does not undermine the validity of a vegan diet as some diets that impose relatively greater negative GHIs upon other animals may produce fewer negative GHIs overall due to their smaller negative GHIs upon moral agents' interests in holistic health. The duty that many people have to adopt a vegan diet does not stem merely from our *prima facie* duty to avoid actions that inflict pain, suffering, and death upon animals, but also from the *prima facie* positive GHI of accepting a taboo on the consumption of animals, regardless of whether the animals in question have been killed for food. This is also why I questioned research that aims to create animals with reduced sentience and research into synthetic flesh.

I emphasise that I do not argue for a universal duty to adopt veganism. *Contra* Francione (2010a, 74; 2010b, 36), veganism is not a 'nonnegotiable moral baseline'. Imagine a population living on a remote island with very poor soil conditions. If it were impossible for the people in question to obtain sufficient quantities of fruits and vegetables without tilling the soil, they could either feed themselves by digging over a lot of land, killing lots of animals in the process, or they could dig over a much smaller area and use some of the mussels who happened to live on the shore. I would argue that adopting the latter diet should at least be permissible as—even though the duty not to eat the mussels may be stronger than the duty to avoid killing any of the organisms that they might kill by tilling and using the arable land—the fact that more organisms with comparable degrees of moral significance would be harmed if they refrained from eating mussels ought to be one of the deciding factors. It is also my belief that no human being should be obliged to toil relentlessly to feed themselves, as we have a wide range of other interests that are very important and that we would not be able to satisfy if we had to 'dig deep' to provide food for ourselves. Taken together, these two considerations seem sufficient to justify the consumption of mussels in this situation. Similar considerations could also be invoked to justify the killing and the consumption of fish, even if soil conditions would need to be less favourable to override the greater moral significance that we ought to grant to fish than that we ought to grant to mussels. Also, if the islanders in question were to stumble upon an animal who had died naturally whilst they struggled to obtain adequate nourishment by other means, it would be appropriate for them to consume the body of that animal in spite of the fact that this might be taboo under more ideal conditions. Whereas this is an imaginary example, the same considerations apply to some groups of people who were mentioned in section 1.1.

When reading these lines, some readers may question whether the human consumption of eggs from rescued hens, obtained justifiably from a farmer who considered that these birds were 'spent', might be considered another legitimate use, even in situations where human health does not depend on such a consumption. Although I must declare that the thought of eating such eggs does not provoke the aversion in me that I feel when I consider eating the hens themselves after their natural deaths or after they have been killed in situations where their killing could be justified on compassionate grounds, I must express my reservations. It would seem to me to be preferable to feed the eggs to the hens themselves after cracking them or after boiling or cooking them so that the hens are able to benefit from reabsorbing the nutrients that they have lost through laying, particularly if we consider that the bodies of modern-day breeds might be strained by the heavy demands of having been programmed to lay large volumes of eggs. Whereas I have sympathy for people who rescue hens from bad farming conditions and have done so myself in the past, another option in situations where the right habitat can be found for these hens is to release them to allow them to roam freely, which may be preferable to confining them to one's land, even if their health prospects might be worse than they would be if they lived under human management.

Another question that is the subject of debate amongst those who think about these issues is whether honey ought to be allowed to be consumed when such consumption is not essential to maintain good health. I know some vegans who eat honey, raising the question whether there is something that sets honey apart from other animal substances. Whereas I am unsure why these people consume honey, I shall explore some arguments that might be advanced to support their position.

The fact that the lives of honeybees may be managed to a lesser extent by human beings than the lives of other domesticated animals may seem relevant to some. Domesticated bees do not seem to mind the fact that they are domesticated as many have the opportunity to leave their hives at any time, unlike many other domesticated animals who may stay for a number of reasons—for example because their movements are restricted by human beings, because they have nowhere else to go, or because they are lured regularly into staying by being provided with shelter and food. This might be a morally significant difference where the systems that are used to keep honeybees do not restrict their movements, but it must also be recognised that many beekeepers confine queens in their hives or clip their wings to reduce the likelihood that they may leave the hive.

Another argument—which I have encountered in this debate—is the view that restoring dwindling honeybee populations may be vitally important to increase the pollination services that honeybees provide for a large number of crops. However, it must also be said that these services are mainly provided by only one of the seven known species of honeybee, the Western or European honeybee (*Apis mellifera*), and that bees pollinate not only valuable crops, but also weeds (Goulson 2003). It is also quite plausible that habitat changes away from monocultures might produce similar benefits, so that the pollination of valuable plants could also be carried out by wild bees and other insects who are now in decline because of these monocultures and of the use of some pesticides (for example neonicotinoids). The fact that a wide range of these other pollinators are dwindling does not provide an outright argument for the keeping of honeybees either, as we have evidence that many wild populations of bees are under strain at least partly because they compete for nectar with domesticated honeybees and are infected by their diseases (Buchmann and Nabhan 1996; Goulson 2003; Goulson and Sparrow 2009; Fürst et al. 2014).

If we assume that my concern about competition with wild species can be managed adequately by keeping domesticated bees in appropriate places or that it is outweighed by the significant crop losses that might result from inadequate pollination, so that the keeping of domesticated bees may be justifiable, it does not imply that taking their honey is justifiable. In many situations, the process of taking honey agitates the bees and—if accompanied by the use of smoke—causes bees to gorge themselves on honey, which might be caused by stress (as bees may expect the imminent arrival of fire in the presence of smoke and respond by filling themselves to prepare for evacuation), and—more importantly—may accidentally kill some bees. Many people who consume honey also sustain the practice of killing queens, who are killed deliberately by many beekeepers when they replace old queens with new ones to maintain fertility in their hives and who regularly kill queens to prevent swarming. For these reasons, I remain unconvinced of the justifiability of consuming honey produced by domesticated bees where these are kept by beekeepers who kill bees either intentionally or foreseeably.

However, this also raises the question whether it would be appropriate to consume honey from beekeepers who do not kill any of their bees intentionally and who also take great care to avoid inflicting both stress and accidental deaths upon their bees, perhaps by—amongst other things—using the 'sun hives' promoted by the Natural Beekeeping Trust (http://www.naturalbeekeepingtrust.org/). The moral argument in favour of the consumption of honey under these conditions would seem to be bolstered by the fact that research with a limited sample of people from Wales showed that people who included the consumption of honey in their dietary records—taken over the course of seven days—lived longer, when followed up over 25 years, than those who did not do so, a finding that remained significant after adjustments were made for a number of possible confounders (Cooper et al. 2010). On this basis, I am inclined to give a positive answer to this question, subject to the condition that the honey that is taken should be genuinely surplus to the bees' own requirements, to avoid bees being fed with sugary solutions that may be less healthy for them.

Some might object that this qualified endorsement is much too restrictive in light of the fact that sugar—a sweetener that many vegans use—is possibly worse not only for human health, but also in that its cultivation kills far more insects than the production of honey does. This may be so, but this is hardly an argument for the use of honey. Rather, it is an argument that vegans must also abstain from the consumption of sugar where its consumption does not yield any health benefits that could be provided by more benign means.

Even if a good case for the consumption of honey might be made in some situations, the fact that those who are committed to qualified moral veganism may, more generally, be justified in eating some animal products in some situations should not be taken to mean that I believe that they are also justified in eating products that contain tiny amounts of products that have been derived from animals who have clearly been used unjustifiably, at least in situations when their ability to enjoy good health does not depend on it. This is at odds with the view of Friedrich (2006, 191), who claims that refusing to eat animal products in some situations, for example when visiting a restaurant where no vegan food is available, might actually cause 'significantly more harm to animals' than eating some foods that do contain animal products. The rationale for this would consist in the fact that the people with whom one eats might be left with the impression that adopting a vegan diet is difficult, and that they would consequently become more hesitant to adopt such a diet themselves.

I think that this possibility is extremely unlikely. If vegans were to adopt diets that were not consistent with their beliefs, their companions might rather be left with the impression that their commitment to qualified moral veganism was only half-baked. Accordingly, anyone who compromises their position every time they walk into a restaurant that does not offer vegan food might communicate to their companions that qualified moral veganism is not a serious ethical position. Unlike what Friedrich (2006, 191) claims, it is not necessarily the case that vegans who go to great lengths to avoid the consumption of animal products pretend that their diets do not cause any suffering. For Friedrich (2006, 191), the question whether a vegan diet should be adopted in any particular situation is one of 'basic math': adopt the diet that causes the least suffering to other animals. I have argued, however, that the question whether a vegan diet should be adopted must depend primarily on the question whether other animals ought to be conceived of as sources of food for human beings, regardless of the fact that, in some situations, eating vegan food may cause more harm to other animals.

2.14 Conclusion

Against the standard picture, I questioned the line that many have drawn between vertebrates and invertebrates, and I argued that all individual entities are sentient. If all living things have health interests, all should be granted a *prima facie* right to those interests not being harmed. Diets that include animal products inflict a lot of pain, suffering, and death on living beings, but the same applies to most other diets. Nevertheless, many diets that include animal products impose a much greater quantity of negative GHIs than many other diets.

In order to stay alive and enjoy good health, human beings must eat sentient organisms or some of their parts. Adopting the view that we should treat like interests alike, but recognising that we have both speciesist and animalist interests, I argued that we ought to embrace qualified moral veganism. This position does not result from the erroneous belief that vegan diets necessarily cause less pain, suffering, and death on moral patients, but results from the belief that human health is, in many situations, undermined by conceiving of other animals as sources of human food. My focus on human health also explains why killing intentionally is more problematic than killing accidentally but foreseeably, a distinction that is considered irrelevant by Cochrane (2012, 96–98) and relevant by Francione (2010a, 72), where the latter refrains from explaining why this might be so. Whereas it does not make any difference for an animal to be killed either intentionally or foreseeably, a virtuous human being will have more problems with the former type of killing of animals. Another virtue that is constitutive of good human health is to show adequate respect for the integrity of nature, which is why I questioned the breeding of animals by artificial selection, the use of genetic engineering, and the creation of synthetic flesh, even if the last technique must be supported to reduce my overriding concern with the infliction of pain, suffering, and death upon animals.

In spite of my considerations, some carnists and vegetarians may remain convinced that human beings do not have any duties towards other animals, or that whatever duties we may have are not so demanding that we should commit to qualified moral veganism. Unless a law existed that demanded carnists and vegetarians to change their ways, forcing dietary change upon them would seem to be hard to justify, particularly if those who would wish to do so did not benefit from being supported by a decent number of people—a reasonable democratic principle. However, when carnists and vegetarians share meals with others, things become slightly more complicated. Most people attach great significance to the practice of sharing meals with each other. Many vegans feel deeply uncomfortable when they share meals with others who consume foods that they disapprove of, or even despise (Adams 2008, 187). The moral response to the death of an animal, and particularly to the deaths of those animals who are biologically close to us, should be one of sadness. It is not normally appropriate to celebrate human togetherness by sharing meals that include the corpses of those whose loss we ought to feel sad about. The corpses of animals who have died are inextricably connected with the animals they once were; their deaths demand a different response. Many vegans may also share my discomfort with sharing meals with vegetarians, where the former believe that the latter eat animal products that have been appropriated unjustifiably. Carnists and vegetarians might retort that vegans are not obliged to share meals with them. Though they are right that vegans could, at least in some situations, eat elsewhere, they should recognise that, if *they* cherish sharing meals with others, vegans might also value some aspects of shared meals, for example the opportunities that these provide to build relationships.

If carnists and vegetarians grant that vegans may have a serious interest in sharing meals with them, particularly in view of the relative shortage of other vegans on the planet, they could argue that, given that vegans do not amend their dietary preferences when they share meals with carnists and vegetarians, carnists and vegetarians should not amend their dietary preferences when they share meals with vegans either. This line of defence, however, is rather weak, for it is unlikely that carnists and vegetarians would object to the consumption of vegan food on moral grounds. Unless carnists and vegetarians could argue convincingly that the consumption of animal products would be required to protect important human interests, an argument which may apply in some situations, the only defence that they would seem to be left with in support of their resistance to dietary change is simply that they prefer the taste of food that contains animal products. They might accept that vegans may be uncomfortable about sharing meals with them, but argue that any moral weight that they may want to give to the interests of those who adopt qualified moral veganism ought to be trumped by their interest in consuming their preferred foods as not doing so would be—in Caney (2008, 539)'s words—'unreasonably demanding'.

I am not persuaded by this argument. The food choices that are made by carnists and vegetarians when they share meals with vegans may demonstrate a lack of (desire to act on our) empathy not only with the nonhuman world, but also with the people with whom they share meals, who may nevertheless be very close to them in many ways, for example by being family members or friends. It is perhaps because the empathy with animals and with their table companions is felt but not acted upon that—in my experience—it is carnists and vegetarians who frequently feel the need to apologise for their food choices to vegans or to sit far away from them at the table, rather than the other way round. More generally, it would seem to be highly appropriate that, when people share meals with each other, those who do not object to consuming particular foods adjust the food items that they eat to accommodate the values of those who do have moral objections where doing so does not undermine a more important moral interest. In chapter four I shall return to this issue in the context of discussing a comment that was made by a vegetarian research participant in one of the studies that I have been involved with: 'Christmas dinner was dreadful'.

CHAPTER THREE

The Politics of Qualified Moral Veganism

3.1 Introduction

Having documented that the negative GHIs associated with the consumption of animal products are wide-ranging and—in many situations—unjustified, I argued in chapter two that we should adopt qualified moral veganism. Many people, however, either willingly or unwittingly make dietary choices that are at odds with this theory. As qualified moral veganism is an ethical position, those who support it must contribute to political and legislative reforms to reduce the likelihood that people will not fulfil their duties when they make choices about what to eat.

This political project is not easy. As the policy-makers with the greatest power tend to be those who are most closely aligned with the status quo, those who seek to persuade other people of the morality of qualified moral veganism face significant resistance. Oppositions may come not only from farmers, but also from politicians, where Clements (1995, 12) has pointed out, in reflecting on the situation in the UK, that 'the National Farmers Union is an extremely powerful body, and it is no accident that many politicians are also farmers'. In fact, those farmers who are the most powerful are those who farm animals as funding provided by the European Union's Common Agricultural Policy has been biased towards those who own large quantities of grassland (Webster 2013, 207; European Commission 2015). Similarly, Joy (2010, 91) speaks of the power of agribusiness in the USA as a 'meatocracy'. This is also why investing one's hope in using the press and media to broadcast views that challenge established ways of thinking in radical ways would be naïve. In their analysis of UK national newspapers for the year 2007, M. Cole and Morgan (2011) reveal that newspapers tend to undermine veganism through ridicule, as well as through portraying vegan diets as impossible to maintain and through presenting vegans as faddists, ascetics, sentimentalists, or even hostile extremists—a general discourse that they label as 'vegaphobia'.

How to cite this book chapter:
Deckers, J 2016 *Animal (De)liberation: Should the Consumption of Animal Products Be Banned?* Pp. 107–129. London: Ubiquity Press. DOI: http://dx.doi.org/10.5334/ bay.d. License: CC-BY 4.0

Those who seek to bring about radical change in relation to the consumption of animal products would therefore be advised to take heed of these challenges, to contribute to identifying them, and to try to address them, knowing that it may be very difficult to curtail the actions of those who either deliberately try to or unwittingly stifle those who espouse views that are radically different from the status quo. If the view is correct that our experiences contribute not only to the formation of our ideas, but also to the formation of our brain structures, entrenched ideas may be very difficult to challenge (Wexler 2006). Once our brain structures have developed in particular ways, it is thought that we then seek information from our environments that accords with those structures, and deny or ignore everything else. This is aptly summarised by Lakoff (2004, 73): 'When the facts don't fit the frames, the frames are kept and the facts ignored' (quoted in Rees 2008).

In spite of these obstacles, this chapter considers three strategies that people with political power might adopt to promote qualified moral veganism. The first option is to educate people about the reasons underpinning qualified moral veganism in the hope that, where necessary, education will trigger behavioural change; the second is to increase the costs of animal products; and the third is to introduce a qualified ban on the consumption of animal products by turning the vegan project into a reality. After discussing these strategies' merits and demerits, I shall engage extensively with three objections that have been raised against the third strategy.

3.2 Educating people about the reasons underpinning qualified moral veganism

A study carried out in 2004 in the state of Victoria (South Australia), which explored, by means of a questionnaire, the attitudes of 415 people towards consuming plant-based foods, found that the strongest barriers that people invoked to the consumption of diets with low quantities of animal products was that they needed more information about such diets (Lea et al. 2006a; Lea et al. 2006b). The same study, however, found that 70% agreed with the statement that such a diet might 'prevent disease in general', but only 35% agreed with the view that it might 'help the environment' (Lea et al. 2006b, 834). Even if awareness of the environmental benefits of such diets was low, about 62% of respondents wanted to learn about such benefits. Similarly, Garnett (2008, 121) has made the more general claim that 'people know little about the ... implications of what they buy and eat', a claim that has also been supported by other empirical research (Joyce et al. 2008).

If many people know relatively little about the positive and negative GHIs of their dietary choices, but nevertheless show a willingness to learn more about them, the first option that policy-makers might pursue is to educate people about these GHIs in the hope that people will change their behaviour where required. This could be done in various ways. One way is to invest in research to expose socio-economic and psychological factors underlying food choice and to increase our knowledge about the positive and negative GHIs of animal products, particularly about the negative GHIs that have been neglected. Another is to invest in the dissemination of acquired knowledge through the press and media with the aim to stimulate people's thinking on these issues and, more generally, to promote the development of people's critical thinking skills that may help them to disentangle conflicting information and lead to changes in their values and behaviour.

There are many reasons, however, why the educational strategy is not sufficient. A first problem is that not everyone has the same educational opportunities. Consequently, educational campaigns are likely to reach some groups more than others, and, as research has found that many highly educated people may be more receptive towards considering dietary changes, highly educated people may be more likely to benefit from educational campaigns, with the result that existing health inequalities may increase (M. Kearney et al. 2000; Wardle and Steptoe 2003; Lea et al. 2006b). Even if educational opportunities could and should be equalised more, it is unlikely that individual differences in the comprehension of health information can be relegated to history. Accordingly, those people with either limited understanding or restricted opportunities to develop their understanding may be unlikely to develop modes of behaviour that accord with qualified moral veganism where they do not already embody these modes. To the extent that the problem posed by a lack of understanding cannot be overcome, some people will forgo opportunities to make positive behavioural changes. Though this does not imply that educational campaigns are wrong, it does emphasise that those who design them must be careful to avoid increasing the gaps between those who adopt relatively healthy diets and those who do not do so.

A second problem is that, even if people develop their understanding about the negative GHIs associated with problematic dietary choices, this new understanding might not be sufficient to propel them towards behavioural change. People's values may remain at odds with the values underpinning qualified moral veganism. Moreover, even if they did alter their values in ways that would support such a position, this might not necessarily result in behavioural change. The fact that 'old habits die hard', or, in other words, that there is 'behavioural lock-in', is a formidable challenge, as is well-known by those who have campaigned to protect people from the effects of passive smoking (Janson 2004). Though the dangers of passive smoking have been known for some time, many smokers who no longer expose others to the effects of second-hand smoke only changed their habits after legal changes had been made to prohibit smoking in public places (Menzies 2011). As with smoking, particular foods also fulfil social, cultural, and religious functions, and people might perceive that the meaning of these functions would be altered by dietary modifications. Research has revealed that the consumption of animal products has been particularly highly prized in Western culture (Twigg 1983; Fieldhouse 1986; Charles and Kerr 1988) and that it represents an important means by which men assert their dominance over women in patriarchal societies (Adams 1990). Consequently, it can be expected that many people who abide by these social conventions and hierarchies would be unwilling to give up the consumption of animal products and that many will either ignore or downplay negative GHIs—a view that has been borne out by empirical research. In the aforementioned study from Victoria, Australia, 30% of respondents to the survey agreed with the statement 'I don't want to change my eating habit or routine', in spite of the fact that many agreed that a diet that is relatively low in animal products might be beneficial (Lea et al. 2006b, 832). Whereas a study in the European Union found that this unwillingness to change was less prominent (J. Kearney and McElhone 1999), research has also found that many consumers dissociate moral issues associated with the production of animal foods from their consumption, which explains why choices in relation to the latter are not necessarily informed by thoughts about the former (Korzen et al. 2011).

Though, in spite of these considerations, people can, and do, change habits without financial incentives (see section 3.3) or the use of legal force (see section 3.4), there is a third, more important reason why educational campaigns may not be sufficient. Many smokers might have had some desire to change for a long time, but they might have been reluctant to change their behaviour on the basis of the view that the benefits for non-smokers would be relatively small if other smokers carried on smoking in public places. A similar 'tragedy of the commons' dilemma (Hardin 1968) operates with the consumption of animal products. While those who eat more healthily may reap some health benefits associated with their dietary changes, the tragedy lies in the fact that they, as well as everyone else, would still be exposed to the wide range of negative GHIs associated with the consumption of animal products that I explored in the preceding chapters.

If people in India, for example, were to decide to adopt vegan diets, perhaps out of a concern with the processes involved with the production of ghee, they would still be exposed to many negative GHIs associated with diets that include animal products. There are many reasons why food is expensive for many people, but I argued in chapter one that an important contributing factor is the high and increasing consumption of animal products. Any Indian people who decide to adopt vegan diets would still be exposed to high food prices, and any slump in the demand for animal products in India might not result in a decrease in the production of animal products, but in producers targeting and finding other consumers who can plug the gap left by Indian vegan people. Therefore, Indian vegans might still experience the negative impacts associated with high food prices, in spite of their efforts to reduce demand. They might also not be able to benefit from eating varied vegan diets, given that world agriculture is currently focused heavily on the production of crops that can be fed to farmed animals and is controlled to a large extent by very powerful companies with greater interests in feeding farmed animals than in feeding people (Loughnan 2012, 228–242). They would also still be exposed to the climate change impacts that result from others consuming animal products. Some harm that they might experience may be much less obvious; for example, they might be left with food that is nutritionally inadequate when they are hospitalised (even if this possibility may be much less likely in India than in many other countries where vegetarianism is less common).

The risk of social harm, for example the psychological harm that is caused to vegans by people who introduce veganism as an interesting subject to talk about whilst consuming animal products, should not be excluded either. Vegans may also find it difficult to find work when they are invited to share meals with potential employers. They might have to 'hunt' for food for a considerable amount of time when they are eating out, interfering with any social duties that they may have. In a culture wherein veganism would be the norm, none of these issues would present themselves. In a culture that regards veganism as no more than an option that people should feel free to take or leave, those who contemplate voluntary change may refrain from doing so out of fear of social isolation. Educational campaigns must be careful to avoid contributing to this by individualising social problems and thus leaving unchallenged the socio-economic contexts wherein people live, a concern that has also been identified in relation to some campaigns to tackle obesity (Deckers 2013a).

Although some campaigns may worsen existing problems, this does not imply that there is no place for appropriate educational initiatives that aim to encourage debate on the consumption of animal products and, more specifically, on qualified moral veganism. Rather than individualising problems, such campaigns should target socio-economic contexts and, particularly, the actions of powerful actors who shape those contexts with the aim to ignore or downplay the concerns of those who are appalled by our global food system. However, it must be recognised that those who fail to minimise negative GHIs may not be persuaded to reduce their negative GHIs merely by being exposed to education. This is why investing resources merely in educational campaigns is insufficient.

3.3 Increasing the costs of animal products

The farmed animals' sector is currently subsidised to produce a wide range of negative GHIs. In many countries, governments privilege the farmed animals' sector over other agricultural sectors. The LEAD study, for example, claims that 'livestock lobbies have been able to exert an over-proportional influence on public policies, to protect their interests', a situation which has resulted in 'the severe under-pricing of virtually all natural processes' associated with the production of farmed animal products (Steinfeld et al. 2006, 222, 228). The European Union, for instance, provides the largest share of its subsidies to its farmers through its Common Agricultural Policy, which was established in 1957 with the aim to increase productivity. About 30% of the European Union's entire budget was spent on 'farmers and market-related expenditure' in 2013, and an additional 9% was spent on 'rural development' (European Commission 2015). These subsidies are not dispensed equally between farmers: those who produce animal products generally receive more than those who produce other foods (Lock and Pomerleau 2005; Weidema et al. 2008). The reason for this relates to the fact that payments are allocated largely in proportion to the size of farms, favouring those with access to large areas of grassland (Webster 2013, 207). A 2012 estimate claims, however, that only 6% of gross domestic product in the European Union was generated from agriculture (European Commission 2012).

Many authors have argued that in order to curtail the consumption of animal products these products should be much more expensive (Walker et al. 2005; Compassion 2007; Lloyd-Williams et al. 2008; Pelletier and Tyedmers 2010). Robert Goodland, for example, advocates the removal of subsidies from the least sustainable forms of agriculture and the introduction of a sliding-scale tax whereby the least sustainable forms of agriculture would be taxed more than the more sustainable forms (Goodland 1997). Similar proposals have been made by others (see e.g. Wirsenius et al. 2011; Nordgren 2012). This scheme could be broadened out into a negative-GHI tax—the introduction of which I proposed elsewhere (Deckers 2010)—that taxes the negative GHIs of all goods in proportion to the risks that they pose to one's holistic health.

Clearly, it is no good to tax goods highly if the tax that is levied on them only cancels out the subsidies that were provided to produce those goods in the first place. Any government initiative that aims to reduce negative GHIs through pricing mechanisms must therefore, as a first priority, ensure that products that produce large quantities of negative GHIs do not benefit from subsidies and that—where the provision of subsidies is a good idea—subsidies are provided to encourage activities that reduce negative GHIs. In this vein, the Australian Government recently introduced Australian Carbon Credit Units (ACCUs). These ACCUs provide farmers with the means to earn carbon credits, which they can earn by reducing greenhouse gas emissions or by storing carbon—for example by planting trees or by incorporating materials that contain carbon into soils—and then sell to those who wish to offset their emissions (DCCEE 2012). This system could be extended to incentivise other activities that reduce negative GHIs.

The most developed proposal along these lines is advanced by Vinnari and Tapio (2012), who argue that governments could increase the security of the supply of food, as well as of other goods, through the development of national stockpiling systems—systems that aim to secure the supply of goods at a national level to guard against natural or social threats to the acquisition of basic goods—composed of those goods that are approved of from an ethical perspective. Governments would agree to buying the cheapest ethically approved goods that had been produced within their country at prices exceeding those that these goods might gain on the global market, and they would then sell these to the highest bidders on the global market. In this way, producers would be provided with incentives to produce those goods that were both approved of and guaranteed to be bought by one's government at a reasonable price. National production would thus be subsidised by one's government as it would probably pay more for the selected products than the price that they might receive on the global market. The authors point out that the introduction of this system would not only lead to a reduction in the consumption of animal products, but also provide greater national food security, protect farmers more against price instabilities, and supply a wider range of foods to the global market as the compositions of national stockpiles would be likely to be more diverse (Vinnari and Tapio 2012, 52). This proposal has received little discussion in the academic literature so far, and it would be interesting to know whether this silence might be related to a perception that developing this kind of governmental intervention is unrealistic in light of our current economic situation or, perhaps, to past experiences with European policies that led to the overproduction of some goods, for example of the 'butter mountains' associated with the Common Agricultural Policy.

Some might oppose the pricing option from the conviction that the poor would be affected more negatively than the rich. As long as we live in a world where great financial disparities exist, those who are poor would be affected more than the rich by price increases in products that are associated with large negative GHIs. However, for two reasons, I do not think that this concern should undermine the value of introducing schemes that would result in products with large negative GHIs becoming more expensive. Firstly, the possibility that the poor might be affected more negatively is an argument for a redistribution of wealth, rather than an argument against pricing negative GHIs. If all the negative GHIs associated with particular products, including their effects on the poor, could be internalised in the prices that people pay, their prices would be just. Whilst this option would allow those who are richer than others the ability to consume more products with relatively large negative GHIs, the fairness of this option in relation to human poverty would depend on whether the scheme increased existing disparities. Whereas the issue of fairness is a legitimate concern if the negative GHIs on the poor are not considered adequately, it is not a necessary consequence of any such scheme. Secondly, the pricing option would lead to some products becoming more expensive, but many other products that are associated with fewer negative GHIs would actually become cheaper. They might become less expensive not only in relative, but also in absolute, terms, as we would no longer be required to spend large sums of money on remedying problems caused by the production of large quantities of goods that are associated with large quantities of negative GHIs.

It is important to recognise, however, that the health concerns posed by products with large negative GHIs may not necessarily diminish by increasing these products' costs. William Rees (2006b) provides the example of the Eastern Atlantic bluefin tuna (*Thunnus thynnus*), whose price has increased significantly but whose bodies continue to be sought in great numbers, in spite of the fact that the populations of this species, as well as those of many other fish, are in sharp decline. In fact, animal products are generally known for their low price elasticities, particularly in relatively well-off countries (D. Chen and Abler 2014). An advocate of the pricing option might try to address this problem by arguing that this does not show that the pricing option does not work, but merely that we must develop better systems to ensure that all negative GHIs are priced fairly.

Adopting the pricing option would transform our present situation, wherein the full costs of many products that result in relatively large negative GHIs are currently not reflected in their prices. However, whereas increasing the costs of animal products might reduce their consumption in capitalist societies, it addresses neither the 'tragedy of the commons' problem identified in section 3.2 that will exist unless all societies cooperate, nor the question of what ought to be done in societies that do not recognise the value of money. Finally, the question must be asked whether raising the prices of animal products is sufficient to address all our moral concerns.

3.4 The vegan project

It would seem odd to wish to stop paedophilia by merely making the price of having sex with children very expensive. Similarly, if animal products should not normally be consumed by human beings, it would seem to be inappropriate to put high prices on the bodies of Eastern Atlantic bluefin tuna, for example, and simply hope for the best. As we possess an animalist interest and as tuna have interests in the enjoyment of things that keep them alive, tuna should be granted rights not to be killed for food by human beings, rights which should be allowed to be violated only in exceptional circumstances, for example when a human being is left at sea with nothing else to eat. As we create laws to counter the actions of paedophiles and many other actions that harm the fundamental interests of human beings, we should also create laws to protect Eastern Atlantic bluefin tuna and—more generally—to prohibit activities that fail to minimise negative GHIs.

When we consider the farmed animal industry, the argument has been made that the negative GHIs associated with the large-scale use of antibiotics in the production of particular farmed animal products are so significant that they justify a ban on the use of prophylactic antibiotics (Anomaly 2010). However, as other aspects of the animal industry do not fare much better as far as their negative GHIs are concerned, it would seem to be appropriate to ban the consumption of animal products for all human beings who would fail to minimise negative GHIs by consuming such products. In earlier work, I referred to the ambition to create international and national laws to introduce such a quali-fied ban as 'the vegan project' (Deckers 2013b). Though it may be—in Caney (2008, 539)'s words—'unreasonably demanding' for human beings to avoid consuming animal products in some situations, in many situations it is not. To the contrary, in many situations it is entirely unreasonable to allow human beings to continue eating animal products. As I have sketched in the preceding chapters, many people who consume animal products fail to minimise nega-tive GHIs through their dietary choices. I have shown that this is so for a num-ber of reasons, including: that they may be more likely to get ill—as will be documented more fully in the appendix—and thus to require treatments that may be funded partly by others; that they are more likely to make other people ill; that their diets require more land and cause more land degradation; that their diets use more water and contribute more to water pollution; that their diets use more fossil fuels and contribute more to climate change and other atmospheric concerns; that they impose more pain, suffering, and death on animals in many situations; and that they cause psychological harm to others who lament the fact that they conceive of the bodies of animals as things that can be routinely eaten.

It is, of course, quite possible that some people will not class the same sorts of things as those that I have mentioned here as negative GHIs or that they will give far less moral significance to some of the negative GHIs that I men-tioned. If the fact that hardly anyone adopts vegan diets can be taken to suggest that people do not attach great moral significance to the concerns that I have expressed in chapter two, many policy-makers might consider a qualified ban to be a step too far from a political perspective. This, however, is misguided, as the question whether we ought to adopt a qualified ban does not depend on the concerns I have outlined in that chapter. Such a ban could also be justified merely on the basis of the narrower negative GHIs associated with zoonoses and with the human use of the environment that I described in chapter one. Those animal products that are associated with those negative GHIs that are widely agreed to exist could, accordingly, be singled out for a ban. For example, many people may agree that climate change is associated with very significant negative GHIs and that drastic action is required to avert dangerous climate change. Accordingly, the policy-makers of nations that fail to minimise nega-tive GHIs in this domain might decide to curtail the consumption of animal products.

Some people who live within those nations, however, may object to a qualified ban on the basis of the view that such a ban would be an unjustifi-able infringement on their personal liberty. My response to this is that such infringements are justifiable provided that those who have legitimate politi-cal power justify the infringement on personal liberty as necessary to safe-guard holistic health. It might be objected that people could do all sorts of things to limit their negative GHIs, and that focusing on the consumption of animal products would be unfair on those who would much rather curtail their negative GHIs in other domains instead. This objection, however, is not compelling. As long as people's interests in holistic health are still being jeopardised, there is a compelling justification to limit negative GHIs. It might still be appropriate to ban the consumption of animal products even in situations where the consumption of animal products does not produce more negative GHIs than the consumption of other products that could be eaten to obtain a similar quantity of health benefits. By analogy, a government that decided to ban car travel inside city centres might not necessarily wrong those who avoided exceeding their fair share of emissions and who contributed little to inner city pollution through the use of their car before the introduction of such a ban. I accept the view that democratic governments should have the authority to make decisions that may curtail the individual liberty of some people to spare others from significant harm, even if the people in question did not cause any of the harm that ought to have been avoided before the introduction of the restriction.

Similarly, it could be argued that adopting a qualified ban on the consumption of animal products would not necessarily restrict the liberty of those who abide by the duty to minimise negative GHIs. Governments might simply adopt the view that the easiest way to tackle irresponsible consumption that harms others is by eliminating those things that we could do without. Since many people fail to minimise negative GHIs, the question whether the consumption of animal products is a domain that justifies such an approach must be debated with extreme urgency. If I were a dictator, I would introduce a qualified ban with immediate effect, provided that I did not think that doing so would increase negative GHIs, for example if there was a good chance that it would trigger a significant amount of violent resistance. As I am not a dictator, and since I do not aspire to become one, it is my aim to contribute to democratic processes that would introduce qualified bans on the consumption of animal products. Even if some people might oppose such a scheme, this does not imply that it would be wrong to implement it. However, great care must be taken to avoid that any well-intended legal changes trigger undesirable negative GHIs, for example through the possibility that some people who oppose such a scheme might resort to violent resistance.

Whereas I shall not elaborate on the sorts of democratic processes that should be adopted to move us in the direction of realising the vegan project, it is nevertheless clear that it is paramount that our increasingly urbanised population be well-informed about the methods that others use to produce their food. Where information that is crucial to make informed decisions is actively hidden, for example by those producers who try to hide how food is produced from the eyes of the public, it has been argued that some legal infringements, for example trespass onto private property, may be required (McCausland et al. 2013). I believe that this is right, and that we should generally prefer non-violent methods to reach our goal.

Some might claim that violent means should also be embraced. They might argue that some human beings are violent towards other animals and that violent actions against these human beings ought to be justifiable where there is a good chance that they might reduce the sum total of violence. I am not persuaded by this line of reasoning as most violent actions against those who are perceived to mistreat animals may alienate those who mistreat them as well as others who are not able to see that this treatment of other animals is as problematic as it is claimed to be by opponents of this treatment. Whilst there may be a place for violence in some situations, for example to block someone who is about to vent their frustration on an animal by hitting the animal, those who support the vegan project must, in order to realise their ambition, be mindful of the fact that public support is unlikely to grow with the use of strategies that may strike large numbers of people as deeply unacceptable.

Meanwhile, supporters of the vegan project would also do well to show their limited support for the most benign ways in which animal foods could be provided for human consumption as long as their ambition has not been realised. In this light, they should, for example, show their support for the consumption of animals who die naturally, or of those who are killed justifiably. They should also support the production and the consumption, by others, of lab-grown flesh if doing so minimises negative GHIs in a particular situation where it is reasonable to believe that it would not jeopardise the ambition to minimise negative GHIs in the long-term. In this respect, it is worth noting that the production of lab-grown flesh has been associated not only with a reduction in concerns related to the human treatment of other animals, but also with a decrease in environmental issues relative to conventional production methods used in the farmed animals' sector (Tuomisto and de Mattos 2011). Even if there is much uncertainty regarding the latter due to the limited technological progress that has been made so far, Tuomisto and de Mattos (2011) expect that the development of lab-grown flesh may be associated with significant decreases in energy use, greenhouse gas emissions, land use, and water use.

In spite of my contention that the consumption of animal products generates many negative GHIs, a total ban on the consumption of animal products cannot be justified. All human beings should be granted a right to health care, which includes a right to food (UN CESCR 1999). For some, this right would be jeopardised unjustifiably by a complete ban. Some people, for example, may have specific physiological demands that may not be able to be satisfied without the consumption of animal products. The high nutrient-density of many animal products, for example, might be critically important for some people who suffer from AIDS and who do not have sufficient access to adequate plant foods (Randolph et al. 2007; Roubenoff 2000). Some people may live in areas where the consumption of alternatives to animal products would produce a larger quantity of negative GHIs—for example those people with limited resources who live at high latitudes where diets that rely solely on plant foods do not provide adequate nutrition or the same amount of food security that is provided by a more varied diet.

3.5 Three objections to the vegan project, and their refutations

In the remainder of this chapter I shall consider three objections that have been raised against the vegan project. The first is that it is pointless to focus on a qualified ban, simply because the vast majority of people are not ready for it. The second is that the vegan project is unacceptable as it would undermine human food security. The third contends that the vegan project alienates human beings from nature.

3.5.1 First objection: People are not ready to adopt a qualified ban, so it is pointless to pursue such a ban

A first objection to my proposal comes from those who think that introducing a qualified ban simply will not work because it does not have enough public support. On this basis, many argue that it would make more sense to focus on small objectives that might gain support, rather than risk putting people off by focusing on objectives that many people will oppose vehemently. Thus, Fetissenko (2011, 150, 155) has argued that arguments that do not focus on narrow personal health and environmental effects associated with the consumption of animal products have 'limited persuasive appeal', and that those people who wish to persuade people to adopt vegan diets might have more success if they focused on those effects and on 'advocating for (slightly) better conditions in which "farm animals" live and die'.

As I write these lines, I am reminded of my visit to Australia in October 2012. At this time, a lot of media attention was given to the fact that many animals were transported over vast distances to the Middle-East and to Malaysia, where they were treated and slaughtered in many ways that Australians did not find acceptable. Apart from this, the only animal issue that gained significant attention was the fact that many Australians still buy eggs from caged, rather than from free-range, hens. If the media's role is merely one of reporting what is going on, it may not be right to blame the media for focusing on these two issues, and to ignore all else. There is no doubt that the reason why the media was highlighting these issues relates to the fact that many organisations that speak up for animals hope to bring about change by means of small, incremental steps. I am not opposed to small changes for the better, but I do believe that there are good reasons to think that many people are actually capable of taking a giant leap forward, at least if they are prepared to be consistent. The reason why I believe this to be the case is that some nations already have some laws in place that, if they were extended consistently from one domain (the use of animals for research) to another (the use of animals for food), would point in the direction of qualified moral veganism.

In this regard, Council Directive 2010/63/EU on the protection of animals used for scientific purposes provides a good example. With this directive, which member states of the European Union were expected to have fully implemented in 2013, the European Union tried to improve the conditions of the use of non-human animals in research. In most European Union law, the articles that form the core of the legal text are preceded by a number of recitals that provide reasons underpinning the law. It is important to recognise that these recitals 'are not considered to have independent legal value', but that they 'can expand an ambiguous provision's scope' and cannot 'restrict an unambiguous provision's scope' (Klimas and Vaiciukaite 2008, 3). Directive 2010/63/EU is a fascinating text, particularly because of recitals 10 and 12. Recital 10 posits that the 'Directive represents an important step towards achieving the final goal of full replacement of procedures on live animals' (Council Directive 2010/63/EU). Recital 12 states that 'the use of animals for scientific or educational purposes should ... only be considered where a non-animal alternative is unavailable' (Council Directive 2010/63/EU). The reason why these recitals are so interesting is that they would have radical implications for the use of animals for food if people were prepared to be consistent. This is clear if we replace a few key words in recital 12: 'the use of animals for' *food* 'should ... only be considered where a non-animal alternative is unavailable'. Indeed, the 'final goal of full replacement' that recital 10 talks about seems to be within the reach of most people who live in the European Union today: most people there have sufficient non-animal alternatives available to feed themselves. If people were consistent, most people who live in the European Union, as well as many who live in other places, would obtain adequate nutrition to maintain good health without the need to consume animal products.

In the core of the legal text, paragraph d of article 38 stipulates that all project evaluations must satisfy 'a harm-benefit analysis ... to assess whether the harm to the animals in terms of suffering, pain and distress is justified by the expected outcome' (Council Directive 2010/63/EU, art. 38, par. d). Though the law does not provide clear guidance on when the harm might outweigh the benefits, it is likely that any research proposal that aims to perform an experiment involving the killing of animals to find out whether people might obtain extra enjoyment (and, if so, how much) from eating animal products compared to eating plant foods would fail any plausible 'harm-benefit analysis' that is in line with the spirit of this law. In situations where other foods could be consumed without increasing negative GHIs, it is hard to think what arguments, other than such an 'extra enjoyment' argument, those who support the consumption of animal products could bring to the table to argue their case. Other goals that could be invoked in the context of research on animals, such as the desire to keep people in their jobs or to provide enjoyment to those who like to experiment on animals, would similarly be unlikely to tip the balance in favour of the benefits for any research ethics committee engaged with such 'a harm-benefit analysis'.

Whereas the critic might object that the law may only be interested in the avoidance of unnecessary harm upon living animals, rather than in the use of animals as such, it must be pointed out that recital 12 does not actually specify whether the restriction would apply to animals who were dead already. However, even if we grant that the law may not intend to curtail the use of animals who have died naturally or who have been killed accidentally, a plausible reading of the reasoning underlying this law supports one of the central objectives of the vegan project: to eliminate the killing of animals where this is motivated by the desire to consume their bodies in situations where human beings are able to enjoy adequate alternatives that produce fewer negative GHIs. It is not consistent to demand that animals should only be used for scientific purposes 'where a non-animal alternative is unavailable', but to allow the use of animals for food merely to satisfy the trivial human interest in eating animal products where better alternatives are available.

Andrew Knight (2011, 16) estimates that at least 126.9 million vertebrates were used in experiments in 2005. This is a small fraction of the number of animals who are killed to provide human food. According to a very conservative estimate by the organisation Animals Deserve Absolute Protection Today and Tomorrow, based on data collected in 2003, more than 150 billion animals are killed for human food every year (ADAPTT 2012). Therefore, more than 1,200 animals are killed to provide food for every animal who is killed for research. Consistency demands that further legal reform be introduced to harmonise our law on the use of animals for research with the vast numbers of animals that human beings use for food, which—as I have documented in the preceding chapters—imposes great harm not only upon nonhuman, but also upon human, animals.

The moral inconsistency that underlies our laws must also be resolved to increase the chance that the harm-benefit analysis that Directive 2010/63/EU talks about be carried out with sincerity. It is highly likely that the lives of animals used in research will continue to be regarded as cheap unless people embrace the vegan project. When many people continue to consume animal products, even where adequate alternatives that minimise negative GHIs are available, researchers who have been trained in the art of justifying their research in terms of need are unlikely to face significant opposition when they argue for the necessity to carry out particular research projects. In this light, it should not come as a surprise that a significant number of those involved in the research industry resist the use of alternatives, are careless in their study designs, and are reluctant to engage in serious study of previous work, resulting in needless duplication (A. Knight 2011, 98).

Though the articles of Directive 2010/63/EU focus mainly on moral concerns with the infliction of pain and suffering, its recitals question the use and the killing of animals for unnecessary research. Moral consistency demands that further European Union legal reform be introduced to prevent billions of animals from being killed completely unnecessarily. Other jurisdictions that agree that animals should not be used for unnecessary research ought to bring about similar reform. An additional moral concern underlying the vegan project—the taboo on using animals who have died naturally, accidentally, or painlessly—may not be supported by the recitals of Directive 2010/63/EU, but a culture that develops strong reservations about killing animals in order to consume them might also be expected to develop strong reservations about consuming animals at all. If the reason why many vegans would not wish to eat animals can be understood not merely in light of a concern with the imposition of pain, suffering, and death upon animals—a necessary aspect of most diets that humans adopt—but also in light of a concern with using animals for food at all, it would be appropriate for adequate legal reform to target the consumption of animal products as such.

Whereas the European Union has not moved into the direction of the vegan project, perhaps partly because of this legal inconsistency, a 2014 legal change in the Indian city of Palitana—a city of around 65,000 people in the state of Gujarat—does appear to be largely in line with what the vegan project seeks to accomplish. To my knowledge, Palitana is the world's first city where the slaughter of animals as well as the sale of flesh and eggs has been banned by local law, effective from 14 August 2014 (Niazi 2014; van Popering 2015). The basis for the ban stems from the ethics of Jainism, particularly from its central focus on its interpretation of the principle of *ahimsa* (non-violence), which has been understood to demand vegetarianism by many, including the circa 200 monks who went on hunger strike to push for this legal change. Whereas the content of people's diets in Palitana may therefore be similar to the content of the diets of those who are moved to qualified moral veganism through considering the arguments developed in this book, the underlying ideology is bound to be markedly different.

In spite of this difference, we should not conclude too quickly that there is no overlap between these ideologies, as the principle that we should try to avoid inflicting pain, suffering, and death upon animals appears to be closely related, even if I know relatively little of Jain ideology, to the principle of ahimsa. Indeed, van Popering (2015) has noted that Jains may even relate positively towards adopting a more general taboo on the consumption of the flesh from animals.

Therefore, I believe that it is justifiable to conclude that there is some evidence to suggest that a growing number of people are ready to take a giant leap forward, a trend that has also been observed in some other countries, for example in the USA and in Australia (Pendergrast 2016). Apart from these signs that the times are changing, there is at least one further reason why it may not be appropriate to focus merely on small, incremental steps. The idea that people should be allowed to use animals for food in situations where doing so cannot be justified might be strengthened by campaigns that merely tinker around the edges. Those who focus their attention on the pushing of deckchairs may lose sight of the possibility that the boat might be sinking. Those who believe that the ship is sinking will hardly be satisfied with an approach centred on the pushing of deckchairs. Accordingly, it is by no means pointless to focus on the adoption of a qualified ban.

3.5.2 Second objection: The vegan project undermines human food security

The second objection is that realising the vegan project would result in a predominantly vegan global agricultural system, and that such a system would compromise the nutritional adequacy of human diets unjustifiably, either by not providing sufficient food for all people who need to consume animal products in order to be healthy now or by jeopardising long-term food security.

In reply to the first concern, it can be noted that many people are likely to fail to minimise negative GHIs by consuming animal products; however, to the extent that they do not do so—say, if they needed to consume animal products because of dire health needs—it could be argued that the farming of animals should still be allowed to cater for their needs. Indeed, I must emphasise that I do not wish to contribute to legal reform that might jeopardise any human being's right to adequate food. However, when it comes to thinking about how this right might be satisfied, it must be pointed out that the demise of the farmed animals' sector may not necessarily be a problem. The consumption of products derived from most farmed animals differs from the consumption of wild or feral animals in a number of morally significant respects: the lives of the latter tend to be controlled to a much lesser extent by human beings; no arable crops must be grown deliberately to feed them; they present no manure management problems; no or fewer drugs are required to treat them; and they pose fewer direct human disease threats as populations tend to be more spread out and further removed from human beings. In light of the concerns I expressed in the previous chapters about the human control of animals and the health issues associated with farming animals, the consumption of products derived from wild and feral animals must be preferred to the consumption of farmed animal products.

Hunting advocates might now warm towards my project, but they might be getting hot too quickly. I am not arguing for an increase in hunting *per se*; rather, I suspect that the numbers of wild and feral animals—who would be able to roam freely to some extent—would increase as the farmed animals' sector contracts, and I would support the killing of these animals for food only to the extent that doing so would be required to ensure that all human beings can be provided with adequate nutrition in situations where this aim cannot be achieved by other means without increasing negative GHIs. I hypothesise that sufficient quantities of animal products would still be available to feed those human beings who must consume animal products out of dire health needs if many relatively affluent countries in temperate climates prohibited the farming of animals. Should the quantity of flesh provided by wild and feral animals not be sufficient, it may then be necessary to allow the farming of some animals for food: the vegan project does not turn its back on those who would compromise their health by avoiding the consumption of animal products.

Whereas it may not intend to ignore some people's nutritional needs, the vegan project has nevertheless been criticised for its failure to buffer human beings sufficiently against the constant threat of food scarcity. Fairlie (2010) devotes several pages of his book *Meat: A Benign Extravagance* to this claim, arguing that a predominantly vegan system would lack the benefits that are brought about, within a mixed system, by the existence of a greater number of a range of farmed animals and of the greater number of the arable crops that are fed to them. These would act as a 'buffer', protecting human beings from food shortages caused by a rising human population, by crop failures, or by the combination of these two factors (Fairlie 2010, 114–118). If this claim is valid, vegan societies might also be free-riding on a general duty to take appropriate measures to secure food for all human beings.

With regard to the population issue, Fairlie (2010, 109–113) points out that a predominantly vegan global society might grow larger than a population that adopted a mixed system. The problem with this is that, unlike societies that slaughter a proportion of their domesticated animals once they reach carrying capacity (as what the Maring of New Guinea do with their pigs) and before the animals start intruding on land occupied by neighbouring societies, such a vegan society would lack the option of slaughtering a significant number of animals to free up space to grow crops to feed the human population more efficiently once it reached global carrying capacity. Though this possibility must be taken seriously, especially since the global human population is already at an all-time high, I do not think that a predominantly vegan global society would necessarily carry on increasing its population until it reached a situation where it would teeter on the brink of exceeding its carrying capacity. Rather, I believe that, in light of my general concern with how human beings control and domi- nate the lives of others, those who advocate for the creation of such a vegan society must also take and support measures to control the human popula- tion so that not only future generations of human beings, but also many other organisms whom we share this planet with, are allowed to thrive.

Even if we accept that a largely vegan population adopting a predominantly vegan agricultural system may not possess the tendency to become any larger than a population dependent on a mixed agricultural system, Fairlie maintains that the former population would still be buffered from food scarcity to a lesser degree by being more vulnerable to crop failures, as the existence of a sizeable number of a range of particular farmed animals protecting humans from the negative impacts of such failures would be lacking. Though in a mixed system some arable crops are grown to feed farmed animals, Fairlie rightly points out that, in times of crop failures, human populations could resort not only to eating the farmed animals, but also to eating the crops that had been destined to feed those animals. In a predominantly vegan system, this option would be almost absent, so that the risk of human starvation through crop failure would be much greater. I share Fairlie's concern with food security, and therefore I would not be willing to advocate the vegan project if it increased our vulnerability to hunger resulting from crop failures. The challenge that remains is to argue that it is possible to establish both global and local vegan projects that do not increase human vulnerability to crop failures compared to mixed systems. I would like to address this challenge by pointing out that there are a number of reasons to believe that, in many locations, the adoption of a predominantly vegan system may be able to provide as much human food security as a mixed system.

Firstly, as mentioned before, it is highly likely that the completion of the vegan project would be accompanied by a significant rise in feral and wild populations of animals. Whereas it may be more difficult to catch, kill, and butcher these animals and to provide the products derived from them to those who need them, their nutritional quality may be better than that of the products derived from farmed animals (Crawford et al. 2010; Hoffman and Wiklund 2006).

Secondly, though the vegan project seeks to limit the number of mixed systems, it does not wish to eliminate them where doing so would increase negative GHIs. Some people in India, for example, lack access to private land where they could grow crops. For them, owning a cow who can graze on public land may mean the difference between life and death (Devendra 2007). It would seem to be highly unethical to deny them the option to use a cow if the socio-political factors that contribute to these people's precarious situations cannot be ameliorated.

Thirdly, even a vegan agricultural system might justifiably use animals in situations where not doing so would increase negative GHIs. In some situations, animals could be kept for traction or transportation, for example. Whilst vegan agricultural systems would not keep animals in order to kill them to provide human food, in times of great need with morally more problematic alternatives, some of these animals' body parts could be eaten after they had died accidentally or naturally or after they had been killed justifiably, for example on compassionate grounds.

Fourthly, some edible arable crops that are grown are not used for food, but for other purposes, for example to produce alcohol. As recognised by Fairlie (2010, 116–117), these crops could be used for food in times of scarcity. In addition, a growing amount of arable land is used to produce alternatives to fossil fuels. Whereas it would be prudent to grow energy crops that could, when necessary, be used for food purposes as well, the GHIs of any proposals to grow and use potential food crops for biofuels must be very carefully considered. As Fairlie (2010, 117) recognises rightly, two major concerns in relation to this are that the energy that is provided by many crops that are currently used for biofuels is rather small and that the distillation processes involved rely frequently on large central facilities. Therefore, a challenge that must be addressed is whether any (parts of) crops that either are already or could be grown for other purposes could be used for food in times of scarcity without increasing negative

GHIs compared to those that would be produced if the land on which they were grown had been used to feed farmed animals. In spite of this concern, I do not think that a predominantly vegan society would necessarily rely more on the production of inefficient biofuels than an alternative society would to maintain the same level of food security. Other strategies could be pursued. Fairlie (2010, 117) mentions the option of 'banking food in state controlled granaries which maintain sufficient surpluses'. More generally, as a result of past technological advances, our abilities to store crops for a long time and to transport them to those who need them have grown considerably. Advocates of the global vegan project should make sure that further research is carried out in these domains and that all available technologies are used in the interests of maintaining or promoting human food security without increasing negative GHIs.

Finally, it is highly likely that the wider adoption of vegan diets would stimulate interest in growing a wider range of vegetables and fruits. This might make the food system more resilient, thus reducing the risks posed by crop failures and by any increases in malnutrition and starvation that might result from these crop failures.

I conclude that the completion of the vegan project would not compromise the needs of those who need animal products out of dire necessity and that it would not jeopardise long-term human food security either.

3.5.3 Third objection: The vegan project alienates human beings from nature

Fairlie (2010, 217) also contends that those who advocate for the vegan project are, allegedly like Singer, 'blissfully ignorant about the perils of growing vegetables'. Fairlie (2010, 219–220)'s claim could be labelled the 'fence' argument as he argues that a vegan agricultural system would require the building of very substantial fences resembling 'the fence around Glastonbury festival'—a large popular music festival held annually in England—to keep out pests. This argument relates to the likelihood that, with the demise of domesticated animals, the number of feral and wild animals would increase, resulting in a greater need to keep them away from the arable crops that are grown for human consumption. Fairlie (2010, 220) contends that 'the fence represents a logical conclusion of the vegan project [and] the most graphic symbol of the rift between humanity and nature'. Thus, the completion of the vegan project would also result in 'millions of people living on the wild side of the fence' losing their livelihoods (Fairlie 2010, 225). Fairlie's 'fence' argument addresses a number of concerns that should be explored. Nevertheless, I think the argument is not without its problems.

The fence that Fairlie dreads would be erected should the vegan project be successful is already there. Domesticated animals must also be fenced in to avoid their encroachment upon arable crops. Admittedly, fences would need to be more robust to withstand the—arguably—greater abilities of wild and feral animals to transcend boundaries, and we would need to have more of them to be able to cope with burgeoning numbers of such animals in a world wherein more space would be occupied by land that was managed to a lesser extent by humans. Fairlie conjures up the image of a relatively small number of large fences surrounding huge nature reserves, as suggested by his use of the phrase 'the fence' in the singular. In reality, it is likely that the system envisaged by the vegan project would consist of a large patchwork of fences erected both within wildlife areas that are relatively free from human activity and outside those areas.

Whereas the ways in which the land would be carved up in a predominantly vegan system might therefore not be as dissimilar from the present situation as he portrays, Fairlie nevertheless asks profound questions about the place that human beings should occupy within the natural world. In Fairlie's opinion, the fences that would be required to support the vegan project would alienate us from the natural world. However, it must be asked whether it is the vegan project or the agricultural project that marks our separation from nature. In fact, our separation may pre-date the time when our species made the transition to a farming way of life. Before the advent of agriculture, hunter-gatherer societies already separated themselves from nature by building shelters. When man ('Adam') and woman ('Eve') were banished from the garden of Eden—as narrated in the Book of Genesis—humans took up agriculture and started building fences to separate themselves further from the rest of nature, or from what is frequently referred to simply as 'nature' or 'the natural world'. Regardless of one's view about the attraction of the garden of Eden—which was not much of a 'garden' anyway—a return to the land of Eden is, at least in the short term, not desirable in light of the size of the expanding human population, at least if we adopt the view that all human beings have a right to adequate nutrition. In other words, it is not desirable for all human beings to become hunter-gatherers again as the collapse of agriculture would—at least in the short term—result in an inability to feed all human beings.

The question remains, however, whether the vegan project alienates us further from nature. Fairlie is not the only one who has made such a claim: a similar one has been made by Pollan (2006, 321–322), who asserts that 'the writings of the animal philosophers' display 'an abiding discomfort not just with our animality, but with the animals' animality, too', and that '[animal philosophers] would like nothing better than to airlift us out from nature's "intrinsic evil"—and ... take the animals with us'. Pollan wrote this comment in the context of a discussion of predation, where his basic argument boils down to this: as some animals predate on other animals, so should we. Similarly, as some of our domesticated animals are predators, we should not deny them the flesh of other animals. The problem with both of these claims is that the conclusions do not follow from their premises. In spite of this, Pollan does raise a fair point that may apply to those philosophers who may call, together with Nussbaum (2004, 317, 315), for 'the gradual formation of an interdependent world in which all species will enjoy cooperative and mutually supportive relations with one another' or 'for the gradual supplanting of the natural by the just', and who would, accordingly, use the fact that 'animals will die anyway in nature' as an argument to justify their being killed by people, where this 'might well be preferable to allowing the animal to be torn to bits in the wild or starved through overpopulation'. Yet, ironically, Pollan (2006, 321) also takes issue with the rawness of amoral nature, as he uses it as an argument for domestication on the same page as his plea for a greater recognition of what nature really is.

Though Pollan (2006, 326) rightly asks vegans to recognise that 'killing animals is probably unavoidable no matter what we choose to eat' and Fairlie (2010, 225) rightly questions the attitudes of those vegans who know very little about what is involved in the production of their food (epitomised perhaps by those who belong to what he calls 'soybean civilisation'), the vegan project might actually connect humans more with 'nature' by a renewed emphasis on growing fruits and vegetables and by questioning the fact that humans have alienated other animals from 'nature'. No participation in 'Pork Camp'—a 'DIY-slaughter' meeting that occurred twice in Germany in 2011—or in Dennis Buchmann's 'Meine kleine Farm'—where consumers can vote on which pig will be slaughtered next and can afterwards buy products made from the pigs—is required to reconnect with nature (Gutjahr 2013). Simplistic proposals to reconnect with nature through embracing new celebrations of carnivory ignore the fact that the farmed animals' sector has taken a great deal of control away from the animals who have been domesticated and who are alienated from the natural environments wherein their wild ancestors used to live. Some domesticated animals would not even be able to live anymore without human assistance. Stark examples are breeds of animals, for example domesticated turkeys and the Belgian Blue breed of cows and bulls, who have largely lost the ability to reproduce without human intervention.

Fairlie is right to suggest that a predominantly vegan agricultural system would not be able to avoid controlling the lives of animals, whose movements must be controlled to protect arable crops. However, the difference between a mixed and a predominantly vegan agricultural system is that in the former system humans set out to control the lives of farmed animals by planning when the latter come into existence, where and how they spend their lives, and when they are killed, whereas in the latter most animals would be either wild or feral and their lives would not be controlled by human beings unless they presented a serious threat to significant human interests, for example when controlling them would be required to protect arable crops. Most animals would be allowed to roam freely unless they presented such a serious threat to important human interests, in which case a predominantly vegan system would have to use measures to control their movements. Whilst this could be done by fencing them out in many situations, in some situations it may be necessary to kill some animals, for example when pigeons pose a significant threat to arable crops and cannot be deterred. In many situations, I believe that—in accordance with the principle of safeguarding nature's integrity—it is better to fence out wild and feral animals than to fence in domesticated animals.

An interesting question remains whether it would also be acceptable to kill wild and feral animals merely on welfare grounds. On this issue, Webster (2013, 46, 197) speaks of 'well-meaning but catastrophic attempts in Europe to manage wildlife reserves with grazing animals that are not harvested for food, because it would not be "natural", but left to die of starvation in a devastated habitat', providing the example of the rewilding project in the Oostvaardersplassen in the Netherlands. To the extent that human beings were responsible for eliminating predators, they would seem to be accountable for the agonising deaths that some animals may suffer as a result of this lack of predators (as some animals may die more slowly than in an environment where they are exposed to predators), which I believe is an argument for killing animals who might be thus affected. However, I am cautious here as we must not fool ourselves into believing that a death caused by a large predator such as a wolf is necessarily better than a death caused by a small predator such as a micro-organism.

Fairlie (2010, 225) envisages that the completion of the vegan project would present someone living in an area that had been designated to become a new wildlife area with the stark choice of 'becoming a tourist guide or vegan gamekeeper' or of migrating to a place where they could become an arable farmer. However, these need not be the only options if relatively wild areas could be created and used for a wider range of other human purposes that would be compatible with nonhuman animals living there. Whereas Fairlie is correct in stating that more land would be set aside for nonhuman animals to roam freely within a predominantly vegan system, a large amount of the land that would be freed up by the demise of domesticated animals could still be managed for human purposes, for example to produce energy alternatives to fossil fuels. In this way, the fact that employment within the farmed animals' sector would diminish could be accompanied by the creation of new labour opportunities. To give some examples, a larger number of people would be involved with the erection of fences and with work in forestry management, and a number of plants that grow either with little or without cultivation and that may be relatively unattractive to or not be used by other animals could be harvested for medicinal or nutritional purposes.

To put it in a nutshell: in spite of the fact that Fairlie is right that more efforts would be required to protect arable land from wild and feral animals, I am not convinced that the completion of the vegan project would alienate human beings further from nature.

3.6 Conclusion

I identified three strategies that governments could adopt to curtail the negative GHIs associated with the consumption of animal products. There is no doubt that greater investment in research and education is required, but there are several problems associated with the ambition to try to bring about dietary change merely through educational campaigns. The first problem that I described is that not everyone has the same educational opportunities, so that well-intended but poorly targeted campaigns may increase any existing health inequalities between those who have particular educational opportunities and those who do not. Though good campaigns could try to decrease this gap, many people with limited understanding of how their food choices affect the health of others are likely to persist in their usual habits. The second problem is that people's values may be so different from those that underlie qualified moral veganism that they would simply refrain from taking personal steps to reduce their negative GHIs or that they may refrain from doing so even if they have similar values. A final problem that I highlighted is that people who commit to qualified moral veganism in a culture wherein this dietary position is not enforced would still be exposed to avoidable negative GHIs, which is why few may adopt such a position in the first place.

The second strategy that could be pursued, to change the financial systems that allocate taxes and to provide subsidies in order to discourage the production of goods that produce unacceptable negative GHIs, may be more likely to result in compliance than the first option because of the significant role that many people attribute to the value of money in capitalist societies. However, international cooperation would be required and it would still not work in societies that do not recognise the value of money. A further problem with this option is that some moral theories, for example the duty-based theory adopted here, do not accept the view that everything should be exchangeable for money. In some situations, it is our duty not to consume animal products, and it is not appropriate to consider that this duty might be dissolved in exchange for money. This is why I defended the third strategy, a qualified ban on the consumption of animal products. Though the vegan project would be justified if my moral theory is accepted, I argued that even if governments were to adopt the view that we have no duties towards other animals, a qualified ban could still be justified merely on the basis of our duties to give some recognition to the human right to health care, as giving full recognition to this right would in fact require that attention is also given to our duties to other animals as good human health cannot be achieved without this inclusion.

I considered three objections against the vegan project, arguing that it is not pointless to focus on a qualified ban, that the ban need not necessarily undermine human food security, and that it does not alienate us from nature. In my response to the first objection I highlighted that there is some evidence that many people are ready to embrace the vegan project provided that they are willing to be consistent, a theme that will be explored further in my next chapter.

CHAPTER FOUR

An Evaluation of Others' Deliberations

4.1 Introduction

If ethics is a search for rules of behaviour that can be universally endorsed (Jamieson 1990; Daniels 1979; Rawls 1971), the values underpinning my own deliberation on the issues explored in this book must be compared with the values underlying the deliberation of others. By considering the challenges raised by others' views, qualified moral veganism might either be revised or, if it survives critique, be corroborated. Though some scholars who work in animal ethics have defended views that are—to a reasonable degree—similar to my own (e.g. Milligan 2010; Kheel 2008; Adams 1990), many people consume animal products where they have adequate alternatives that, in my view, would reduce negative GHIs. This raises the question whether qualified moral veganism overlooks something of importance—the fact that so many people act in ways that are incompatible with qualified moral veganism provokes the following question in me: Am I missing something?

The ambition of this chapter is twofold. Its first aim is to analyse the deliberations of two widely different groups of people on vegetarianism, veganism, and the killing of animals. By describing the views of others as accurately as I can, I aim to set aside my own thoughts on the matter temporarily—to the extent that doing so is possible—to throw light on where others might be coming from. The second aim of the chapter is to evaluate these views. By doing so, I hope that the reader will be stimulated to reflect upon their own dietary narratives through critical engagement with the views of others. At the same time, I hope that further light will be shed on the question whether the vegan project might stand a chance of gathering support from large numbers of people.

How to cite this book chapter:
Deckers, J 2016 *Animal (De)liberation: Should the Consumption of Animal Products Be Banned?* Pp. 131–157. London: Ubiquity Press. DOI: http://dx.doi.org/10.5334/ bay.e. License: CC-BY 4.0

4.2 Methodology

The views of two distinct groups of people are being reported and evaluated in this chapter. The groups are distinct as they are situated at opposite ends of the socio-economic spectrum of the current UK population. The first group comprises academic scholars and students, none of whom are specialised in animal ethics. Many of them are paid relatively high wages and/or come from families with relatively high incomes. The second group comprises people who—with the exception of one (a nurse)—lack academic qualifications and live in relatively deprived areas.

The first ('academic') group comprises a small sample of academic scientists and students from Newcastle University, an academic institution situated in the north-east of England. Six scientists who worked in disciplines related to environmental science were recruited to participate in the 'Deliberating the Environment' research project, funded by the Economics and Social Research Council's Science in Society Programme and carried out by me in collaboration with four colleagues (Derek Bell, Mary Brennan, Tim Gray, and Nicola Thompson) at Newcastle University. Twenty-one students were recruited from those who took a module on environmental ethics, and the recruited students included both single and joint honours (second-year) BA students in Philosophical Studies (2003–2004). Both scientists and students agreed to their data being published, and, whilst scientists agreed to being interviewed, students agreed to complete a questionnaire with a range of questions about environmental issues. The questionnaire contained the following questions that were relevant for the purposes of this chapter: 1) 'Are you a vegetarian/vegan? Why/ why not?'; and 2) 'Do you think you should be a vegetarian/vegan? Why/why not?' Henceforth, the answers to these questions will be indicated by the numbers 1 and 2 respectively. None of the students were vegans, but three identified themselves as vegetarians at the time of the study.

The scientists participated in a series of deliberative exchanges with six individuals who were part of the second ('non-academic') group and who lived in relatively deprived communities in the Newcastle area. The latter were recruited from the electoral register by being sent a letter asking them to participate in the research project. We defined a deliberative exchange as a one-to-one deliberation or conversation between two persons from different social groups, facilitated by a researcher. All participants consented to interviews—which were carried out in 2003–2004—being recorded and transcribed, and to data being used in publications. Five exchanges were held on the theme of 'animals and biodiversity'. For this exchange theme, non-academics were respectively paired up with academics as follows: Jane and Barry, Henry and Eric, Gail and David, Keith and Alice, and Fiona and Craig. Real names have been replaced by fictitious names to preserve the anonymity of the interviewees; the same fictitious names were used in an article that analyses and evaluates some of these people's views on genetic engineering (Deckers 2005b). The exchanges were facilitated by a researcher, Nicola Thompson, who asked a range of questions on the theme, including the questions whether the participants ate animal products and why they did or did not do so. None of the participants in these exchanges identified themselves as either being vegetarian or being vegan.

The second ('non-academic') group also includes six slaughterhouse workers who worked in a slaughterhouse in Oldham (Greater Manchester) in 2005, when they were interviewed for a documentary about their jobs that was shown on BBC Two on 4 July 2005 and was produced and directed in 2005 by Brian Hill, from Century Films. Whereas I had no involvement in these interviews, the data provide a great additional resource to stimulate reflection on the vegan project for three reasons. Firstly, unless there is a large discordance between their actions and their thoughts, the views of slaughterhouse workers might be expected to be greatly at odds with the vegan project as slaughterhouse workers engage routinely in actions that the vegan project seeks to prohibit. Secondly, their moral reflection on these actions is unlikely to be suppressed to the same extent as that which has been documented for many other people who may rarely or never be exposed to the concrete realities of slaughterhouses (Adams 1990; Franklin 1999; N. Williams 2008). Thirdly, critical engagement with the views of these workers might help those who are working in this or in other slaughterhouses to deal with the psychological harm that may be caused by their work, both the understanding and the discussion of which have been held to be inadequate (Dillard 2008). In this regard, it is noteworthy that I am not aware of any other study that has critically engaged with the views of the workers interviewed for this film.

The data were categorised using thematic analysis (Bryman 2008, 554–555). Repeated listening to and readings of the interview data revealed that the data could be categorised in a number of themes. The iterative comparison of the views of academic staff, students, and local citizens revealed the following themes in relation to the question of how participants either approved of or rejected the consumption of animal products and the production process:

- Liking the taste of products derived from animals
- Taste trumps thoughts
- Health reasons
- Our bodies have been designed to eat animal products
- Since some animals eat other animals, we should be free to do so too
- Animals have been designed to be eaten
- Animals owe their lives to the fact that we eat them
- Tradition
- Questioning the exploitation of animals

The iterative comparison of the views of the slaughterhouse workers who contributed to the film revealed that their views could not easily be categorised into the same themes. Rather, the following themes emerged:

- Power: being allowed to do something that not many people are allowed to do
- Sincerity: facing up to 'reality', in contrast to others
- Fun: making and having fun
- Skill: killing better than others who do not do so properly
- Religion: being justified by Yahweh, God, or Allah

In the following sections I shall discuss how these themes emerged from the data; in addition, poignant statements will be quoted to illustrate the themes and participants' views will be evaluated.

4.3 Thematic analysis and evaluation of the views of academic staff, students, and Newcastle residents

4.3.1 Liking the taste of products derived from animals

Several participants tried to justify their dietary choices by expressing that they liked the taste of 'meat'. Some expressed unease about this taste, but added that they liked meat 'too much to give it up'. A male student, for example, wrote the following:

- 'I was a vegetarian for 11 years, but gave up because I liked the smell of bacon, and wanted a bacon sandwich.'

Such a perspective was also present in the exchange amongst Newcastle citizens and academic staff. Craig, for example, replied as follows to the question why he ate animals: 'cause it tastes good'. The importance of taste as a barrier towards adopting vegetarian diets has also been found in other studies (Lea and Worsley 2003). In a study that compared vegetarian and non-vegetarian English teenage girls, one comment by a girl echoed what this male student wrote: 'I've tried being vegetarian but I didn't manage for very long. Just waft a bacon sandwich under my nose and I change my mind' (Kenyon and Barker 1998, 193).

While I agree that the fact that something tastes good can be a powerful incentive to (want to) eat it, the question must be asked whether it provides a sufficient justification to reject qualified moral veganism. Human flesh might taste good to some people; however, we do not think that someone's taste for human flesh provides a sufficient justification for killing human beings to satisfy that desire, at least not when humans can live healthily without eating human flesh. The same applies in relation to the consumption of human beings who die naturally. If my argument in chapter two fails, so that no moral distinction between eating plants and eating nonhuman animals can be made, the argument could be made that, as we should not refrain from eating plants, we should not refrain from eating nonhuman animals either. This argument would seem to hold up for those who remain unconvinced about there being a moral distinction between eating plants and eating nonhuman animals.

However, in view of some other things that participants said, it is difficult to maintain the view that any of them genuinely adopted the view that no moral distinction between eating plants and eating nonhuman animals should be made. In light of this, I find it difficult to understand how mere flavour could provide a moral justification for rejecting qualified moral veganism. Presumably, some people may adopt the view that eating nonhuman animals poses more concerns than eating plants but that the difference is insufficiently great to justify qualified moral veganism. Likewise, it might be argued that the fact that killing animals is a foreseeable consequence of motorised transport is insufficient to undermine the use of such transport. The problem with this view is that the concerns that I have identified in chapters one and two seem much more significant than the experiences that humans gain from eating animals' flesh, particularly where it requires that animals be killed for food. Whereas human beings stand to lose much from forgoing motorised transport, I think that human beings do not forgo any important interests by abstaining from the consumption of animal products in situations where they could eat other things that produce a smaller quantity of those things that I have argued to be negative GHIs.

4.3.2 Taste trumps thoughts

Some participants agreed with this argument in theory, yet failed to adopt the philosophy in practice. The clearest accounts on this were provided by two students, who thought that they were wrong not to adopt qualified moral veganism but explained their failure to adopt such a stance by reference to the good taste of animal products. The following two accounts are quotations from the two students, a female and a male student, respectively, in response to the relevant questions (1 and 2):

- '(1) No, was vegetarian once—but chicken is just too good. (2) Try not to think about it when I'm eating—no, we shouldn't eat animals.'
- '(1) No, I don't want to give up milk—dairy cows suffer more than livestock—therefore there's also no point in me giving up meat. (2) Yes, clearly it's wrong to keep an animal just for my own gain.'

I agree with the two students' answers to the second question, apart from the fact that qualified moral veganism does not support the general statement that 'we shouldn't eat animals' if 'we' is taken to stand for all human beings. I disagree, however, that these moral perceptions should be trumped by the fact that one likes something or does not want to give something up. In order to continue with their eating habits, it appears that these students had to try to dissociate the product from the production process. Whilst no participants apart from the students thought that they ought to adopt vegetarianism, attempts to dissociate animals from the products that are made from them were made by participants in both groups.

The clearest expression of such dissociation came from Barry, who tried to reconcile consuming and (his aversion towards) killing animals as follows during the deliberative exchange:

• 'I don't police the streets of Newcastle ... I pay for a policeman to do it. ... Just so, we have people to slaughter animals, so that we can eat them.'

In sharp contrast, Gail said that she had been a vegetarian, a choice she had made under the influence of the boyfriend she had been dating at the time but also on the basis of the feeling underlying the following rhetorical question:

• 'I couldn't [kill animals] so why should I make someone else do it for me?'

In spite of this contrast between Barry and Gail, whereby the former appeared to be much more convinced that it was acceptable to support the actions of others who do things that one would not be comfortable doing oneself, both agreed that this feeling of unease should not undermine their choices to consume animals, with the latter claiming that she 'love[d] meat'.

The question must be asked, however, whether Barry and Gail were right to support the actions of others by purchasing food items the production of which they were morally concerned about. Barry's analogy does not seem to be appropriate as it is unlikely that Barry had much choice in deciding whether to pay the police unless he had been prepared to break the law—whereas he would not need to break the law if he wanted to abstain from consuming animal products. Another reason why I doubt its appropriateness relates to the fact that Barry is likely to have lacked enthusiasm for policing the streets of Newcastle himself, but there was no indication that he objected to others doing so. His personal dislike of the idea that policing the streets of Newcastle might be a suitable job for him, therefore, was not based on a moral objection to the streets being policed at all. This contrasts sharply with his dislike of animals being slaughtered for food, which was clearly based on a moral unease with the idea of anyone carrying out such a slaughter. It would have been interesting to challenge Barry on this, for example by asking him whether he would also be happy with the idea of children working in sweatshops so that we can wear the clothes that they make. The sheer fact that it is others who do things that we find morally objectionable cannot therefore be used to dissolve our moral culpability where we support their doing so. This is clearly so where the goods and services that are provided by others are actively sought out, as is the case in situations where people rely on others to slaughter the animals whom they eat; apart from the two students mentioned earlier, the participant who came closest to expressing such a view was Keith, who expressed that he wished that he could become a vegetarian—adding, upon being asked whether he would have problems with killing animals:

- 'Yeah I would, no doubt about it ... we do tend to turn a blind eye, you get other people to do it.'

A more ambiguous account was provided by Fiona where she responded to the question whether she had ever killed animals:

- 'It's hypocritical really I mean I would eat it, so if there was nobody around to do it for me I [would] probably end up doing it.'

4.3.3 Health reasons

It is possible, however, that participants adopted the view that it is not just taste that matters, as many also expressed the view that they included animal products in their diets for health reasons. In that case, participants' views must not necessarily be understood as a rejection of qualified moral veganism, but only as a reflection of the fact that they perceived that they had to eat animal products in order to remain healthy; they might have agreed that adopting a vegan diet would be ideal, but have thought that—in practice—many people, including themselves, would not manage to remain healthy on such a diet. While the data collected in this study fail to provide convincing evidence for the view that any of our participants supported qualified moral veganism, eight students referred to health reasons to support the consumption of animal products.

Two students (one male and one female) associated abstaining from (some) animal products with feelings of physical weakness, writing (respectively) as follows:

- 'I've tried it for two weeks but I was feeling weak. I believe we are meant to be omnivores.'
- 'I used to be vegetarian but I got ill and decided that though I hate how animals are treated I would rather eat them than continue being ill.'

To justify their food choices, students also referred to specific nutrients and food categories which they thought were either present or lacking in particular diets. One female student wrote that 'some animal protein is necessary', another simply wrote 'essential food groups' on her paper, and a male student wrote that he required 'quality protein'. Similarly, two students (one female and one male) thought that vegetarian or vegan diets were very limited and would compromise their health, writing (respectively) as follows:

- 'I like meat far too much to ever give it up, plus I don't eat fruit so I'd be severely undernourished if I didn't [eat meat].'
- 'You can't survive on carrots all your life.'

The deliberative exchanges contained similar claims. For example, Barry—who also claimed that vegetarianism was a fad (see further below)—said:

- 'Every time I eat veg, I always have to go and eat something properly afterwards.'

Keith was more cautious:

- 'Vegetarians do have quite a bit of difficulty in getting all the other nutrients, don't they?'

If these participants are correct that it is not possible to remain healthy on vegan diets, it is quite understandable why many people do not commit to adopting such diets. It would seem to be difficult to expect people to commit to adopting a diet that might undermine their health. Accordingly, those who accept either that a taboo on the consumption of animal products would be desirable or that there is a moral distinction between killing animals and killing plants for food might argue that some animals should be allowed to be eaten or—in situations where no animals would be available who had died naturally, accidentally, or mercifully—to be killed for food, even if both actions might be perceived to be necessary wrongs to safeguard the greater good of human health. The likelihood that at least some other animals may not be able to anticipate that they are going to be killed and, a fortiori, that some may not feel wronged by humans taking their products—for example eggs and milk—whilst they are alive would seem to provide arguments for using such animals or at least the products derived from them in situations where, by refraining from doing so, humans would undermine their own health. Such an argument would be sound for anyone who accepts that the potential moral loss associated with eating the products from another animal would be less morally significant than the loss that the human animal would incur should they suffer from bad health as a direct consequence of a refusal to eat animal products.

The question must be asked, however, whether these participants were justified in believing that their health would be undermined by the adoption of a vegan diet. In the appendix I shall argue that medical evidence supports the view that carefully chosen vegan diets are adequate for most, if not all, people. Whilst it must be emphasised that such diets should include other things than just 'carrots' or 'fruit', the view that any animal products should be included within the 'essential food groups' lacks scientific support. Nevertheless, it must be recognised that an adequate vegan diet may not be within everyone's reach. This might have been the case for Keith, if he lived in an area where the cost, at the point of purchase, of an adequate vegan diet was higher than the cost, at the point of purchase, of an adequate omnivorous or vegetarian diet and if he was not able to afford to adopt the former diet. However, research has shown that the likelihood that it would be more expensive for Keith to adopt an adequate vegan diet might be rather small (Berners-Lee et al. 2012). It must also be considered whether the perception that one might be 'weak' on a vegetarian or vegan diet simply reflects the culture that prevails in many societies. In this culture, eating animals is associated with strength, whereas eating other foods is associated with weakness (Charles and Kerr 1988). To add flesh to this point, I shall mention a comment that I recall was made by a supporter when I scored a goal for my football team a few years ago: 'Not bad for a vegetarian.'

4.3.4 Our bodies have been designed to eat animal products

Some participants associated their choice to eat animal products with particular assumptions about the essence of the human body. Both a male and a female student wrote that it is in 'our nature to eat animals'. Two female students, as well as several participants in the deliberative exchanges, also referred to particular beliefs about our evolutionary history:

- Students: 'We are designed to eat meat'; 'we did not evolve as herbivores, and it is not a bad thing to eat meat.'
- Barry: 'Vegetarianism … goes against evolution.'
- Eric: 'We've evolved as omnivores.'
- Alice: 'We were evolved to eat meat.'
- Henry (a similar claim was made by Gail): 'We've always been carnivorous, haven't we?'
- Keith: 'We're hunter-gatherers by nature and it's been bred into us for probably millions of years and it's a hard thing to break isn't it?'
- Jane: 'We've always been meat eaters … so … [we] … 've got to eat meat.'

Whilst it is correct that the bodies of many human beings can digest foods that are derived both from plants and from animals, I do not think that this provides a justification for rejecting qualified moral veganism. We could also eat the flesh of humans who had either died naturally or been killed to provide us with their flesh, but the sheer fact that we could do so does not justify the view that 'it is not a bad thing to eat' them, at least in normal situations. With regard to the drinking of milk, there is controversy on the issue whether human bodies are well-adapted to drinking the milk from other animals. Around four billion people are, to various degrees, 'lactose-intolerant' (Campbell and Matthews 2014), a term that has been claimed to spring from a 'Western bias' as such 'intolerance' is not an aberration given that many human beings lose the enzyme to digest milk during their childhood (Norris and Messina 2011, 43). However, the fact that many people's bodies tolerate drinking milk from other animals does not make it a logical necessity that we ought to do so. If human bodies had been designed in such a way that we could not thrive without eating animal foods, the argument could be made that we ought to do so, a conclusion that would follow logically if the assumption that we should not jeopardise our ability to thrive is accepted. However, people who are able to thrive by eating plant foods and are able to access them without much difficulty cannot justify the consumption of animal products by claiming that doing so would be necessary to maintain their health.

4.3.5 Since some animals eat other animals, we should be free to do so too

The female student who said that it is in 'our nature to eat animals' added the following words:

- 'Cats eat mice, why shouldn't humans eat chickens etc.?'

A similar comment was made by Fiona, who responded as follows to the question why she ate animals:

- 'Animals eat other animals and we're a form of animal ... we are omnivorous therefore I don't see a problem with eating animals although I don't like to kill them.'

A similar assumption might underlie Craig's response, which immediately followed that of Fiona's: 'it's just part of life'. Likewise, Eric expressed the view that 'we're part of the animal population'. The problem with these claims is that it is not clear why the question of how we ought to behave should be based upon what other animals do. Some spiders eat their species members, but this does not provide a justification for the view that we should likewise eat our species members. It is not clear why we should model our behaviour on our perceptions of how some other animals behave.

4.3.6 Animals have been designed to be eaten

Some participants put the emphasis on their perception of what other animals might have been designed for. A male student tried to justify eating animals as follows:

- 'If we're not meant to eat animals, why are they made of meat?'

This is not much of a justification as the fact that we can eat something does not imply that we ought to eat it. Apart from the fact that the different body parts that constitute the bodies of animals are reduced here to their use value for humans by using the notion of 'meat', a further objectification might underlie the choice of the words 'made of'. This terminology may suggest that their bodies are manufactured, in a similar way to how complex machines are built from simple components. The assumption that animals should be eaten by humans because they are edible may also underlie Fiona's attempt to justify eating animals by a reference to her belief 'in the food chain', a comment that was made by three students as well. The problem with this argument is that humans are also 'made of meat' that contains valuable nutritional components that can be digested by other humans. In addition, our bodies or remains will one day be consumed by other organisms. Indeed, we are part of the food chain too. However, the argument that we ought to eat humans simply because we are made of the right stuff fails to satisfy logic as well as the standards of acceptability that many people might hold. Therefore, it is not clear why the sheer fact that other animals are constituted of components that we could eat should, *ipso facto*, be a reason for eating them.

While the data did not bear this out, but merely hinted at it, some participants might have thought that some Grand Designer had designed things to be that way and that we should play our roles in accordance with the will of that Designer. The problem with this view is that the same argument could be used to justify any behaviour, for example killing other humans in order to eat them. However, someone who took this line of defence to justify homicide would not be exculpated. The question must be asked why we should exonerate, on the basis of their belief in a much-disputed metaphysical idea about the Chain of Being, those who kill animals for food when they have the opportunity to avoid doing so. With regard to this belief in a Chain of Being, some people might argue that we have much more ground to accept the view that animals are violated unjustifiably when we kill them for food in situations when we could have killed plants instead, at least when this could be done without producing unacceptably large health, social, or ecological costs. Similarly, I do not think that we should prioritise any interest we might have in such a religious conception over our interest in abstaining from the consumption of animal products in general.

4.3.7 Animals owe their lives to the fact that we eat them

A female student wrote the following:

- 'Fields wouldn't have cows in if farmers didn't breed them, and farmers wouldn't breed them if we didn't eat them. My father's a farmer and I'm proud to have lived on a farm.'

Another female student expressed a similar view by writing that 'cattle [are] bred specifically to eat and for milk.' Eric and David made the same claim in an attempt to justify the butchering of animals. These participants are right that many animals and breeds would not have existed if they had not been bred specifically to provide food for humans. I am not convinced, however, that this provides a justification to continue breeding and killing animals where refraining from doing so would not be associated with significant moral problems. True, many animal breeds might become extinct if humans decided to stop breeding them. This theme was elaborated on by Eric, who claimed that 'vegans have a slightly strange position' as he was not sure what they would do with all the animals who have been bred for their products. Presumably, and interestingly, Eric was aware of the fact that many vegans want their dietary stance to be adopted by many humans, which would indeed raise the problem of what should be done with farmed animals, at least if many humans decided to turn to vegan diets relatively quickly. David claimed that, if the view that animals should not be 'kept'—a view that he attributed to the 'Animal Liberation Front'—was passed into law, '90% of the cows would be dead within the next week, because there'd be no reason for having them any longer'. A similar concern was introduced by Jane in a different exchange.

In my view, this need not be the inevitable outcome. Should humans stop farming animals, some animals might be able to adopt a feral existence, while many others might need to be looked after by farmers for the rest of their lives. Once there would no longer be an economic incentive to breed animals, it is likely that many farmers would no longer want their animals to reproduce. The question must be asked if this would be a significant loss. Many animals have been bred to acquire some features that humans take interests in, but these features are not always in the animals' best interests. For example, cows who are classed within the Belgian Blue breed are highly prized for the low fat content and quick development of their musculature, but many need human intervention, frequently by caesarean section, in order to give birth. In light of this problem and of the human health costs associated with the farming of cows, for example its contributions to climate change and to zoonotic and other diseases, I would argue that the extinction of the Belgian Blue should not be regarded as morally problematic.

Neither should the probability that many fields might no longer have cows in them concern us, especially in light of the fact that a huge amount of tree planting would be highly desirable to sequester carbon from the atmosphere and to provide more alternatives to fossil fuels. In addition, if we consider the violent ways in which many animals are treated, I think that it would have been better had the animals not been born in the first place; I would conclude the same thing with regard to human beings who are born in squalid conditions or with regard to the imaginary scenario wherein humans would be born and raised in good conditions but killed before they became aware of the fact that they were going to be killed, as appears to be the case for many animals who are killed for food by humans. The validity of this analogy hinges on my assumption that breeding human children for human consumption, provided that they are killed before they are able to contemplate what they have been bred for, is not that much different from breeding other animals in order to kill them for human consumption, particularly if the animals in question are closely related to us.

4.3.8 Tradition

Both Jane and a male student wrote that 'we have always eaten meat' to justify their choices to eat animals. While it is unclear why Eric (who said that 'vegans have a slightly strange position') said that he did not 'understand the foundation of veganism' and why Barry said that vegetarianism is a 'fad'—a claim he made twice in quick succession—these claims might be related to the possibility that they thought that the lack of a strong vegan or vegetarian tradition might be deemed morally relevant. Eric also said that he 'couldn't eat dog', a statement that might be influenced by the lack of a recent tradition of eating dogs in the UK, as well as by the habit of speaking about animals in abstract terms—hence the word 'dog' rather than 'dogs'—when their bodies are being considered for human consumption.

A psychological reason might explain why some people refer to historical practices to reject qualified moral veganism. Qualified moral veganism does not imply that it would always be wrong to kill animals in order to eat them, unlike, for example, denying women the right to vote. Many people might find it more difficult to decide on what is right and wrong in relation to practices that are right in some contexts, but not in others. In other words, a practice that may be justified in some situations might be perceived to be not so bad compared to a practice that should not be tolerated under any circumstances. Such a psychological inability to dissociate oneself from particular practices that would have been acceptable for a long time, even in recent history, and that might still be acceptable in particular contexts today, might also account for why Keith made the claim that I cited before:

- 'We're hunter-gatherers by nature and it's been bred into us for probably millions of years and it's a hard thing to break isn't it?'

Keith appears to acknowledge that eating animal products is not a biological necessity, but his attachment to a long cultural tradition as well as his perception that practices that have been regarded as acceptable for a long time cannot be all that bad seem to stand in the way of his wish to adopt vegetarianism. This line of reasoning can also be found in academic work on the subject. Webster (2013, 15), for example, writes that 'it is a fact of life that most of those who can, will eat food from animals'. Whereas the fact that we are entrenched in our cultures and the fallacy of overgeneralisation might explain why people refer to tradition to explain their practices, the explanation fails to provide a good reason to reject qualified moral veganism. The possibility that an activity that can be right in some situations might be perceived to be better than an activity that is always perceived to be wrong does not provide a good justification for engaging in that activity in situations where it is not right to do so.

A different psychological mechanism might be at work as well: resistance to that which is new. Consuming animal products is so much part of the dominant culture in the UK that any suggestion that it might be problematic is perceived to be a threat to that culture, and to one's identity within it. I mentioned earlier on that Barry expressed that vegetarianism is 'a fad' and that Eric did not understand the 'foundation of veganism'. Barry also appeared to associate vegetarians with extremists, as well as with the Animal Liberation Front; in the same exchange, Jane replied 'they can go ahead and be vegetarians' to the question of what she thought about vegetarianism, having expressed before that 'they're always trying to turn us vegetarian'—whereby the word 'they' lacked identifiable referents. Steiner (2013, 215) has interpreted—correctly in my view—such dissociations as follows: those 'who react in this way seem to be exhibiting a desire to incriminate the vegan messenger for taking some kind of moral high ground, thereby countering an authentic moral appeal with an ad hominem dismissal'; he adds that he 'cannot help but wonder whether such a reaction is born of a repressed intimation that the ... consumption of animals is at odds with our cosmic kinship with them'.

The dominant culture is also strengthened by particular rituals that are used to maintain or strengthen tradition. What is problematic about these rituals for people who reject some aspects of the dominant culture is that they not only socialise people into the ideology of that culture, but also serve to strengthen bonds between members of that culture and weaken bonds with those who are classed as outsiders. In research carried out in the early 1980s about food choices where women who lived in the north of England and who had at least one child were interviewed, it was found that 'the food involved in the Christmas ritual is fundamentally a celebration of the coming together of family members' and that 'self-indulgence rather than self-denial is the order of the day' (Charles and Kerr 1988, 26). The consumption of animal bodies was felt to be particularly important at this time of the year, with one poor woman describing how she saved up for a whole year in order to be able to afford to buy body parts from animals in a special shop: 'We went to Dewhurst's in town. We got everything, it was lovely to have meat you know. We even got steak, so you can tell it was a treat, a real treat ...' (Charles and Kerr 1988, 27). This goes some way towards explaining why the Christmas ritual may be associated with deeply conflicted feelings for those who do not identify with the dominant culture's focus on the consumption of foods derived from animals as important status symbols that serve to establish and reinforce personal and social identities. In this light, a remark by Gail—who had been a vegetarian in her youth—is telling:

• 'Christmas dinner was dreadful.'

Whilst I appreciate the fact that 'old habits die hard', the perception that something has always been done does not imply that it should be deemed to be either good or bad. Not so long ago, women in the United Kingdom and in many other countries lacked the right to vote. Some who wanted to keep the status quo at the time this was changed referred to tradition as well. However, few people who live now are likely to think that this tradition should have been honoured. The question must be asked why the tradition of eating the bodies of some animals (yet not the flesh of others, for example dogs, who are not eaten in many societies) should be honoured. Many people who lived in the past might have consumed animal products out of nutritional necessity, rather than from the conviction that there is no moral difference between the consumption of animal products and the consumption of other organisms. The fact that many people are able to enjoy adequate nutrition nowadays without consuming animal products, without significant moral costs, undermines the relevance of a 'traditional' reason to consume such products.

4.3.9 Questioning the exploitation of animals

Whereas none of our interviewees adopted vegetarian or vegan diets, some expressed feelings of unease about the felt need to reconcile particular feelings for animals with the practice of eating them. Alice expressed that people should not be cruel towards animals, and that veganism was 'very admirable', but it was not clear whether this perception related to a concern over the exploitation of animals. She added that she did not eat a lot of 'meat' and that it would be difficult for her to get a 'balanced diet' if she did not do so occasionally; however, she also questioned whether this might just be an 'excuse'. Having expressed that he 'love[d] beef' and that he 'was brought up on farms', Henry recounted the story of a cow who had been regarded as a pet by both his father and himself and who had died after choking, saying:

• 'Cried me eyes out when that cow died ... but fair enough if it was sold at the butcher's shop the following week ... I would have still had some.'

In the same exchange, Eric, the scientist who said that he did not understand the 'foundation of veganism' and 'couldn't eat dog', related Henry's memory directly to a childhood experience that he went on to recount. After Eric's father had killed the chicken that Eric's mother had looked after for months on Christmas Eve, Eric's mother had refused to eat the chicken. Eric added that he had visited countries where dogs were eaten and that he had asked the people he was with: 'tell me if we're being served dog cause I don't want to offend anybody but I really can't bring myself to eat it'. Eric also appeared to relate his unease with the words that he added: 'look in that garden, all these kids they're playing with the dogs'. He then went on to generalise this feeling to the consumption of all animals who were considered to be 'pets'.

Whereas I can understand the view that we may have feelings and responsibilities for companion animals that we do not have for other animals, I do not accept the assumption that killing animals who are not regarded as companion animals in order to eat them should be relatively problem-free. In this regard, Eric appeared to be aware of his inconsistency, saying that he would not want to eat 'cat' and 'horses' either, but that he could not see why people who 'eat a sheep or a pig ... shouldn't eat a horse or a dog'. However, the question whether an animal was a companion animal was not the only question that mattered to him; he added that he could not eat animal products from animals who had not been 'looked after properly', providing the example of 'veal':

- 'I couldn't stand the thought of calves being crated ... and in the dark.'

This was contrasted with an example of an animal whom he would eat:

- 'I would much rather eat a pheasant that's had a wild life and been shot.'

The view that killing animals might be associated with cruelty was most prominent in the views expressed by students. A female student who was neither vegetarian nor vegan expressed the view that 'some of the forms of killing animals are cruel'. Three students identified themselves as being vegetarians, and related their choices to adopt vegetarianism to concerns with the killing of animals. Two female students wrote as follows:

- '(1) I am a vegetarian. I don't like the thought of animals being killed for my food. (2) I think it is a personal choice. I don't feel people who eat meat are wrong.'
- '(1) I'm a vegetarian. I have been all my life. I do not agree with the often inhumane way in which they are killed. (2) I think that it is a matter of personal beliefs, but I do think that if you eat meat, it should be free range and well-treated.'

Though the moral concern with killing animals was more prominent amongst students' questionnaire responses, the view that killing animals might be problematic was not entirely absent amongst our interviewees. Jane said that she had once killed a frog while stepping on the animal, which gave her 'the most ghastly feeling', while Henry expressed the view that humans sometimes killed for 'enjoyment' and that that 'should be stopped or cut down a bit'. Fiona said that she did not have 'a problem with eating animals although [she did not] like to kill them', and David made a very similar claim where he said, in relation to killing animals: 'I would have difficulty [doing it] ... despite being brought up on a farm where we did kill things, I didn't personally but others did'. He also recounted the story of one of the pigs of the farm where he was brought up who was killed on his village green, adding: 'that sticks in my memory very, very clearly'. Whereas he did not find the fact that he ate animals who had been killed (where it might not be ethically required for him to do so for health or other reasons) inconsistent with the fact that he had a problem with killing them, he was keen to point out that others, including his daughter (who was 'extremely carnivorous but would not go ... near an animal being slaughtered') might not be consistent:

- 'What I do find hypocritical is ... people who eat meat ... but then complain when they actually go to a butcher's shop ... about seeing it when it's red.'

At the same time, he expressed the view that many people are prone to this kind of hypocrisy. I quite agree with him here, but I am disappointed that he only recognised its presence in others. Surely, it is wrong to seek the benefits from actions that one considers to be morally wrong.

Much of the literature in what Haynes (2008) refers to as the 'animal welfare science community' has focused on the moral problem of inflicting pain and suffering, where concerns associated with killing *per se* are dissociated from the narrow definition of 'welfare' that is adopted. What the data that I have examined here have in common with one of the reasons why I adopt qualified moral veganism is the view that animals do not usually fare well by being killed, regardless of whether the killing inflicts pain or suffering on them. Therefore, these data question the killing of animals for food in situations where convincing justifications for doing so are lacking. One difference between these views and my view is that I think that the negative value associated with killing animals for food when it is not in the animals' interests should be given much more weight. A further problem that I have specifically with the views of our vegetarian students is that many vegetarian diets are not free from the moral concerns that these students identified: many cows and chickens who are used by vegetarians to provide milk and eggs for them are still being killed once farmers are convinced that it is more cost-effective to replace them, and in many situations male calves and chicks are killed without good justification as well. Even if his view that he could live healthily 'without destroying life' was misguided, one male student might have been aware of this connection, although it is unclear why he did not adopt qualified moral veganism:

- 'I am a vegetarian hoping to become a vegan, because I can have a healthy life without destroying life, and it pains me to see animals exploited.'

A final observation is that the two female vegetarian students felt the need to make a distinction between what they thought to be ethical for themselves and what they thought might be ethical for others to do by contrasting their 'personal' views with the views that others may have. I think that at least three possible interpretations can be offered why students might have decided to cast their opinions in this way. In one interpretation, the addition of the word 'personal' could be perceived to be trivial or superfluous, as all decisions that are made by personal agents are personal. A second interpretation is that the word is added to show respect for the views of others, to signify something like: 'I might perceive something to be wrong, but I appreciate that others have different opinions, and I do not want to state categorically that they are wrong.' In other words, by using this word, students might express agreement with Pyrrhonian moral scepticism or a similar meta-ethical stance. I endorse this type of stance, and I have engaged with it elsewhere (Deckers 2007). A third interpretation is that students thought that their views were ethical, but that they felt uncomfortable about presenting them as ethical views, preferring to cast them merely as matters of taste as would those who adopt a relativist or radical scepticist position.

If ethics, however, can be defined as the search for, and the articulation of, values that can be universalised, this third interpretation is problematic. It is understandable, however, why students might have been inclined to present their positions outwardly as if they were based on a relativist meta-ethical position while they might have inwardly been convinced of Pyrrhonian moral scepticism. By presenting their moral positions as mere matters of taste, they may adopt a strategy that might make it more likely that they will not be belittled or marginalised by the dominant culture, which suppresses those who challenge the continued existence of that culture. This third interpretation may be the one that is correct. It clearly is the correct way to interpret the view of a male contributor to an on-line forum that was analysed in another study (Fox and Ward 2008, 425): 'I never call myself a vegan or vegetarian. I tell people that I have food allergies and I have to eat like this for my health.' This interpretation might also explain why many more people adopt vegetarian diets than adopt a more morally consistent vegan diet (van der Kooi 2010). Only the former are increasingly socially accepted within some countries, for example in the UK; people who adopt vegan diets, by contrast, are marginalised in many countries (McDonald 2000; M. Cole and Morgan 2011).

4.4 Thematic analysis and evaluation of the views of Oldham slaughterhouse workers

I shall now turn to the views of workers in a slaughterhouse in Oldham, who were interviewed about their jobs and their political views for a documentary broadcast in 2005 on BBC Two. My attention is focused in particular on evaluating their views about killing animals for food. A thematic analysis of their views revealed that they entertained positive perceptions about their jobs by associating the killing of animals with power, sincerity, fun, skill, and religion.

4.4.1 Power: Being allowed to do something that not many people are allowed to do

Arran was a slaughterman, that is, someone who is allowed to kill animals, a position that not all slaughterhouse workers had, but that many aspired to. When Arran was asked about his job, he reminisced about the time when he was taken into the slaughterhouse by his dad; when he saw men with 'blood over their aprons', he thought 'that looks pretty interesting' and wanted to become a slaughterman too. Arran added that, in his job, 'you can get away with murder every day and not get arrested for it'. Patch, however, was a cleaner and said that he would like to be a slaughterman, a position which he identified with being 'the ringmaster'.

While Arran's identity was clearly influenced by the desires to be like his father and to kill others, I do not think that these should trump qualified moral veganism. Many of the animals who were killed by Arran were not destined to be eaten by people whose health might suffer otherwise. Accordingly, it is hard to conceive how Arran might have failed to maximise positive GHIs by refraining to kill animals. Perhaps Arran's choice to work in the slaughterhouse was influenced by the thought that it might have been hard for him to find other work. This may have been so, but I do not think that any negative GHIs that may be associated with being out of work ought to be considered to be so significant that the negative effects produced by the killing of animals in these circumstances ought to be trumped by them. The fact that Arran compared his job with 'murder' is interesting as it suggests that he did perceive a moral similarity between what he did and homicide. If Arran had moral problems with killing human beings—and I assume that he had—the question must therefore be asked why he did not experience similar problems with the killing of other mammals.

Though I would agree that there is a moral distinction between both practices, in line with my commitment to speciesism, I do not think that the difference is sufficiently great to warrant a rejection of qualified moral veganism. When I was young, I was told (at least once) by a fellow pigeon-fancier that I was 'not a man' if I could not bring myself to kill pigeons. As has been documented by many studies (Adams 1990; Sobal 2005; Ruby and Heine 2011), the meaning of what it is to 'be a man' has been associated with the ability to kill other animals and with the permission to eat their bodies in many cultures. This clearly operates here as well. The concept of 'being a man' seemed to be very much tied up with the role of 'slaughterman' amongst workers in the slaughterhouse. Cleaners like Patch, who engaged in tasks that have traditionally been associated more with the role of women in many societies, aspired to be slaughtermen, and were ordered around and bullied by the slaughtermen who worked in the slaughterhouse. In this respect, it is no coincidence that Patch identified the role of slaughterman with the position of a 'ringmaster' in a circus. Patch might have felt that cleaners like him were being ordered to do things by the ringmaster, suggesting that he identified in some way with circus animals who are taught to obey orders. There is a strong current in Western culture that identifies women more with other animals and that elevates men to a position that is quite separate from, and superior to, the position occupied by women and other animals (Adams 1990). The fact that women may not feel the same pressure to 'be [like] a man' might also account for the fact that studies have shown that women are more likely than men to avoid eating the bodies of animals (Kalof et al. 1999; Wardle et al. 2004; Lea et al. 2006a; DeLeeuw et al. 2007). However, I do not think that the highly questionable positive value associated with occupying any of these identities should trump the positive values underlying qualified moral veganism.

4.4.2 Sincerity: Facing up to 'reality', in contrast to others

In the documentary, Arran added the following words immediately after drawing the aforementioned comparison between killing animals and murder:

- 'It sounds pretty sick but it is not. Some people might think it is pretty sick but they don't think like that when it's on their plate on Sunday.'

With these words, Arran might be expressing that he feels good about the work he is doing, and he might be adopting the view that some other people are inconsistent by valuing his work negatively whilst valuing the products of his work positively. Arran's perception is supported by research that shows that many people hold contradictory beliefs about the ethics of eating animals (Povey et al. 2001; Berndsen and van der Pligt 2005; Macnaghten 2004). Arran resolved this perceived contradiction by contesting the negative value that he perceived other people might associate with his work.

Arran's perception that other people did not value his work was shared by Taylor and Eddy. As Arran, Taylor appeared to be aware of people's inconsistencies, suggesting that people were in denial over the process that led to the product:

- 'People think they are already dead when they come in when you tell them you work in the slaughterhouse.'

Taylor also contrasted his willingness to work in the slaughterhouse with his perception that none of the children who attend private schools would want to work in the slaughterhouse. Interestingly, this disdain for a particular class of people was shared by a scientist who—paradoxically—belonged to that class (at least provided that being educated to postgraduate level and climbing to the rank of academic professor are sufficient conditions to belong to that class), who claimed that vegetarianism was 'a fad ... a middle class thing'.

My view, by contrast, is to think that those who value slaughterhouse work negatively are right to do so, but that they are wrong to value the products of the slaughterhouse positively, at least in situations when humans could eat other foods at a smaller moral cost. The inconsistency perceived by slaughterhouse workers in the general discourse of others is not absent from academic work either. Webster (2013, 213, 221, 15, 145), for example, has spoken positively of 'vegans' as showing 'respect in the most profound form' and has spoken of the abattoir as 'the most brutalizing environment', but at the same time he has endorsed the consumption of animal products in many situations and has written that 'it is a fact of life that most of those who can, will eat food from animals' and that 'it is certain that consumption of pig meat will increase'.

4.4.3 Fun: Making and having fun

Whilst he was filmed standing alongside a cow who had been killed seconds before, Arran said the following words:

- 'Oh my God, somebody killed Daisy.'

Once again, Arran might be expressing a certain discontent with the perceptions of those who like to think of cows as bucolic animals, the iconic images of cows that are fostered in much of the children's literature. He might think that people with such perceptions fail to face up to the reality that they support in their eating practices. Arran might also think that there is something problematic about killing cows in particular situations, as suggested by the words 'oh my God'. At the same time, the abstract image of 'Daisy the cow' might help Arran to cope better with the concrete reality of his work. The practice of making fun of those who live with inconsistencies might be another coping mechanism: the thought that he has managed to resolve something that he perceives others not to have managed to resolve might give Arran a temporary release from having to live with the uncertainty of the morality of what he does.

A similar strategy might underlie the statements he made whilst slitting the throat of a sheep ('This is the fun part.') and whilst standing next to a pig who was suffering a heart attack whilst coming off a lorry ('poor little bastard'). Arran's word combination in the latter case shows both empathic association and dissociation. His choice of words suggests the feeling of some compassion towards the animal, but it is also interesting to note that he might associate the pig with the opposite of what he might aspire to be, or of how he might wish to be perceived by others: rich, big, and not a bastard. Whilst he might not have made a conscious decision to do so, Arran's words may also distance him from the pig by portraying the pig as something else than what the pig really was, as the pig may not have been poor, nor little, nor a bastard.

A similar coping strategy might be adopted by Eddy when he pronounces the words 'happy birthday' whilst killing a cow. It is unlikely that it was the cow's birthday, and, even if it was, it is unlikely that Eddy would have known it was. Eddy might have said these words to provide himself with a temporary release from the negative emotions he associated with what he was doing at that particular time. Through conjuring up images of birthday parties in his head, Eddy might have learned to associate positive feelings with some of the activities that he might have felt to be problematic, thus hoping that somehow, through association, those activities would turn out to be more positive than they in fact are.

Some workers also seemed to make a game out of stunning sheep, with one person saying 'didn't even see it coming' whilst he firmly planted over a sheep's head a metallic device through which he released an electric charge. Having played football most of my life, I know how pleasurable it can be to outmanoeuvre others through the use of a bit of skill—which I do not possess in great quantities—and in that sense I can appreciate that some people might obtain pleasure out of being able to catch sheep by surprise. People have also been reported to enjoy other practices that involve the killing of animals, including fox hunting (Marvin 2005). What I do not share, however, is the view that the mere production of such feelings should be allowed to trump the positive value associated with allowing the animals to be. More generally, I do not think that making fun of animals or having fun whilst killing them are sufficient reasons to reject qualified moral veganism.

4.4.4 Skill: Killing better than others, who do not do so properly

The role that is played by tradition in maintaining and consolidating certain practices was mentioned earlier on. I also mentioned that not all the slaughterhouse workers interviewed in the documentary were allowed to be slaughtermen. In order to become a slaughterman, it was necessary to show sufficient skill in the art of killing, but it was also necessary for workers to learn by heart what was presented as the 'slaughterman's motto', which is also known as the 'slaughterman's creed':

'Thine is the task of blood.
Discharge thy task with mercy.
Let thy victim feel no pain.
Let sudden blow bring death;
Such death as thou thyself would ask for.'

While I acknowledge that there are morally distinct ways in which animals can be killed, I question whether the perception that the killing might have been done properly should be sufficient to reject qualified moral veganism. The use of the words 'thine', 'thy', 'thou', and 'thyself' is significant here. It might help slaughtermen to convince themselves that what they do is right: by being able to recite a formulaic sentence that repeats archaic words, they might feel supported in their practices from the conviction that they are participating in a tradition, perhaps even in some kind of religion, that binds different slaughtermen together, both across space and across time. However, the felt need to adopt this ritual chant, which includes the disputed claim that 'no pain' might be felt if things are done properly, suggests that it might function as an attempt to ameliorate a practice that is perceived to be quite problematic.

Though one of the functions of the motto might be to unite slaughtermen, it did not remove all perceptions of difference between them. Arran was aware of the fact that some people might perceive him to be cruel, yet he defended himself against this charge by claiming that the Jewish slaughtermen were cruel as they used different slaughtering methods. The charge was reversed by Danny, a kosher slaughterman, who claimed that non-Jewish slaughtermen had to learn to slaughter animals 'in a humane way'. While it is beyond my expertise to decide which method of slaughter might be the best, nothing seems to me to be 'humane' about slaughtering animals merely for the purpose of their being eaten by people who could eat healthy alternatives without increasing negative GHIs. By criticising the methods that are used by others, slaughtermen might try to forget the problematic methods that they use themselves to kill animals, as well as the fact that they slaughter animals at all.

4.4.5 Religion: Being justified by Yahweh/God/Allah

This distinction between kosher and other methods to kill animals takes me to the role played by religion. The slaughterhouse included workers representing the three monotheistic religions that are dominant in British society today, namely Judaism, Christianity, and Islam. However, the interviews hardly brought out Christian influences.

The Christian tradition might underlie a claim that was made by Arran, where he said the following:

• 'If you look carefully you can see their souls escape through the door, that's why we've got that hole there.'

It was fairly clear that Arran was mocking—while he was aware of the idea, he did not seem to use the Christian idea that something of the animal might resurrect to a new life after death as a justification for his practices. Both a Jewish slaughterman (Danny) and a Muslim slaughterman (Mohammed), however, tried to justify what they did by a reference to religion. They referred to their religions when they made the following claims:

- Danny: 'Human beings are on a higher level, a higher plane compared to animals.'
- Mohammed: 'If all veins in the neck are cut, it is, by the name of Allah, 100% halal.'

With regard to the Christian reference, I do not adopt the view that any Christian would make a good case for homicide should they try to justify that practice by reference to their belief in the resurrection. While the killing of another animal might not be morally on a par with homicide, I do not think that killing animals in general can be justified merely by reference to a belief in the resurrection. Neither do I accept Danny's view that humans 'are on a higher level' than 'animals'. Though I agree with the view that humans should be given more moral significance than other animals, this view does not imply that we 'are on a higher level' than 'animals', as we are animals. Perhaps it can be said that many human beings are capable of reaching a level of self-awareness that no other animals are capable of reaching, but I write these words with some hesitation. Human beings certainly do not operate at a 'higher level' in every respect; bats, for example, are most definitely better at echolocation. More importantly, I do not think that the belief that human beings should be granted special moral significance justifies a rejection of qualified moral veganism. Rather, I adopt the view that human moral agents must cultivate an interest in not eating animals and an interest in not killing animals for food that should normally be prioritised over any interest we may have in not killing plants for food. A deep analysis of the data reported here suggests that many people agree on this at least where it concerns the theoretical interest in not killing animals for food, even if they might not follow this through consistently in their eating and working practices.

In this light, it must be questioned whether any moral weight should be given to the belief that a certain practice might be justifiable on the basis of a belief in some greater being, for example Yahweh, God, or Allah. Imagine that I adopted a belief in the 'X' religion, a religion which justified the killing of human children for human consumption—the X religion might say, for example, that we should accept children as gifts from the deity of the X religion, some of which children we should consume whilst expressing our gratitude to the great Giver. Few people would adopt the view that we should tolerate such practices out of respect for the views of those who adopt the X religion. The question must be asked, therefore, how much moral weight we should give to those who justify the killing of animals for food in the name of their belief in some greater being. Gorringe (2011), for example, has tried to justify his practice of killing sheep for food through the Christian conviction that sheep are 'gifts'. For my part, the belief that we violate an animal's right to life unjustifiably when we kill that animal, where this is not carried out to serve the best interests of the animal concerned or to safeguard really important human interests that could not be protected otherwise, should trump any belief, religious or otherwise, that it might be acceptable to kill that animal. Conceiving of animals as 'gifts' seems nothing other than a gross distortion of reality: animals do not give themselves up to be consumed by human beings, and their bodies are, therefore, not to be considered as 'gifts'.

Incidentally, if we bear in mind that the scriptures that are held sacred by the three religions concerned were written a long time ago, it should not surprise us that they contain texts that support the killing of animals for food. Then, life may have been a struggle for a significant proportion of the human population. Now, life is a doddle for many of us. Indeed, it was not until relatively recently that many people gained the opportunity to remain healthy on diets that did not include animal products, largely because of the advantages of mechanised agriculture and modern storage technologies. Even so, it is worth pointing out, for those who adopt the view that the answers that were provided by the authors of these texts in response to issues that they struggled with at the time ought to determine which answers we ought to give to (remotely) similar issues today, that the Hebrew texts that are cherished by all three religions do not justify the eating of animal products in any straightforward manner. The final editor of the Book of Genesis, for example, may have struggled with the issue before the book was treated as a text that should no longer be changed, as the deity only gives fruits and vegetables for human consumption in Genesis 1.19 and Genesis 3.18, whereas the consumption of animals is only presented as being granted divine approval after the flood has taken place, in Genesis 9.3. Some might argue that this single mention is sufficient, but this seems to me to be a very lazy way out. Regrettably, it appears to be a popular option amongst many Christians in the USA (DeLeeuw et al. 2007). Some religious people, however, may not wish to dispute that we should cause as little harm as possible and that, in many situations, we cause more harm by eating animals than by eating plants. If those who are inspired by these religious texts really do want to stick to a literal reading, I would recommend that they read Ecclesiastes 7.21, which recommends that we 'do not pay attention to everything folk say'; religion should therefore not necessarily be an obstacle to qualified moral veganism.

4.5 Conclusion

In this chapter I analysed and evaluated the views of some academic scientists and some students from Newcastle University and of some men who worked in a slaughterhouse in Oldham on vegetarianism, veganism, and the killing of animals for human food. The identities of most of these people seem to be constituted at least in part by the adoption of certain beliefs that serve to dissociate people from other animals. In addition, the identities of slaughterhouse workers appear to be constructed partly by a range of associations and dissociations with the views and roles of others. Earlier research has also claimed that people's attitudes and actions are strongly affected by the roles that people have in society (S. Knight et al. 2009), yet I believe that it would be wrong to claim that these slaughterhouse workers, as well as other participants in these studies, had values that differed radically from the values held by many others, including by those who support qualified moral veganism; much of the evidence reveals some common ground.

Even if the data are less clear about the consumption of animal products *per se*, many people seem to agree that, in many situations, there is something that is morally problematic about killing animals in order to eat them. However, the positive value of allowing animals to be is suppressed by many other values, for example by the positive value that is attributed to the thought that killing animals or eating animal products are necessary either to build or to strengthen one's identity; in my view, this is where things go wrong. More generally, I believe that we ought to cultivate an interest in abstaining from the consumption of animal products and grant this interest such moral weight as to adopt qualified moral veganism. Of all the other interests that we may bring to bear on the issue, that interest which is rooted in our fear of death, or 'thanatophobia', might be the most fundamental. Whereas qualified moral veganism does not deny that it may be necessary to kill animals for food in some situations, it would be wrong for us to think that we might be able to ward off or transcend our mortality by killing and consuming other animals, or—as has been put eloquently by Christman (2008, 313)—by 'follow[ing] the path of Gilgamesh in relying upon the lifeblood of animals to protect us from the whims of the cosmos'. Those who remain unconvinced may nevertheless be inspired by this beautiful poem, written by Jane Legge (1969, 59), and quoted by Cora Diamond (1978, 472–473):

Learning to be a Dutiful Carnivore

Dogs and cats and goats and cows,
Ducks and chickens, sheep and sows
Woven into tales for tots,
Pictured on their walls and pots.
Time for dinner! Come and eat
All your lovely, juicy meat.
One day ham from Percy Porker
(In the comics he's a corker),
Then the breast from Mrs Cluck
Or the wing from Donald Duck.
Liver next from Clara Cow
(No, it doesn't hurt her now).
Yes, that leg's from Peter Rabbit

Chew it well; make that a habit.
Eat the creatures killed for sale,
But never pull the pussy's tail.
Eat the flesh from 'filthy hogs'
But never be unkind to dogs.
Grow up into double-think-
Kiss the hamster; skin the mink.
Never think of slaughter, dear,
That's why animals are here.
They only come on earth to die,
So eat your meat, and don't ask why.

I am not convinced that the views expressed in samples of two different socio-economic groups in contemporary British society undermine qualified moral veganism, and I conclude that this position stands firm in light of the various problems that beset other positions. Many people appear to have significant concerns with the infliction of pain, suffering, and death upon animals in order to eat the products that we can derive from their bodies. Though the questions that were asked in the empirical studies that have been analysed in this chapter did not ask specifically whether people also had concerns about eating animals who either had died naturally or had been killed accidentally or mercifully, no enthusiasm for eating the bodies of these animals could be identified. Further research is needed to discuss qualified moral veganism explicitly and with more diverse groups of people—in this way, it may become clear whether I have ignored something of great moral importance that would result in my rejection of this position.

Conclusion

In this book I have argued that, in many situations, the human consumption of foods derived from animals fails to minimise negative GHIs, thus jeopardising the satisfaction of one or more of the following interests:

1/ an interest in avoiding the consumption of animals, including those who die naturally or accidentally, which is based on a more general animalist interest.

2/ an interest in avoiding the consumption of animals who are closely related to us, which is based on a more general evolutionist interest.

3/ an interest in avoiding the consumption of animal products where such consumption relies on the intentional infliction of pain, suffering, and death upon animals.

4/ an interest in avoiding the consumption of animal products where such consumption relies on the intentional infliction of pain, suffering, and death upon animals who are closely related to us.

How to cite this book chapter:
Deckers, J 2016 *Animal (De)liberation: Should the Consumption of Animal Products Be Banned?* Pp. 159–165. London: Ubiquity Press. DOI: http://dx.doi.org/10.5334/bay.f. License: CC-BY 4.0

5/ an interest in avoiding the consumption of animal products where such consumption relies on the intentional infliction of pain, suffering, and death upon animals with relatively great capacities for richness of experience.

6/ an interest in avoiding the consumption of animal products where such consumption relies on actions that pose relatively high risks of inflicting accidental pain, suffering, and death upon animals.

7/ an interest in avoiding the consumption of animal products where such consumption relies on actions that jeopardise the integrity of nature.

8/ an interest in holistic health.

Those who agree that the first of these interests is sufficiently important so that it is not—in Caney (2008, 539)'s words—'unreasonably demanding' to protect it may adopt the view that we ought to adopt a *prima facie* duty not to consume animals. I have also argued that this interest, as well as all the others apart from 8/, may conflict with some other moral interests, for example with our interest in eating, and that in some situations these other interests ought to prevail (for example in a situation where one can choose between starvation or consuming an animal). This is why the duty to adopt moral veganism, derived from interests 1/ and 3/, must be qualified. In situations where the consumption of animals ought not to be avoided, I have argued that, *ceteris paribus*, we should try to abide by 2/.

Those who reject either the existence or the moral relevance of 1/ and 2/ may nevertheless adopt the view that, where it does not serve the best interests of the animals concerned, the intentional infliction of pain, suffering, and death upon animals is worse than the intentional infliction of pain, suffering, and death upon other organisms. On this basis, even those who do not agree that it is better not to consume animals who die naturally or accidentally might agree with 3/ and forgo the consumption of most animal products. Whereas I would not agree with their rejection of 1/ and 2/, even these putative opponents will come close to embracing qualified moral veganism, given that chapter two documents that most animal products that are consumed are derived not from animals who die naturally or accidentally, but from animals who are bred in order to provide flesh, milk, and eggs and who are disposed of when they either have fulfilled or no longer fulfil (to an accepted standard) these external purposes.

However, consistency demands that, in the absence of overriding moral considerations, those who reject 1/ and 2/ but not 3/ (out of a concern about the intentional infliction of pain, suffering, and death upon animals where this does not serve their best interests) will agree not only to consuming animals who die naturally or accidentally, but also to consuming animal products that are derived from animals on whom pain, suffering, or death is inflicted intentionally in situations where the consumption of any alternative foods that are available would inflict more intentional pain, suffering, and death upon animals. The same applies to those who reject 1/ and 2/ but support 4/ and 5/, with the qualification that the moral equation would be based not only on the number of intentional injuries and deaths, but also on relative degrees of biological relatedness (4/) and of capacities for richness of experience (5/).

Vegans who reject 1/ and 2/ might retort that their diets are justified as they would only impose pain, suffering, and death upon animals accidentally, unless the imposition was in the animals' best interests. The problem with this view is that I argued (in sections 3.5.2 and 3.5.3) that many vegan diets also rely on the intentional killing of animals (for example through the use of pesticides) and that we have good reason, for example to safeguard human food security, not to ban the intentional killing of animals, to protect the fruits and vegetables that are grown for human consumption, even if such intentional killing should only be committed where the animals jeopardise a significant proportion of our crops. Whereas we should always be mindful of other options, for example the option to move slugs and snails to other parts of our gardens or to create habitats that encourage the presence of predators who eat these animals, in some situations the intentional killing of animals may be justified where such a killing is not in their best interests.

Those who reject either the existence or the moral significance that I attributed to 3/ may nevertheless adopt 4/ and/or 5/ and attribute special moral significance to nonhuman animals who are closely related to us and/or to nonhuman animals who are thought to possess relatively developed capacities to enjoy rich experiences. Interest 4/ would explain why killing an adult chicken for food may be more troubling than killing a mature mussel, but interest 5/ would explain why killing a one-day-old chicken embryo may be less troubling than killing an adult mussel. My view is that both the criterion of relative biological relatedness and that of relative experiential complexity are important when it comes to determining the relative moral significance of different nonhuman animals, but that more deliberation is required on their relative importance.

The same applies for adjudicating the relative importance of 4/ or 5/ versus 6/. Whereas I have argued that the intentional killing of animals for food is more problematic than the accidental but foreseeable killing of animals, the fact that the former type of killing can be controlled implies that it can be performed relatively quickly, minimising concerns about the infliction of pain and suffering, which is an argument in its favour. A further argument in its favour is the fact that a much larger number of animals are killed in most arable farming processes than in the killing of one cow, for example, to provide the same quantity of food. Whereas these arguments do not alter my position, neither do I adopt the view that we should be allowed to risk imposing accidental but foreseeable deaths on *any* number of animals to avoid intentionally killing one animal for food.

The relevance of interest 7/ was considered (in sections 2.11 and 2.12) in relation to biotechnological projects that seek to alter animals through genetic engineering, as well as to develop in-vitro flesh. Whereas I contended that the latter ought to be developed to feed domesticated cats and that its development may also minimise negative GHIs associated with the human consumption of animal products in a less-than-ideal world compared to other strategies that should be pursued, I also argued that both, but particularly the former, present a threat to 7/. We undermine the integrity of nature not only through these new biotechnological developments, but also through more conventional ways in which we interfere with nature, for instance through selective breeding. This is also why it is not because animals who are farmed or kept as companions might do well in some situations that their dependency on human beings does not present any moral concern. Some animals may fare better by living independently, but even their not doing so does not imply that freeing them from human domestication would necessarily be wrong, as interest 8/ should be our overriding concern, which is why we must give due consideration to 7/. As we must give some consideration to the moral interest of safeguarding the integrity of nature for our own health, the welfare of other animals should not be the only thing that we should think of when we contemplate weaning other animals off their dependency on humans. When we keep our focus on holistic health, it should also be clear that our psychological health is best served by not conceiving of other animals as sources of food where our physical health does not depend on doing so. Prioritising principle 8/, therefore, demands that we strike the right balance between all the morally relevant interests that should come into play when we consider our fundamental interest in eating.

Those who are not troubled by the way in which many human beings regard and treat other animals may be inspired to rethink by considering the following fictitious story. Imagine that human beings had already managed to build spaceships 100,000 years ago and that a group of them had decided to fly off to an imaginary planet that was not too dissimilar from how earth is now. Imagine that some had recently returned to earth. Though we recognised that these creatures were very similar to those who had never left, we were also aware that they were not quite the same, and that it was very difficult for us to communicate with them. This was not merely due to the fact that they spoke a different language that was very difficult for us to get to grips with, but also due to the fact that it became apparent to us that they were much smarter than we were. The 'supersmarts' were not only physically different from other humans by having—amongst other features—bigger ears and eyes, as well as smaller mouths, but they also possessed some curious talents, including the abilities to predict the future much more accurately than we could, to plan for the future in much greater detail, and to control their environment to a much greater extent. As they had many different interests from ours, they preferred to mix with other supersmarts, even if they also appreciated interacting with us. Attempts at interbreeding, however, had not been successful.

If some accounts that I engaged with in this book were accepted, it might be said that we ought to ascribe greater moral significance to the supersmarts than to members of our own species because of their greater capacities to have rich experiences (which I assume to come with their greater intelligence). In this book I have argued that I do not agree with a moral theory that attributes differential moral significance merely on the basis of differences in capacities to enjoy rich experiences. Whereas I have no doubt that we ought to ascribe great moral significance to the supersmarts, I do not think that we ought to prefer the satisfaction of their interests to the satisfaction of those of members of our own species.

The question that is at least as troublesome, however, is what moral significance the supersmarts should bestow upon us. If they were to model their behaviour on what many human beings currently do with other animals, it may be expected that they would use us for their own purposes—which would perhaps include us being farmed—as well as compromise our vital interests in many ways, even to satisfy their own relatively trivial interests. It seems to me that those who object to being treated like this by the supersmarts likewise ought to object to animals who are closely related to us being used in similar ways by human beings, for what we might be to the supersmarts may not be much different from what these animals are to us. As all organisms that are alive today descend from a common ancestor, every speciesist should also be an animalist, and, as it would be rather bizarre for the supersmarts to adopt the view that there was a large gap in moral significance between them and us, so it is most strange indeed for human beings to act as if a large gap in moral significance ought to exist between us and other animals who are closely related to us.

Whereas many people may have similar values, or morally relevant interests, to mine about how we should relate to other animals, relatively few people adopt qualified moral veganism. This may be caused either by failures to act on one's deepest values or by the fact that some of these values or feelings are not one's deepest. If the latter applies, it may be difficult for people to be convinced by qualified moral veganism. Similarly, a person who was not moved by the virtue of consistency—if such a person were to exist—would not understand any moral argument that was based upon it. However, even people who do not appreciate that we may have duties towards other animals might still adopt the view that we have duties towards human beings. It is my view that interest 8/ can only be given the protection that it deserves if we also tend to the other listed interests, but even those who reject 1/ to 7/ may be swayed where they adopt an interest in human health conceived more narrowly than 8/. Indeed, as I argued in the first chapter, the fact that many omnivorous diets produce more negative GHIs than many vegan diets may be a cause for concern for those human beings who agree that some things, for example dietary gas emissions, can be classed as negative GHIs and that they may fail to minimise them due to their diet. Even people who do not care about other animals may therefore have good reasons to adopt vegan diets.

In chapter three I argued that we must take seriously our duty to allow no more than those negative GHIs that are required to safeguard our interests in holistic health and that people with political power and governments that are serious about the duties that I have outlined in this book must act appropriately. I distinguished three strategies that governments could adopt to curtail the negative GHIs associated with the consumption of animal products, including starting and supporting educational campaigns, changing financial systems to incentivise activities that produce positive GHIs and discourage those that produce negative GHIs, and creating legal reform to introduce a qualified ban on the consumption of animal products. The phrase 'vegan project' refers to the ambition to contribute to global legal reform to introduce such a qualified ban. I have argued in this book that a total ban on the consumption of animal products cannot be justified, but that it is ethical to prohibit the consumption of animal products for the majority of human beings in most situations. Importantly, I argued that even governments who are not prepared to adopt the view that we have any duties towards other animals might still be justified in passing legal reform to create a qualified ban on the basis of a duty to give some recognition to a narrowly conceived notion of a human right to health care.

I refuted three objections against the vegan project in section 3.5, arguing that it is not pointless to focus on a qualified ban, that adopting a qualified ban need not necessarily undermine human food security, and that such a ban would not alienate us from nature. Both existing law and—as I argued in chapter four—the values that many people already adopt could be mobilised in support of the vegan project.

Throughout this book I have assumed that carefully chosen vegan diets can be healthy, in a narrow sense, by being nutritionally adequate and that there is no reason to think that the majority of the human population would experience great difficulties in adopting such diets. Without these assumptions, it would be difficult to argue that vegan diets ought to be the default diets for the majority of the human population, as I do not wish to advocate diets that compromise people's nutritional needs. Whereas our duty to strive for holistic health demands that due consideration be given to the moral duties argued for in this book, in the appendix to this book I shall adopt a much narrower health focus by exploring how vegan diets might affect the nutritional status of those who adopt them. The treatment of this important matter has been reserved for the appendix as it may not appeal to many readers who may be interested in the moral argument but who may prefer not to delve into a detailed assessment of the highly complex nutritional literature. Even those who do not accept that any duties that we may have towards others include a duty to adopt qualified moral veganism may still be persuaded to adopt vegan diets by the argument that I shall make in the appendix: people who adopt vegan diets may be healthier than many others, and many people who adopt vegan diets may not find it too difficult to ensure that they are well-nourished. Nevertheless, to avoid deficiencies, many vegans may need to pay particular attention to ensuring that they consume foods or supplements that contain adequate amounts of vitamins B12 and D, iodine, and omega-3 fatty acids. In addition, vegans with specific dietary needs must tend to these needs. Young and old people, for example, must eat sufficient foods that are relatively rich in calories and relatively easy to digest, such as cooked foods.

Whereas the appendix to this book does not undermine my enthusiasm for the vegan project, it does not remove the fact that our relationships with other animals can be very complex and that it may not always be easy for us to decide what is best for us to do. To use an example from another domain, I used to live in a house that I shared with my family as well as with mice for a number of years. We were not happy to share our living space with the mice, but neither were we happy to oust them from the place where they had chosen to live. We lived on the first floor and the second floor of the house, whereas the mice occupied the space between the two floors, as well as the loft. Both these spaces were inaccessible to us. Now and again, one mouse strayed, which resulted in their being trapped in a 'humane trap', but I was not so sure whether it really was humane for mice to be trapped in that way. This doubt was partly related to the problem of what to do with them afterwards. If we released them nearby, they might return, in which case they might again visit the places where we did not want them. If we released the mouse further away, we thought that there was a good chance not only that it would not be welcomed by the mouse in question, but also that it might cause significant pain and suffering and death to any offspring who might die whilst awaiting the return of their mother, for instance. We resisted trapping any mice other than those who strayed into unwanted territory, but we did pay a price for our reluctance. Occasionally, some died in places that could not be accessed by us, resulting in the stench of the decaying body filling the house for a duration of anywhere between two and six weeks. Sonic devices might have helped to deter mice from living inside our house, but we did not try this method, opting for a reasonably comfortable co-existence. However, in light of the fact that the efficacy of these sonic devices is questionable (Aflitto and DeGomez 2014), I can understand anyone who, in similar circumstances, would wish to trap mice—and I am not entirely convinced that 'humane' traps are better than lethal traps.

Many questions remain, yet I hope to have developed a theory on the duties that we may have in relation to the consumption of animal products that will also inspire people to question many other ways in which people engage with other animals. For now, I rest my case: yes, it might be kind to avoid eating animal products in many situations, as it really is kind to be kind to our kind.

Might a Vegan Diet Be Healthy, or Even Healthier?

1 Introduction

Most great apes consume a wide variety of plant foods (Nestle 1999, 214; Milton 1999). The Western lowland gorillas who live in the Central African Republic, for example, have been observed to eat over 200 different plants and more than 100 varieties of fruit (Popovich et al. 1997). Many of these plants foods are low in calories, so that the great apes must eat large quantities of them.

The human ape is an exception. With the emergence of *Homo erectus* about 1.8 million years ago, a transition took place towards diets that were nutritionally dense, which facilitated a significant expansion in brain size (Leonard 2014). Another factor that facilitated a further increase in brain size was the introduction of cooking about 250,000 years ago. When they started cooking, human beings benefited not only from easier mastication, but also from a greater digestibility of, and an increase in energy derived from, food (Carmody and Wrangham 2009). Whereas cooked foods did not only include animal products, it is thought that our gathering and hunting ancestors may have obtained more than half of their daily energy from animal foods (Cordain et al. 2000; Mann 2000). As animal foods provide more energy than plant foods per unit of weight, this fact need not contradict what Nestle (1999, 215) has claimed, namely that, up to when our ancestors started farming about 10,000 years ago, there is 'substantial support for the predominance of plant foods in hunter-gatherer groups living in areas where plants could grow'. Whereas no milk other than human milk may have been consumed before farming was introduced, there is sufficient evidence to support the view that hunter-gatherer societies consumed a greater proportion of animal foods than subsistence farming communities later did (Leonard 2014): without modern technology,

How to cite this book chapter:
Deckers, J 2016 *Animal (De)liberation: Should the Consumption of Animal Products Be Banned?* Pp. 167–190. London: Ubiquity Press. DOI: http://dx.doi.org/10.5334/bay.g. License: CC-BY 4.0

it was difficult for most sedentary populations to adopt dietary patterns that contained large quantities of animal foods.

Modern science and technology have allowed many populations to become more sedentary, to escalate the production of plant foods (through mechanical and chemical agriculture), to use newly acquired genetic knowledge to create modified feed crops and animal breeds in order to increase the quantity of animal products, and to develop intensive production systems of animal products (also known as factory farms or confined animal feeding operations—'CAFOs') as well as refrigeration and modern methods of transportation. Consequently, current diets of Western people in particular tend to include large quantities of animal products. These tend to be higher in total and saturated fats, as well as lower in mono-unsaturated and n-3 fats, than the animal products consumed by hunter-gatherer communities (Leonard 2014).

What we are currently witnessing is the globalisation of this typical Western diet through the influence of multinational corporations and of other market forces such as the acquisition of new capital by many populations, for example by many people living in China: until recently, many Chinese people could not afford to eat many animal products on a regular basis, and Chinese people were also much less exposed to the economic and political influences of large agricultural corporations that promote the consumption of such products. The recent increase in the consumption of these products in China was also facilitated by political shifts to a particular version of communism, followed by the rise of capitalist ideology, both of which undermined Buddhist questioning of such consumption. China's neighbouring country, India, has a long vegetarian tradition rooted in Hinduism and Buddhism, which emphasises the principle of ahimsa (non-violence) and a reverence for cows, in spite of the fact that some milk products have been consumed for a long time—incidentally, not without controversy, as the consumption of milk products was opposed by the Buddha's cousin, Devadatta (6th century BCE), and by those who followed his teachings (Simoons 1994, 6, 8). Like China, however, India is now moving rapidly away from its largely plant-based dietary tradition (Kasturirangan et al. 2014).

Even if their number is rising, it is nevertheless still the case that very few Western people adopt a vegan diet, and the number of people elsewhere who adopt dietary patterns that are totally or largely vegan is diminishing rapidly. There is no doubt that the moral case against veganism would be strengthened if it could be shown that vegan diets are unhealthy. Similarly, one might expect that the moral case in favour of such diets would be stronger if it could be shown that such diets are healthier than alternative diets. This is why I shall explore the healthiness of vegan diets in this appendix. Unlike in the main parts of this book, the concept of health is understood here in a narrow sense: the pivotal question that will be addressed is whether vegan diets are nutritionally adequate for those who adopt such diets, irrespective of their healthiness for others.

Before I embark on this task, it must be pointed out that any research into the nutritional value of vegan diets is hampered by several problems. One problem is the fact that many people who adopt these diets live in countries (for example India) where little attention has been paid to nutritional research, and few financial resources allocated to its funding. Another is that many people have traditionally adopted vegan diets out of necessity rather than out of choice. Up until recently for most, and even today for some, people ate what they ate because they lacked access to a diverse range of foods and, in many situations, found it harder to obtain animal products than to obtain other food. If many studied vegan populations adopt very restrictive diets because of pressing personal, social, or ecological constraints, it will be easy to find examples of deficient vegan diets, but much harder to find convincing evidence of the nutritional adequacy of such diets. The adoption of a very restrictive vegan diet may also be a symptom of a food disorder, for example anorexia. A further problem is the existence of a cultural bias against vegan diets (Sabaté 2003, 503S): as a result of this bias, dominant factions of societies that possess financial resources to study nutrition resist funding research that might undermine the status quo.

In spite of these obstacles, some research into the nutritional risks and benefits associated with vegan diets has taken place; I shall first engage with the question whether vegan diets could be healthy, and then move on to discussing the question whether well-planned vegan diets might actually be healthier than other diets.

2 Might vegan diets be healthy?

Many nutritionists claim that vegan diets can be healthy; the American Dietetic Association (ADA), for example, has argued that 'appropriately planned … vegan diets … are appropriate for individuals during all stages of the life cycle' (ADA 2009, 1266). To address this question in detail, however, it is necessary to focus on those dietary components that have frequently been suspected to be deficient in vegan diets. The components that deserve special scrutiny are: protein, calcium, vitamin B12, vitamin D, essential fatty acids, zinc, iodine, and iron.

Protein

Peas, lentils, and beans are good sources of protein that are readily available and relatively easy to grow in many parts of the world. It is important that vegans consume protein foods that contain the full range of essential amino acids overall; although there is no need for the full range of essential amino acids to be part of every meal (ADA 2009, 1268; McEvoy and Woodside 2010, 87), it is clear that we do need all essential amino acids to be healthy, which is why diets that rely on a very limited range of protein sources must be avoided. Although concern has been expressed over some populations that rely heavily on staples with limited quantities of protein, such as taro, cassava, and yams,

Millward (1999, 259) has argued that 'cereal-based diets, especially those based on wheat and maize, supply protein levels considerably above the requirement level'. However, there is no evidence to suggest that those who consume relatively small quantities of cereals are likely to have deficiencies, provided that they consume other foods that contain significant quantities of protein. Overall, there is no evidence to suggest that vegans who eat a good range of plant foods are likely to lack in protein (Messina et al. 2004).

Calcium

Fruits and vegetables that contain relatively large amounts of potassium and magnesium decrease bone calcium resorption, whereas diets that include relatively large amounts of nuts and grains increase such resorption by producing a high renal acid load, mainly caused by residues of sulfates and phosphates (ADA 2009, 1269). Green leafy vegetables that are low in oxalate, including broccoli, kale, spring greens, and cabbage, tend to be high in calcium, as well as in vitamin K, another important contributor to bone health (Messina and Mangels 2001, 663). The study of the Oxford-cohort of the European Prospective Investigation into Cancer and Nutrition (the 'Oxford-EPIC cohort') found that adult vegans who consume more than 525 mg of calcium per day do not show higher fracture rates than omnivores (P. Appleby et al. 2007). There is no evidence that well-planned vegan diets fail to provide sufficient calcium, but there is evidence that diets that include adequate amounts of calcium and vitamin D are protective of bone health (Tang et al. 2007).

Vitamin B12

No plant foods are known to produce vitamin B12, or cobalamin, but those who eat plants inadvertently eat B12 as this vitamin is produced by micro-organisms (particularly *Pseudomonas denitrificans* and *Propionibacterium shermanii*) who live in symbiosis with many plants. The presence of vitamin B12 is essential for cell growth, and crucial for a healthy nervous system. Vitamin B12 deficiency leads to elevated plasma homocysteine (Hcy) concentrations (hyperhomocysteinaemia), a risk factor for neurological disorders and cardio-vascular problems, including pernicious anaemia and haematological disease (megaloblastic anaemia with demyelination of the central nervous system) (McEvoy and Woodside 2010, 90; Waldmann et al. 2005). Whereas our intestinal bacteria can synthesise B12, it is generally assumed that we should also consume products containing B12 (Li 2011).

Some studies have found that some vegans had inadequate intakes of B12, where particular concerns have been raised over the B12 status of older people due to their limited absorption capacity and of pregnant women due to their higher demands (Majchrzak et al. 2006; Waldmann et al. 2005; Donaldson 2000; ADA 2009; Piccoli et al. 2015). This is not a reason to eat flesh, as B12 binds with the protein in animal foods, impeding absorption, which is precisely why older people are better off with vegan sources of B12 (Norris and Messina 2011, 31). Since the haematological symptoms of vitamin B12 deficiency may go undetected for a long time due to a high consumption of foods containing folate (folic acid), of which many vegans consume rather a lot through the consumption of things like oranges, green leafy vegetables, and beans, vegans must be very careful to ensure that their consumption of B12 is sufficient (ADA 2009, 1269). Many products, including cereals and yeast extracts, now exist that have been fortified with B12 produced through industrial fermentation of bacteria. In his assessment of the evidence, Sanders (1999, 267) has written that, provided that 'these foods are consumed regularly, the hazard of vitamin B12 deficiency is easily avoided'.

Norris and Messina (2011, 32) usefully point out that the human body only absorbs a tiny amount of B12 every time the vitamin is consumed, which is why they recommend the adoption of any one of these strategies for optimal consumption: 1/ two daily servings of fortified foods, providing 1.5 to 2.5 micrograms each; 2/ one daily supplement of at least 25 micrograms; 3/ one supplement of 1,000 micrograms twice weekly.

Vitamin D

Inadequate levels of vitamin D have long been known to contribute to bone problems such as rickets, but more recently have also been found to contribute to a range of other conditions, including fibromyalgia, rheumatoid arthritis, multiple sclerosis, depression, cancer, hypertension, and diabetes (Norris and Messina 2011, 47). Adequate exposure to sunlight can provide the body with all the vitamin D it needs, but overexposure must be avoided as ultraviolet irradiation is a significant contributor to skin cancer. Those people who are not regularly exposed to sunlight, as well as those whose bodies are limited in the uptake of vitamin D, such as older and dark skinned people, must therefore consume products that have been fortified with vitamin D or take supplements (Craig 2009, 1629S; Stacey et al. 2005, 1444; Holick 2007). Vitamin D3 (cholecalciferol), used as a supplement, is usually derived from lanolin (sheep's wool) or fish oil, and is also found in some lichen and extracted from them by some companies, but the consumption of vitamin D2 (ergocalciferol)—produced from the ultraviolet irradiation of ergosterol from yeast—has been shown to be as effective in providing the human body with vitamin D (Holick et al. 2008).

Plasma 25-hydroxyvitamin D concentrations were measured in 2,107 participants of the Oxford-EPIC cohort, showing that vegans had lower concentrations of vitamin D, particularly during the winter months (Crowe et al. 2010). Whereas most participants in this study had concentrations that were deemed to be adequate, it is nevertheless very important to recognise that many people who live far away from the equator and who do not expose themselves frequently to sunlight (because of spending much time indoors and clothing) fail to meet recommended levels. This may be why Craig (2009, 1630S) has expressed the view that a daily supplement of 5–10 micrograms of vitamin D would be 'highly desirable for elderly vegans'; however, some recent studies suggest that a higher dosage may be required to maintain optimal blood levels, which is why Norris and Messina (2011, 47) recommend 25 micrograms or 1,000 International Units (IUs) daily for people who do not benefit from adequate sun exposure.

Essential fatty acids

Omega-3 (or n-3) and omega-6 (or n-6) fatty acids are widely regarded to be beneficial for human health. The two most important ones of these are two short-chain polyunsaturated fatty acids: α-linolenic acid (ALA), which the body can use to create other fats within the n-3 fatty acid family, and linoleic acid (LA), which the body can use to create other fats within the n-6 fatty acid family. These two fatty acids are called 'essential' because they cannot be synthesised by the human body, but are required for healthy functioning. They must therefore be supplied by our diets. Enzymes in our bodies convert these short-chain fatty acids to long-chain n-3 and n-6 polyunsaturated fatty acids. ALA is converted (incidentally, not only by humans, but also by many other animals, including fish) to eicosapentaenoic acid (EPA), docosahexaenoic acid (DHA) and docosapentaenoic acid, with stearidonic acid (SDA) as an intermediate in the pathway; LA is converted to arachidonic acid (Saunders et al. 2012a).

The palaeolithic diets that were adopted by hunter-gatherers are estimated to have had an n-6:n-3 ratio of 1:1 to 2:1. Many people who live today, by contrast, overconsume LA (C. Williams and Burge 2006). The n-6:n-3 ratio of typical Western diets has been estimated to be around 15:1 to 17:1 (O'Neill 2010, 200). This is a serious problem, as overconsumption of LA impairs ALA conversion. Many people also underconsume ALA, which may cause deficiencies in the particularly important EPA and DHA (B. Davis and Kris-Etherton 2003). High intakes of trans-fatty acids, alcohol, and caffeine, as well as imbalanced diets and illness in general, may produce the same deficiencies in EPA and DHA. Such deficiencies are believed to cause cardio-vascular disease and cancer, as well as exacerbated pain associated with a range of conditions (Simopoulos 2002; von Schacky 2009; Christophersen and Haug 2011). They may also cause cognitive decline, age-related macular degeneration, and depression (Saunders et al. 2012a, 24S).

A clear message emerges from this. Vegans must make sure to consume adequate amounts of ALA, and avoid high consumption of products that inhibit the conversion of ALA, including products that contain relatively large quantities of LA. Accordingly, a recent study recommends that at least one unit of n-3 be consumed for every four units of n-6 (Saunders et al. 2012a, 24S). The authors of the study also recommend an ALA intake of 2.6 g/day for men and 1.6 g/day for women, whilst recommending the following daily intakes for infants and children: 0.5 g at 0–6 months; 0.5 g at 7–12 months; 1 g for children aged 1–3; 1.6 g for children aged 4–8; 2 g for boys aged 9–13; 2.4 g for boys aged 14–18; and 1.6 g for girls aged 9–18 (Saunders et al. 2012a, 24S). The main reason for the gender differences relates to the fact that males tend to convert ALA less efficiently (Childs et al. 2008).

Plant foods that are high in omega-3 fatty acids include chia, flax, canola (rapeseed), hemp, walnuts, perilla, and olive oil (Saunders et al. 2012a; O'Neill 2010, 201). Blackcurrant seed oil, derived from the seeds of *Ribes nigrum*, is rich not only in omega-3 fatty acids, but also in SDA, and the same applies to oil derived from plants belonging to the *Echium* genus, a collection of species within the *Boraginaceae* family (Li 2011). Genetically engineered soybeans that contain SDA have also been recommended (Saunders et al. 2012a), but their inclusion within a diet would depend on their acceptability, a debate that I touched upon briefly in section 2.11 and that I shall not engage with any further here. To ensure adequate consumption of ALA, Norris and Messina (2011, 89) recommend that adults consume three to four daily servings from this list: '1 teaspoon canola oil, 1/4 teaspoon flaxseed oil, 2/3 teaspoon hempseed oil, 1 teaspoon walnut oil, 2 teaspoons ground English walnuts or 2 walnut halves, 1 teaspoon ground flaxseeds, 1/2 cup cooked soybeans, 1 cup firm tofu, 1 cup tempeh, 2 tablespoons soynuts'.

People with increased needs (for example pregnant and lactating women) and people with compromised conversion rates (for example people with diabetes or hypertension, and older people) may also benefit from consuming limited amounts of DHA- and—where available—EPA-fortified foods and DHA-supplements derived from microalgae (which can retro-convert to EPA inside the human body), as well as from consuming brown algae (kelp) oils (Saunders et al. 2012a; ADA 2009, 1268, 1271; Craig 2009, 1629S; Geppert et al. 2005). Norris and Messina (2011, 58, 55) write that vegans over the age of 60 'should consider' a daily DHA (or a combination of DHA and EPA) supplement of 200 to 300 milligrams, a supplement dose that they are also 'inclined to recommend' at a frequency of every two to three days for those who are younger.

Although it may be unlikely to happen, overconsumption of DHA-rich products must be avoided, as this may raise total and low density lipoprotein (LDL) cholesterol, cause prolonged bleeding, and reduce immunity (Craig 2009, 1629S; Geppert et al. 2005; Sanders et al. 2006).

Zinc (Zn)

Provided that it is present in the soil, many plant foods contain zinc. Plants that tend to be high in zinc are cereals and legumes. Unrefined whole grains provide higher concentrations than refined grains, as zinc can be found particularly within the outer layer of grains (Saunders et al. 2012b, 17S). Various ways to increase zinc uptake have been described, including soaking and sprouting beans, seeds, and grains, as well as leavening bread and consuming foods that contain citric acids (Lönnerdal 2000). Zinc absorption can be reduced by phytates (phytic acids), protein, and insoluble fibre, as well as by some minerals, including iron, calcium, and potassium (Li 2011). Whereas whole grains are higher in phytates than refined grains, the relative greater effect of phytates in the former is more than compensated for by the fact that whole grains are higher in zinc (Messina and Mangels 2001, 664). A study that compared 25 vegans with 20 omnivores found that the inhibitory effect of phytate failed to compromise zinc status as the bodies of people who take in little zinc appear to be able to increase zinc absorption and retention (Haddad et al. 1999).

As an aside, whereas it is good to be mindful that potassium may inhibit the absorption of zinc, it is nevertheless important to secure a sufficient intake of potassium as well. The following are listed as good sources of potassium by Norris and Messina (2011, 76): beet greens, spinach, Swiss chard, cooked tomatoes and tomato juice, bananas, sea vegetables, orange juice, and legumes.

Iodine

Iodine deficiency affects more than two billion people. It is the leading cause of preventable mental retardation worldwide. Foetuses and breastfed children are particularly vulnerable as they depend on maternal iodine intake for thyroid hormone synthesis, which is essential for human neurological development. Thyroid iodine uptake is inhibited by perchlorate—an ubiquitous environmental contaminant—cigarette smoke, cruciferous vegetables (of the family *Brassicaceae*), and seaweeds of the genus *Laminaria* (including kombu) (Leung et al. 2011, e1304; Lightowler 2009, 433–434); there is also concern over the inhibitory effects of particular isoflavones found in soya and flaxseed. Both the underconsumption and the overconsumption of iodine can cause goitre (an enlargement of the thyroid gland) and hypothyroidism, but the latter can also cause hyperthyroidism (Norris and Messina 2011, 70–71). A small American study found, however, that in spite of the fact that a cohort of Boston-area vegans had relatively low urinary iodine levels, these low levels were not associated with thyroid dysfunction (Leung et al. 2011).

Provided that they have access to adequate nutrition, vegans should not suffer from iodine deficiencies. Iodine can be provided through plants grown on iodine-rich soil, the consumption of seaweed, and the consumption of iodised salt. As levels of iodine in seaweed vary considerably and are therefore unreliable, and as the overconsumption of salt must be avoided, Norris and Messina (2011, 72, 89) recommend the use of supplements as their favourite strategy, where their recommendation for adults is that they take supplements of 75 to

150 micrograms three to four days per week in order to meet a recommended daily allowance of 150 micrograms, whereas lower levels of 90 micrograms daily are recommended for very small children and higher levels of up to 290 micrograms daily for lactating women. They also recommend one quarter of a teaspoon of iodised salt per day as an alternative to supplementation. The development of a global strategy to ensure routine, adequate iodisation of foods which are commonly used that guards at the same time against excess intake of iodine, which negatively affects the thyroid gland (Lightowler 2009, 431), would seem to be appropriate in view of the scale of the problem of iodine deficiency. Some localities have already developed guidelines; in the USA, for example, vegan pregnant and lactating women have been recommended to supplement their diets with 150 micrograms of iodine daily (Leung et al. 2011, e1303).

Iron

Foods contain iron in two forms: haem iron and non-haem iron. Vegan foods only contain the latter, which is less easily absorbed by the body. Whereas iron deficiency can be a problem for vegans, it is more likely to be a problem for omnivores who consume large quantities of milk than for diet-conscious vegans. Good vegan sources of iron are dried fruit, sea vegetables, leafy green vegetables, and beans (Norris and Messina 2011, 64, 70). Vegans who consume a good range of fruit and vegetables in addition to foods that contain relatively large amounts of iron are unlikely to be affected by a deficiency as many fruits and vegetables contain large quantities of vitamin C, as well as other organic acids, which enhances iron absorption. Retinol, carotenes, and alcohol have also been reported to increase iron absorption, whereas inhibitors include oxalates, phytates, and calcium, as well as the polyphenolics that are present in tea, some herbal 'teas', coffee, and cocoa (Ma et al. 2005; Siener et al. 2006; Hallberg and Rossander 1982; Li 2011; McEvoy and Woodside 2010, 88; ADA 2009, 1268). It is for this reason that Norris and Messina (2011, 70) recommend that people who drink tea and coffee only do so between meals rather than with their meals. As low iron status is moderately common in premenopausal women, these women need to make sure that their diets include good sources of iron, together with vitamin C to aid absorption (Key et al. 2006, 37). At the same time, there is evidence of the human body's ability to adapt to low iron intake by increasing absorption and decreasing losses (Hunt and Roughead 1999; Hunt and Roughead 2000).

Taking stock

The account presented above shows that vegan diets can fulfil all the nutritional requirements that are needed to support good health. Nutrients that present particular concerns are vitamin B12 and omega-3 fatty acids as few vegan foods that are currently used for human consumption contain these. Accordingly, vegans must make sure that they consume adequate portions of such foods. A nutrient that I have not mentioned, but that may be a concern, is selenium (Norris and Messina 2011, 76): as the selenium content of soil varies across the world, vegans must ensure that they do not restrict their diets to foods that are grown on soils that have low selenium levels. All in all, vegan diets can be adequate for all human beings, including children. Although small children with reduced stomach capacities may need to eat regularly and must ensure that they eat foods that are sufficiently high in energy density to provide sufficient calories, that are relatively easy to digest (for example by including cooked rather than raw foods), and that are not excessive in fibre (Messina and Mangels 2001, 662), many nutritionists adopt the view that vegan diets can be adequate for all human beings (Messina and Mangels 2001; Norris and Messina 2011; Van Winckel et al. 2011; ADA 1997).

3 Might vegan diets be healthier than other diets?

The claim has also been made that well-planned vegan diets may be healthier than other diets (Norris and Messina 2011, xv; B. Davis and Melina 2014, 29). It is this claim that I shall explore in the remainder of this appendix. One way in which this claim could be examined is by focusing on mortality differences between vegans and others. The problem, however, is that no studies exist of populations where omnivores share similar genetic profiles, similar lifestyle patterns, and similar social and environmental factors with a significant number of vegans. Nevertheless, a meta-analysis of seven prospective cohort studies—that is, studies which compare, usually over a long time, those who remain healthy with those who become ill—from the UK, Germany, California, the USA, the Netherlands, and Japan, including 124,706 participants, compared vegetarians with omnivores and found that all-cause mortality was 9% lower amongst vegetarians (T. Huang et al. 2012).

Whereas the fact that vegetarians benefit from increased longevity does not imply that this would also be the case for vegans, there is evidence that people who consume large quantities of fruits and vegetables—foods that tend to be more prominent in vegan diets—live longer than those who do not do so. Some evidence for this is provided by a Finnish study of 2,641 men who were aged between 42 and 60 and whose diets were assessed by four-day food intake records between 1984 and 1989. With a mean follow-up time of nearly 13 years, the study found that, after adjustment for major risk factors for cardio-vascular disease, those within the highest fifth for intake of fruits (including berries) and vegetables had a relative risk for all-cause death that was 34% lower than that of those in the lowest fifth (Rissanen et al. 2003). Several other studies found a positive association between diets that are relatively high in the consumption of fruits and vegetables, such as the traditional Mediterranean diet of people who lived in Pioppi (Italy) up to about four decades ago, and a reduction in mortality (Keys 1995; Benzie and Wachtel-Galor 2010). As diets that include a large proportion of fruits and vegetables have been shown to be healthier than diets that include relatively few of these foods, it has been estimated that a large number of premature deaths could be prevented amongst populations that consume large quantities of animal products by increasing the consumption of plant foods (Scarborough et al. 2012a).

In the remainder of this appendix I shall focus on studies that provide evidence for a difference between vegan and other diets in relation to the morbidity factors of obesity, bone health, cardio-vascular disease, diabetes, cancer, diverticular disease, Parkinson's disease, and insulin-like growth factor 1 (IGF-1) and mTORC1 related diseases.

Obesity

Several studies have shown that vegan diets are associated with a reduced incidence of obesity as they tend to include fewer trans-fats (which are found mainly in processed foods with partially hydrogenated fats), fewer saturated fats (which can also be found in fully hydrogenated vegetable oils), and more dietary fibre (Rizzo et al. 2013; ADA 2009, 1274; McEvoy and Woodside 2010, 84; Spencer et al. 2003; Davey et al. 2003; Haddad et al. 1999). Obesity is a known risk factor for a wide range of health conditions, including cardio-vascular disease, type 2 diabetes, some cancers, and dyslipidaemia (WCRF/AICR 2007, 374–376). In addition, HIV patients may avoid or reduce lipodystrophy problems by adopting vegan diets (McCarty 2003b). In recent years, many companies in the dairy industry have responded to the challenges associated with rising rates of obesity by producing and promoting low fat alternatives. In spite of the reduction in fat, these products still contain large amounts of calories that are turned into fatty tissues if they are surplus to human energy requirements, thus contributing to increases in weight (Lanou 2009).

Bone health

The Oxford-EPIC study found that UK vegans had a 30% increase in fractures compared to other dietary groups in the UK and that 45% of the vegan group consumed less than 525 mg of calcium per day, compared to only 6% in the other dietary groups (P. Appleby et al. 2007). When vegans whose consumption averaged more than 525 mg of calcium per day were compared with other groups, however, fracture rates in this specific vegan group were about the same as those in the other groups.

Cows' milk is frequently recommended for bone health. However, in a study of 72,337 postmenopausal women that followed up participants for hip fractures for 18 years, it was found that neither a high calcium diet nor cows' milk consumption was associated with a reduced risk of hip fracture (Feskanich et al. 2003). An earlier, retrospective study found that hip fractures are higher in countries with high protein consumption from animal products (Abelow et al. 1992).

This finding tempted Lanou (2009, 1639S) to speculate that high consumption of animal products may undermine bone health. For three reasons, it is hard to conclude this from the Abelow et al. (1992) study. Firstly, the study estimated protein consumption for whole populations, rather than for the study groups; estimated intakes of animal protein may therefore differ greatly from what those who suffered hip fractures actually consumed. Secondly, the interpretation ignores that many countries where relatively large quantities of animal products are consumed tend to have high life expectancies (Kannus et al. 1996); the fact that rates of hip fractures are higher in countries where lots of animal products are consumed may therefore simply be explained by the fact that life expectancies are higher within those countries. Thirdly, the possibility that cultures that rely heavily on animal products may have different lifestyle factors that contribute to fracture risks should not be ignored (Calvez et al. 2012).

In spite of these reservations, limited evidence in support of Lanou (2009)'s hypothesis comes from a more recent, prospective study, which is interesting as it makes a direct comparison between fracture rates and bone mineral density loss in vegans and omnivores. The study, which took place in Ho Chi Minh City (formerly Saigon), compared the rate of femoral neck bone mineral density loss and morphometric vertebral fractures of 88 vegan and 91 omnivorous women over the age of 50 two years after baseline measurement. Groups were matched at baseline, but the vegans had significantly lower dietary intakes of calcium and vitamin D, as well as of total protein and fats. In spite of their lower consumption of calcium and vitamin D, this study found that there was no difference in fracture rates between vegans and omnivores, but that 'higher intakes of animal protein and lipid' (fat) were associated with greater bone loss (Ho-Pham et al. 2012, 75), a finding that the authors relate to earlier research that attributes a causal role in bone loss to the presence of high levels of acid in animal protein (Barzel and Massey 1998). Given the small number of participants that were involved and the specific genetic, cultural, and environmental context, it is not possible, however, to conclude that vegans are more likely to have healthier bones that are less prone to fractures than omnivores.

Further research has also revealed that high consumption of protein may be a risk factor for fractures not *per se*, but only when it is combined with low consumption of calcium (Burckhardt 2013). On the other hand, through increased consumption of fruits and vegetables, vegans tend to have a lower renal acid load, which reduces urinary calcium excretion and bone resorption (New 2003). In this respect, high consumption of vegetables and fruits with high potassium, magnesium, and vitamin K contents may be particularly desirable

(Calvez et al. 2012; Tucker et al. 2001; Booth et al. 2000; Feskanich et al. 1999). A further reason why vegans may be protected relates to the fact that vegans do not consume preformed vitamin A, which is known to cause a reduction in bone mineral density if it is consumed in large amounts (Burckhardt 2015).

Whereas bone health is not necessarily undermined by low calcium intakes, it must be emphasised that calcium is the main mineral in human bones. Adequate consumption of calcium is one factor that contributes to good bone health, even if it does not guarantee it as the rate at which calcium is absorbed is determined largely by other dietary factors. One of these factors is vitamin D status, the importance of which was highlighted earlier. Another is adequate protein consumption. The importance of the latter is borne out by a study of 1,865 women from Canada and the USA who were followed up over 25 years, where, of the 40% who adopted a vegetarian diet, those with the highest protein consumption had the lowest risk of wrist fractures (Thorpe et al. 2008).

Cardio-vascular disease

Cardio-vascular diseases are the most common causes of mortality. Most cardio-vascular diseases result from venous or arterial blockages (thrombosis). These occur by a rupture of atherosclerotic plaque and result in tissue damage from blood starvation. Cerebrovascular and ischaemic heart diseases are the two most common types of cardio-vascular disease.

A meta-analysis that included 124,706 participants recruited for seven prospective cohort studies that compared vegetarians with omnivores in the UK, Germany, California, the USA, the Netherlands, and Japan found that vegetarians had a 29% lower mortality risk for ischaemic heart disease (T. Huang et al. 2012). This is in line with findings from a meta-analysis of five prospective studies that compared data for 76,172 people from Germany, the UK, and the USA, which found that the mortality rate from ischaemic heart disease was 24% lower in vegetarians than in non-vegetarians after a mean follow-up of just over ten years and a half (Key et al. 1999). Although the death rate for ischaemic heart disease was slightly higher for the vegans than for the vegetarians in this latter meta-analysis, the risk ratio for death from cerebrovascular disease for vegans was only about half that for those who ate animals' flesh at least once a week.

Two large, and ongoing, cohort studies in particular have been widely reported with regard to diet-associated cardio-vascular disease risk. The first is the Oxford-EPIC study; the second a study ('the AHS-2 study') from the USA and Canada with a cohort of 73,308 Seventh-day Adventists who were recruited at churches between 2002 and 2007 and followed up over more than five years (Orlich et al. 2013).

The Oxford-EPIC study has documented that self-reported hypertension was lowest amongst vegans, whilst a study of blood pressure in a sub-cohort of

8,663 participants who reported not to suffer from hypertension found that the 612 vegans in that sub-cohort showed lower systolic and diastolic blood pressures than people in any other dietary category in that sub-cohort, which could only partly be attributed to differences in body mass, i.e. the fact that the vegans tended to be leaner (P. Appleby et al. 2002). In 2013, the authors of the study reported that a vegetarian group (which included vegans), which comprised 34% of a total sub-cohort of 44,561 people living in England and Scotland, had a 32% lower risk of ischaemic heart disease after a follow-up of just over 11 years than the omnivores in the same sub-cohort when adjustment for all confounding factors apart from body mass index (BMI) was performed, and a 28% lower risk when BMI was factored in (Crowe et al. 2013).

Similar findings are reported in the AHS-2 study (Orlich et al. 2013). Compared to the group of omnivores, deaths from ischaemic heart disease and cardio-vascular disease were, respectively, 10% and 9% lower amongst the group of 3,533 'vegan'—defined here as those who reported to consume animal products less than once a month—women, whereas the group of 2,015 'vegan' men experienced risk reductions of, respectively, 55% and 42%. For a sub-group of this cohort, comprising 500 white subjects, it was found that the group of 49 'vegans' had a 63% lower risk of suffering from hypertension (where someone suffering from hypertension was defined as someone who either took medication for it or someone who had a systolic blood pressure exceeding 139 mmHg or a diastolic blood pressure exceeding 89 mmHg), which was only partly accounted for by differences in body mass (where 'vegans' tended to be leaner) (Pettersen et al. 2012).

Whereas the Oxford-EPIC and the AHS-2 studies concern Western populations, similar results were obtained in a Chinese study, where healthy men who consumed no animal products other than milk were found to have lower risks of cardio-vascular disease than omnivorous men (Yang et al. 2012).

Why is it that vegans may be less prone to cardio-vascular disease than omnivores? Both obesity and hypertension may play a role in this difference, as both high BMI and high blood pressure have been associated with elevated risk. Another reason relates to levels of cholesterol. Low density lipoprotein (LDL) and high density lipoprotein (HDL) are the main cholesterol components that are found in our blood; a low level of the former and a high level of the latter are generally thought to benefit cardio-vascular health. LDL can oxidise, promoting plaque formation and hardening of the arteries, but this can be undermined by high levels of HDL. Vegan diets may protect against cardio-vascular disease because they do not contain animal products, which tend to be relatively high in substances that elevate LDL cholesterol, including total and saturated fat (Fung et al. 2010; Bernstein et al. 2010; Norouzy et al. 2011). Vegan diets are also generally higher in fibre, which has been found to reduce LDL cholesterol (Jenkins et al. 2001). In relation to this, research has found that the consumption of whole grains, which—unlike refined grains—include the bran, germ, and endosperm, and are relatively rich in fibre, reduces cardio-vascular risk factors (Liu et al. 1999; Park et al. 2011). Vegan diets also tend to be relatively low in bio-available phosphate, where high phosphate levels are associated with increased risk (McCarty 2003a). Vegans must be careful, however, to avoid overconsumption of refined carbohydrates (as for example white-flour products, white rice, and sugar), as this reduces HDL, which removes excess LDL cholesterol from the bloodstream (O'Neill 2010, 202–203). As mentioned before, they must also be careful to maintain adequate levels of vitamins B12 and D, as well as a good balance of n-6 over n-3 fatty acids, as deficiencies in these domains have been associated with elevated risks of cardio-vascular disease (Li 2011; Woo et al. 2014; Bouillon and Verlinden 2014).

Vegans may benefit not only from lower LDL levels, but also from the fact that they tend to remove detrimental components ('atherogenic remnants') more quickly from the blood (Vinagre et al. 2013). In addition, several studies have associated reduced risks of cardio-vascular disease with high intakes of fruits, vegetables, and nuts (Finks et al. 2012; Takachi et al. 2008; He et al. 2006; Mozaffarian et al. 2011; Hu 2003; Jenkins et al. 1997; Sacks et al. 1999). This stems at least in part from the fact that diets that are high in nuts and in plant sterols are known to reduce total and LDL cholesterol levels (Katan et al. 2003; Mukuddem-Petersen et al. 2005; Sabaté et al. 2010).

Diabetes

Although some studies have linked the development of type 1 diabetes to the consumption of dairy products (Dahl-Jørgensen et al. 1991; Banwell et al. 2008), a meta-analysis of studies pointed out that no causal link has been established (Agostoni and Turck 2011). However, a more recent study suggests that consumption of cows' milk very early in life may trigger type 1 diabetes if it is accompanied by exposure to enterovirus infections in early life (Lempainen et al. 2012).

More evidence exists on the positive benefits of vegan diets for the prevention and treatment of type 2 diabetes, as well as of the associated cardio-vascular diseases (Kahleova and Pelikanova 2015; Tonstad et al. 2009; Marsh and Brand-Miller 2011; Salas-Salvadó et al. 2011). As weight is a major risk factor for the development of this condition, vegans are less likely to develop type 2 diabetes because of their lower weight (Fung et al. 2004; Trapp and Levin 2012). However, several studies show that there are other factors why vegan diets may prevent type 2 diabetes, such as the fact that no red and processed flesh is consumed, and that more whole grain foods and nuts may be consumed, all of which factors have been associated with reduced diabetes risk (Pan et al. 2011; Marsh 2011).

Vegan diets have also been shown to help in the treatment of type 2 diabetes by lowering total and LDL cholesterol and by controlling lipid levels, for example by reducing triglycerides, a type of fat that is also associated with a greater risk of heart disease (Jenkins et al. 2006; Barnard et al. 2006; Barnard et al. 2009, 1594S; Tonstad et al. 2009; Vinagre et al. 2013). Many vegan diets have a low glycaemic index (GI) and a fairly low glycaemic load. The GI is a measure of the effect of carbohydrate-containing foods on blood glucose response (i.e. how quickly the body converts carbohydrates into energy) after their consumption (Jenkins et al. 1981), and the glycaemic load is the product of the amount of foods consumed and their glycaemic index (Finks et al. 2012, e70). People who consume large quantities of foods that have a high GI are thought to be at increased risk not only of diabetes and cardio-vascular disease, but also of a number of conditions—sometimes grouped under the label of 'metabolic syndrome'—including obesity, hypertriglyceridemia, and low HDL cholesterol (Finley et al. 2010; Ludwig 2002; Finks et al. 2012). It has also been found that obesity reduces tolerance of diets with high glycaemic load (Liu et al. 2000). In relation to diabetes, diets with high GI values are associated with greater insulin resistance and a greater incidence of hypoglycaemia amongst those who are treated with insulin (Willett et al. 2002; Ebbeling et al. 2007).

In a randomised controlled trial of a duration of five months, whereby 99 people with diabetes were divided into a group of 49 who were asked to follow a vegan diet and a group of 50 who were asked to follow a diet recommended by the American Diabetes Association, the overall GI of the vegan group's diet was significantly lower than that of the other group's diet (Turner-McGrievy et al. 2011). The associated reduction in body weight, together with the reduced fat content (and the associated reduction in intramyocellular lipid—a contributor to insulin resistance) and increased fibre content of the vegan diet, was thought to result in better glycaemic control (Turner-McGrievy et al. 2011, 1472). The vegan group also managed to reduce their medication significantly more than those who belonged to the other group, a significant finding in light of the fact that some hypoglycaemic drugs contribute to weight gain (Barnard et al. 2006; Barnard et al. 2009). All this does not imply that one's dietary glycaemic index is necessarily lowered by the adoption of a vegan diet, as Norris and Messina (2011, 185) rightly point out that 'the key is to choose carbohydrate-rich foods with low GIs, which means eating more unprocessed, whole plant foods in place of refined carbohydrates'.

Cancer

It is highly probable that many vegan diets are less likely to cause cancer than other diets are. The Oxford Vegetarian Study and the Oxford-EPIC study provide evidence for this claim (Key et al. 2009a). The former study recruited 11,140 vegetarian and non-vegetarian participants throughout the United Kingdom between 1980 and 1984. The latter study recruited a much larger number of participants between 1993 and 1999, and is part of a much larger, multicentre, prospective study with 519,978 subjects overall, carried out in

23 centres from 10 European countries (Denmark, France, Germany, Greece, Italy, the Netherlands, Norway, Spain, Sweden, and the United Kingdom). Data from the Oxford Vegetarian Study and the Oxford-EPIC study were combined, resulting in a cohort of 61,566 people (15,571 men and 45,995 women) who were followed up to 2007; participants were separated into three dietary groups on the basis of their answers to four questions, collected by means of an intake questionnaire: 32,403 omnivores, 8,562 fish eaters (who did not eat any other animals' flesh), and 20,601 vegetarians (Key et al. 2009a).

Before looking at the evidence of this combined study, it must be recognised that this study is not free from methodological concerns. Since it is a longitudinal study, it is quite possible that dietary patterns varied significantly over the large number of years that participants were followed up. A second problem is that actual diets may differ from reported diets. From a personal lunch-time conversation with a participant in the EPIC study, I found out, for example, that he had chosen the vegetarian group, whereas he actually ate fish. A third problem is that the more subtle distinctions between the kinds of foods that people eat are ignored by the fact that the questionnaire only aimed to distinguish between three dietary categories, omitting a vegan diet category. A fourth problem is that participants appeared to be particularly health conscious whichever diet they adopted, as death rates were significantly lower (at 52% of the general population's death rates in the Oxford-EPIC study) than that in the general British population (Key et al. 2009b). These problems impair the ability to generalise results from this study group to other people.

In spite of these difficulties, it is significant that the study found that the overall cancer incidence amongst vegetarians was about 12% lower than the incidence amongst omnivores (Key et al. 2009a), which is in line with the 18% reduction that was found in a recent meta-analysis of seven prospective cohort studies that compared vegetarians with omnivores in the UK, Germany, California, the USA, the Netherlands, and Japan (T. Huang et al. 2012). The combined Oxford study found lower incidences in the vegetarian group for ovarian and bladder cancers, as well as for cancers of the lymphatic and haematopoietic tissues and for stomach cancers (of which there were only 49 cases), but the risk of cervical cancer—of which there were only 50 cases—was more than twice as high in the vegetarian group than in the group of omnivores. The authors speculate that this higher observed incidence of cervical cancer might be related to non-dietary factors, for example differences between groups in attendance for cervical cancer screening. They did not find a significant difference between dietary groups in relation to the incidence of colorectal cancer, which contrasts with a study that aggregated EPIC data from 10 European countries, which found that high consumption of red and processed flesh was associated with a higher risk of colorectal cancer (Gonzalez and Riboli 2006, 229). Similarly, an expert systematic review in the USA deemed that the evidence of the increased risk for colorectal cancer associated with consuming red and processed flesh was convincing (WCRF/AICR 2007, 116, 382). The same review judged that there was limited evidence for a positive association between the consumption of red and/or processed flesh and increased risks of cancers of the oesophagus, stomach, pancreas, lung, endometrium, and prostate (WCRF/AICR 2007, 116). Another expert review adds breast, bladder, and oral cancer (Anand et al. 2008).

The link between the consumption of animal products and cancer has also been studied by Ganmaa and Sato (2005), who correlated the incidence rates for breast, ovarian, and corpus uteri cancers (using data detailing cancer incidence between 1993 and 1997) with food intake in 40 countries—even if food consumption was merely estimated by means of 1961–97 FAOSTAT data. They found a positive link between the consumption of animal products and these hormone-dependent cancers, a finding that is corroborated by other studies (Larsson et al. 2006). Ganmaa and Sato (2005) express particular concern with the consumption of milk from pregnant cows. As many cows in the dairy industry are almost continuously pregnant, their milk expresses high levels of oestrogen and progesterone (hormones which are known to stimulate the mammary gland), which are hypothesised to increase the risks associated with these cancers (Ganmaa and Sato 2005).

In many situations, men may not benefit from the consumption of dairy products either. A World Cancer Research Fund (WCRF) and American Institute for Cancer Research (AICR) joint expert review concluded that 'there is limited evidence suggesting that high consumption of milk and dairy products is a cause of prostate cancer', but also that cows' 'milk probably protects against colorectal cancer' (WCRF/AICR 2007, 129). This is more or less the opposite of what was found in a longitudinal study of 4,383 English and Scottish children who participated in a family food study between 1937 and 1939: no positive link between high cows' milk consumption and prostate cancer risk was found, but the study did find a near-tripling in the odds of colorectal cancer amongst those who had been raised in households with high dairy consumption (van der Pols et al. 2007). Some other studies, however, also found a positive link between high consumption of dairy and prostate cancer risk (N. Allen et al. 2008; Chan et al. 2005; Torfadottir et al. 2011). Much has been written on the latter issue, but little clarity has been provided because of the high likelihood of confounding factors. An analysis of pooled data from 45 observational studies, supported by a grant from National Dairy Council (Rosemont, Illinois), found no increased risk (Huncharek et al. 2008).

Apart from the fact that no dairy products are consumed, many other reasons have been provided in support of the view that vegan diets are cancer-protective. One is the fact that vegans are less likely to be obese (WCRF/AICR 2007). Expert reviews also indicate that diets that are high in fruits and vegetables are associated with decreased cancer risk because of the higher levels of health-promoting substances (such as ascorbic acid, carotenoids, and flavonoids) and a lower level of some carcinogenic components that have been found in some animal products, such as dioxins (WCRF/AICR 2007; Craig 2009; Dewell et al. 2008; ADA 2009).

A significant concern with many studies that explore relative cancer risks of different populations is that they fail to distinguish between vegetarians and vegans. Consequently, relatively little is known as yet about the benefits or disadvantages of vegan diets. The vegetarian group in the study that combined data from the Oxford Vegetarian Study and the EPIC-Oxford cohort, for example, included both vegetarians and vegans, resulting in a failure to identify the relative cancer risk of the latter (Key et al. 2009a). To alert the reader to this issue, the authors write that to explore the hypothesis that the consumption of dairy products may increase prostate cancer risk 'we would need to examine the cancer rates among vegans', but they are not consistent in their failure to separate vegans from vegetarians as they add that 'there are currently too few cancers [amongst vegans in their study] to be informative' (Key et al. 2009a, 195); what they may have meant to say is that there were too few vegans in the study to allow for generalisations to be made about vegan diets. As stated in the paper, however, the claim is informative. In spite of the fact that generalisations from studies of small populations are inappropriate, the fact that very few cancers were identified amongst vegans must be considered to be good news. In 2014, the Oxford team did report findings separately for the 2,246 vegans who were part of a sub-cohort of 61,647 British people who were followed up for almost 15 years (Key et al. 2014). During this time, there were 4,998 incidents of cancer, and the incidence was 19% lower in the vegan group than in the omnivorous group. Another study that has looked at vegans as a separate group is the AHS-2 study, which has reported a 16% reduction of risk amongst vegan Adventists compared to omnivorous Adventists (Orlich et al. 2013).

Overall, it is safe to conclude that many vegan diets are associated with a lower incidence of cancer than many other diets, even if the jury is still out on what the ideal diet might be to protect against cancer (Norris and Messina 2011, 176–178).

Diverticular disease

Diverticular disease includes two diseases of the colon (large intestine or large bowel): diverticulosis (the presence of pockets or pouches) and diverticulitis (infected or inflamed pockets or pouches). A study published in 1979 explored the incidence of diverticular disease in two groups of southern English people who did not experience any symptoms of the disease: 56 vegetarians were compared with 264 non-vegetarian volunteers. When radiographs of the participants' colons were analysed by a consultant radiologist who knew neither the participants nor their diets, 12% of the former group and 33% of the latter group were diagnosed to suffer from diverticular disease (Gear et al. 1979). In the Oxford-EPIC cohort, a sub-cohort of 15,459 participants, combining vegetarians and vegans, was found to have a 30% reduced risk of diverticular disease compared with the sub-cohort of 31,574 omnivores (Crowe et al. 2011). When the vegan participants were isolated from the vegetarians, the researchers found a 72% lower risk for the former compared to the omnivores in the study. While these findings have primarily been associated with the fact that vegetarians and vegans tend to consume more fibre, different studies (with, arguably, participants less health-conscious than participants in the Oxford-EPIC studies) found that, after adjusting for differences in dietary fibre between study participants, high consumption of total fat or of red flesh (Aldoori et al. 1994), the consumption of flesh from sheep and cows as well as milk products (Manousos et al. 1985), and the 'long-term and frequent' consumption of flesh (Lin et al. 2000) were linked with diverticular disease. Whereas only the Aldoori et al. (1994) study was a prospective cohort study—the ones by Manousos et al. (1985) and by Lin et al. (2000) being small case-control studies—these findings lend strong support for the view that vegan diets that tend to be high in fibre are much less likely to cause diverticular disease than many omnivorous diets.

Parkinson's disease

On the basis of population-based studies, McCarty (2001b) found that Parkinson's disease was less prevalent in sub-Saharan Africa, rural China, and Japan. A similar observation was made by de Lau and Breteler (2006), who report that the incidence of Parkinson's is lower in East Asian populations, including Chinese, Taiwanese, and Japanese populations, than in Western populations. McCarty (2001b) also reported that the incidence of Parkinson's amongst African Americans was very similar to that of white Americans, suggesting that the low incidence of Parkinson's amongst sub-Saharan Africans may not stem from genetic factors. As sub-Saharan and East Asian populations consume relatively few animal products, McCarty (2001b) suggests that vegan diets may be protective and that they may even be therapeutically beneficial through a number of mechanisms, including the promotion of vascular health and blood-brain transport of L-dopa, as well as through caloric restriction, which was found to protect the central dopaminergic neurons of mice. A different study, funded by Syngenta Crop Protection, reviewed the epidemiological literature, as well as the literature on risks and protective factors, concluding that little is known as yet about the aetiology of Parkinson's disease, but that there is some evidence that the consumption of dairy products increases risk (Wirdefeldt et al. 2011). A very small Indian study, however, did not find a reduction in Parkinson's for those who adopted a vegetarian diet (Behari et al. 2001). In his review of the literature, Giovanni (2009, 326) comments that 'data regarding the prevalence of Parkinson's disease in vegetarian or vegan groups or relative clinical findings are not available as yet'. Accordingly, the view that a vegan diet might be protective of Parkinson's is no more than an interesting hypothesis at the present time.

Insulin-like growth factor 1 (IGF-1) and mTORC1 related diseases

Insulin-like growth factor 1 (IGF-1) is a growth-stimulating hormone that is found in the human body. 'mTORC1' refers to mammalian target of rapamycin complex 1, a nutrient-sensitive enzyme that responds to a range of signals in the human body, including IGF-1.

Overproduction of IGF-1 has been associated with many diseases (Hoppe et al. 2006). IGF-1 is a key factor involved with episodes of rapid growth during childhood; the growth acceleration hypothesis claims that IGF-1 contributes to the development of a range of diseases that may not manifest themselves until much later in life (Singhal and Lucas 2004). Diets that increase IGF-1 levels in the blood have also been associated with some cancers, including colorectal and breast cancer (O'Neill 2010, 200).

Studies that compared vegan with other study participants have found that vegans had lower levels of IGF-1 (Fontana et al. 2006; N. Allen et al. 2002). Two cross-sectional analyses of the EPIC-study found that the production of IGF-1 was particularly stimulated by the consumption of dairy products (Norat et al. 2007; Crowe et al. 2009). The same conclusion was reached in a much larger study that combined findings from 15 cross-sectional studies and 8 randomised controlled trials (Qin et al. 2009). Dairy products have come under increased scrutiny not only because of their role in IGF-1 stimulation, but also because they, as well as animals' flesh, contain large quantities of calories and leucine. Together with products that have a high glycaemic load (including hyperglycaemic carbohydrates), products that are high in calories and leucine and that stimulate IGF-1 are thought to play a major, synergistic role in the activation of mTORC1 (Melnik 2012). This has been held to cause or worsen acne, a skin disease that prevails amongst more than 85% of teenagers in Western countries, and that is absent amongst people who eat palaeolithic diets, such as the inhabitants of Kitava, one of the Trobriand Islands of Papua New Guinea (Melnik 2012, 20–21; Lindeberg et al. 1999). Increased mTORC1-signalling has also been linked with a number of other Western health concerns, including obesity and type 2 diabetes (Shaw and Cantley 2006; Zoncu et al. 2011). Men who suffer from severe, long-lasting acne have also been found to have an increased risk of developing prostate cancer later in life (Sutcliffe et al. 2007). Laboratory experiments, including experiments with mice, have suggested that this may stem from the possibility that long-term hyperstimulation of mTORC1-signalling promotes the development of cancer tumours (Nardella et al. 2009; Wang et al. 2011).

Critical scrutiny of the Kitavans' diet around 1990 reveals that they ate a diet that contained mainly tubers that provide carbohydrates with a low glycaemic index (such as yam, sweet potato, taro, and manioc), as well as fruits, vegetables, coconuts, and fish (Lindeberg et al. 1999, 1216). In a randomised controlled trial with patients who suffered from ischaemic heart disease combined with either glucose intolerance or type 2 diabetes, such a diet has also been shown to improve glucose tolerance more than a Mediterranean-style diet that included whole grains and low-fat dairy products (Lindeberg et al. 2007). Compared to a Swedish control group, it was also found that Kitavans consumed a much smaller amount of mono-unsaturated fats and a higher amount of n-3 fatty acids (Lindeberg et al. 1999). In light of these studies and the connection between mTORC-1 and a range of Western diseases that are rare or absent amongst Kitavans, the adoption of a vegan diet that is similar to the palaeolithic diet that was adopted by the Kitavans around 1990 has been recommended (Melnik 2012). One reason why such a diet is low in foods with a high glycaemic index is that it contains little fructose—which is present in many processed foods through the widespread use of high fructose corn syrup (Melnik 2012, 29; McCarty 2011; Seneff et al. 2011).

A vegan diet that is similar to the traditional Kitavan diet may also protect against a number of ageing-associated diseases, including Alzheimer's disease (Seneff et al. 2011; McCarty 2001a; McCarty 2003c). Alzheimer's disease patients have been shown to have elevated levels of IGF-1 (Melnik 2011). This may help to explain why, when 2,148 New Yorkers without a diagnosis of dementia who were at least 65 were followed up over a period of nearly four years, it was found that the incidence of Alzheimer's was greater amongst those who ate the largest quantity of animal products (Gu et al. 2010).

Other benefits and concerns

A further benefit for young children is that a vegan diet avoids the consumption of cows' milk, which not only is low in iron, but also causes occult intestinal blood loss in about 40% of children below the age of one, and which contains high quantities of calcium as well as casein and other proteins that all inhibit the absorption of dietary non-haem iron (Ziegler 2011, 38S–40S). Casein has also been found to inhibit the absorption of zinc (Lönnerdal 2000). These concerns may help to explain why nutritionists do not recommend the consumption of cows' milk for children below the age of one (Millward and Garnett 2010, 104). Middle ear infection (otitis media) has also been found to be more severe and more common amongst children with cows' milk allergies (Juntti et al. 1999). Such allergies are by no means restricted to children as many people are lactose intolerant, lacking sufficient quantities of the lactase enzyme within the lining of the small intestine to allow the body to absorb lactose, whilst some people are also allergic to other components in dairy products (Millward and Garnett 2010, 104–105). In light of their hypothesis that the continued production of lactase throughout adulthood may only have developed in northern Europeans about a thousand years ago, Norris and Messina (2011, 43) argue that the concept of 'lactose intolerance' stems from a Western bias as good lactose tolerance may be the exception, rather than the rule.

Limited evidence has been presented to support the view that vegan diets may also reduce the risk of cataracts, dementia, gallstones, kidney disease, and rheumatoid arthritis (B. Davis and Melina 2014, 72–80). As many toxic substances accumulate inside the bodies of animals, vegan diets also tend to have lower levels of many toxic substances, including biodegradation-resistant organic environmental pollutants, such as polychlorinated dibenzo-p-dioxins (PCDDs), polychlorinated dibenzofurans (PCDFs), and polychlorinated biphenyls (PCBs), as well as of toxic heavy metals, such as mercury (Schecter et al. 1997; O'Neill 2010, 201).

In spite of these benefits, recent research that included a sample of 422 vegans from the Oxford-EPIC cohort revealed that vegans had relatively high circulating concentrations of uric acid, which may contribute to the development of gout, chronic kidney disease, cardio-vascular disease, and cancer; these high concentrations of uric acid are attributed to the exclusion of dairy products and to low calcium consumption (J. Schmidt et al. 2013). The authors are cautious, however, about the possible existence of causal connections between uric acid and these diseases, and they add that concentrations can be lowered through increased calcium consumption.

An additional concern for people with small stomach capacities, such as small children, is that vegan diets can be bulky due to increased consumption of dietary fibre, which can cause early satiety. Accordingly, McEvoy and Woodside (2010, 86–87) advise that vegan children take frequent meals and snacks, and that foods that are high in fat, such as nuts and nut butters, be used to provide sufficient calories and protein. For those who suffer from nut allergies, however, adequate substitutes must be used.

4 Conclusion

After a brief introduction, I argued in the second part of this appendix that vegan diets can be nutritionally adequate, but that vegans must make sure to consume foods that contain adequate amounts of vitamin B12 and omega-3 fatty acids as the former cannot be obtained from plants and the latter are present in significant quantities only in a few common vegan foods. The former can be obtained by consuming products that contain the B12 vitamin. Adequate consumption of the latter is facilitated by the consumption of plants and plant foods that have relatively high levels of omega-3, such as chia, flax, canola (rapeseed), hemp, walnuts, perilla, olive oil, blackcurrant seed oil, and plants in the *Echium* genus, as well as by the consumption of brown algae (kelp) oils. People with specific dietary requirements, such as young and old people, must make sure that they eat sufficient foods that are relatively rich in calories and relatively easy to digest, such as cooked foods.

The question whether vegan diets might be healthier than other diets was addressed in the third part. The evidence to support the possibility that vegan diets might be healthier is limited. Factors that complicate the development of our understanding include the facts that relatively few people adopt vegan diets, that some people's adoption of vegan diets may be triggered by psychological illness, and that many are biased against vegan diets. In spite of these limitations, there is sufficient evidence to conclude that many diets that are high in fruits and vegetables are associated with many health benefits, including reductions in cardio-vascular disease and some types of cancer.

Whereas this appendix has discussed scientific evidence for and against vegan diets, it has not answered the question of what a good vegan diet is, at least not in detail. For those who seek more practical advice on what kind of vegan diet to adopt to meet nutritional requirements, I recommend the books *Becoming Vegan* (B. Davis and Melina 2014) and, particularly, *Vegan for Life* (Norris and Messina 2011).

References

Aarestrup, F., Agerso, Y., Gerner-Smidt, P. et al. 2000. Comparison of antimicrobial resistance phenotypes and resistance genes in Enterococcus faecalis and Enterococcus faecium from humans in the community, broilers, and pigs in Denmark. *Diagnostic Microbiology and Infectious Disease*, 37, 127–137. DOI: http://dx.doi.org/10.1016/S0732-8893(00)00130-9

Abelow, B., Holford, T., Insogna, K. 1992. Cross-cultural association between dietary animal protein and hip fracture: a hypothesis. *Calcified Tissue International*, 50, 14–18. DOI: http://dx.doi.org/10.1007/BF00297291

Adams, C. 1990. *The sexual politics of meat: A feminist-vegetarian critical theory*. New York: Continuum.

Adams, C. 2008. *Living among meat eaters: The vegetarian's survival handbook*. New York: Lantern Books.

Afjal Hossain, M., Imran Reza, M., Rahman, S. et al. 2012. Climate change and its impacts on the livelihoods of the vulnerable people in the southwestern coastal zone in Bangladesh. In: W. Leal Filho (ed.). *Climate Change and the Sustainable Use of Water Resources*. Berlin: Springer, 237–259. DOI: http://dx.doi.org/10.1007/978-3-642-22266-5_15

Aflitto, N., DeGomez, T. 2014. Sonic Pest Repellents. http://arizona.openrepository.com/arizona/bitstream/10150/333139/1/AZ1639-2014.pdf. (Accessed 20 September 2015.)

Agostoni, C., Turck, D. 2011. Is cow's milk harmful to a child's health? *Journal of Pediatric Gastroenterology and Nutrition*, 53, 594–600.

Aiello, A., King, N., Foxman, B. 2006. Ethical conflicts in public health research and practice. Antimicrobial resistance and the ethics of drug development. *American Journal of Public Health*, 96, 1910–1914. DOI: http://dx.doi.org/10.2105/AJPH.2005.077214

Aiking, H., De Boer, J., Verreijken, J. (eds.) 2006. *Sustainable protein production and consumption: Pigs or peas?* Environment and Policy. Volume 45. Dordrecht: Springer. DOI: http://dx.doi.org/10.1007/1-4020-4842-4

Aldoori, W., Giovannucci, E., Rimm, E. et al. 1994. A prospective study of diet and the risk of symptomatic diverticular disease in men. *The American journal of clinical nutrition*, 60, 757–764.

Aldrich, S., Walker, R., Simmons, C. et al. 2012. Contentious land change in the Amazon's arc of deforestation. *Annals of the Association of American Geographers*, 102, 103–128. DOI: http://dx.doi.org/10.1080/00045608.2011.620501

Alexandratos, N., Bruinsma, J. 2012. *World agriculture towards 2030/2050: the 2012 revision. ESA Working paper No. 12-03.* Rome: FAO.

Ali, A., Cheng, K. 1985. Early egg production in genetically blind (rc/rc) chickens in comparison with sighted (Rc+/rc) controls. *Poultry science*, 64, 789–794. DOI: http://dx.doi.org/10.3382/ps.0640789

Allen, C. 2013. Fish cognition and consciousness. *Journal of agricultural and environmental ethics*, 26, 25–39. DOI: http://dx.doi.org/10.1007/s10806-011-9364-9

Allen, N., Appleby, P., Davey, G. et al. 2002. The associations of diet with serum insulin-like growth factor I and its main binding proteins in 292 women meat-eaters, vegetarians, and vegans. *Cancer Epidemiology Biomarkers & Prevention*, 11, 1441–1448.

Allen N., Key T., Appleby P. et al. 2008. Animal foods, protein, calcium and prostate cancer risk: the European Prospective Investigation into Cancer and Nutrition. *British Journal of Cancer*, 98, 1574–1581. DOI: http://dx.doi.org/10.1038/sj.bjc.6604331

American Dietetic Association 1997 Position of the American Dietetic Association: Vegetarian diets. *Journal of the American Dietetic Association*, 97, 1317–1321. DOI: http://dx.doi.org/10.1016/S0002-8223(97)00314-3

American Dietetic Association. 2009. Position of the American Dietetic Association: Vegetarian diets. *Journal of the American Dietetic Association*, 109, 1266–1282. DOI: http://dx.doi.org/10.1016/j.jada.2009.05.027

Anand, P., Kunnumakkara, A., Sundaram, C. et al. 2008. Cancer is a preventable disease that requires major lifestyle changes, *Pharmaceutical research*, 25, 2097–2116. DOI: http://dx.doi.org/10.1007/s11095-008-9690-4 , DOI: http://dx.doi.org/10.1007/s11095-008-9661-9

Anil, A., Whittington, P., McKinstry, J. 2000. The effect of the sticking method on the welfare of slaughter pigs. *Meat Science*, 55, 315–319. DOI: http://dx.doi.org/10.1016/S0309-1740(99)00159-X

Animals Deserve Absolute Protection Today and Tomorrow. 2012. *More than 150 billion animals slaughtered every year.* http://www.adaptt.org/killcounter.html. (Accessed 31 July 2012.)

Anomaly, J. 2009. Harm to others: The social costs of antibiotics in agriculture. *Journal of Agricultural and Environmental Ethics*, 22, 423–435. DOI: http://dx.doi.org/10.1007/s10806-009-9160-y

Anomaly, J. 2010. Combating resistance: The case for a global antibiotics treaty. *Public Health Ethics*, 3, 13–22. DOI: http://dx.doi.org/10.1093/phe/phq001

Anthony, R., Gjerris, M., Röcklingsberg, H. 2013. Fish welfare, environment and food security: a pragmatist virtue ethics approach. In: H. Röcklingsberg, P. Sandin (eds.). The ethics of consumption. Wageningen: Wageningen Academic Publishers, 257–262. DOI: http://dx.doi.org/10.3920/978-90-8686-784-4_41

Appleby, M., Walker, A., Nicol, C. et al. 2002. Development of furnished cages for laying hens. *British Poultry Science*, 43, 489–500. DOI: http://dx.doi.org/10.1080/00071660220000004390

Appleby, P., Davey, G., Key, T. 2002. Hypertension and blood pressure among meat eaters, fish eaters, vegetarians and vegans in EPIC-Oxford. *Public Health Nutrition*, 5, 645–654. DOI: http://dx.doi.org/10.1079/PHN2002332

Appleby, P., Roddam, A., Allen, N. et al. 2007. Comparative fracture risk in vegetarians and nonvegetarians in EPIC-Oxford. *European Journal of Clinical Nutrition*, 61, 1400–1406. DOI: http://dx.doi.org/10.1038/sj.ejcn.1602659

Armand-Lefevre, L., Ruimy, R., Andremont, A. 2005. Clonal comparison of Staphylococcus aureus isolates from healthy pig farmers, human controls, and pigs. *Emerging Infectious Diseases*, 11, 711–714. DOI: http://dx.doi.org/10.3201/eid1105.040866

Aston, L., Smith, J., Powles, J. 2012. Impact of a reduced red and processed meat dietary pattern on disease risks and greenhouse gas emissions in the UK: a modelling study. *BMJ open*, 2(5). DOI: http://dx.doi.org/10.1136/bmjopen-2012-001072

Atkinson, S., Velarde, A., Llonch, P. et al. 2012. Assessing pig welfare at stunning in Swedish commercial abattoirs using CO_2 group-stun methods. *Animal Welfare*, 21, 487–495. DOI: http://dx.doi.org/10.7120/09627286.21.4.487

Audsley, E., Angus, A., Chatterton, J. et al. 2011. *Food, land and greenhouse gases. The effect of changes in UK food consumption on land requirements and greenhouse gas emissions. A report prepared for the United Kingdom's Committee on Climate Change.* Revised report. Cranfield: Cranfield University.

Balaban, P., Maksimova, O. 1993. Positive and negative brain zones in the snail. *European Journal of Neuroscience*, 5, 768–774. DOI: http://dx.doi.org/10.1111/j.1460-9568.1993.tb00541.x

Baluška, F., Mancuso, S. 2009. Deep evolutionary origins of neurobiology: Turning the essence of 'neural' upside-down. *Communicative and Integrative Biology*, 2, 60–65. DOI: http://dx.doi.org/10.4161/cib.2.1.7620

Baluška, F., Mancuso, S., Volkmann, D. et al. 2009. The 'root-brain' hypothesis of Charles and Francis Darwin: Revival after more than 125 years. *Plant Signalling and Behavior*, 4, 14–20. DOI: http://dx.doi.org/10.4161/psb.4.12.10574

Bankowski, Z. 2001. Law, love and legality. *International Journal of the Semiotics of Law*, 14, 199–213. DOI: http://dx.doi.org/10.1023/A:1011205710567

Banwell, B., Bar-Or, A., Cheung, R. et al. 2008. Abnormal T-cell reactivities in childhood inflammatory demyelinating disease and type 1 diabetes. *Annals of neurology*, 63, 98–111. DOI: http://dx.doi.org/10.1002/ana.21244

Barnard, N. Cohen, J., Jenkins, D. et al. 2006. A low-fat vegan diet improves glycemic control and cardio-vascular risk factors in a randomized clinical trial in individuals with type 2 diabetes. *Diabetes Care*, 29, 1777–1783. DOI: http://dx.doi.org/10.2337/dc06-0606

Barnard, N., Cohen, J., Jenkins, D. et al. 2009. A low-fat vegan diet and a conventional diabetes diet in the treatment of type 2 diabetes: a randomized, controlled, 74-wk clinical trial. *American Journal of Clinical Nutrition*, 89S, 1588S–1596S. DOI: http://dx.doi.org/10.3945/ajcn.2009.26736H

Baroni, L., Cenci, L., Tettamanti, M. et al. 2007. Evaluating the environmental impact of various dietary patterns combined with different food production systems. *European Journal of Clinical Nutrition*, 61, 279–286. DOI: http://dx.doi.org/10.1038/sj.ejcn.1602522

Barr, S., Laming, P., Dick, J. et al. 2008. Nociception or pain in a decapod crustacean?. *Animal Behaviour*, 75, 745–751. DOI: http://dx.doi.org/10.1016/j.anbehav.2007.07.004

Barzel, U., Massey, L. 1998. Excess dietary protein can adversely affect bone. *Journal of Nutrition*, 128, 1051–1053.

Basurko, O., Gabiña, G., Uriondo, Z. 2013. Energy performance of fishing vessels and potential savings. *Journal of Cleaner Production*, 54, 30–40. DOI: http://dx.doi.org/10.1016/j.jclepro.2013.05.024

Bates, J., Jordens, J., Griffiths, D. 1994. Farm animals as a putative reservoir for vancomycin-resistant enterococcal infection in man. *Journal of Antimicrobial Chemotherapy*, 34, 507–514. DOI: http://dx.doi.org/10.1093/jac/34.4.507

Bateson, M., Desire, S., Gartside, S. et al. 2011. Agitated honeybees exhibit pessimistic cognitive biases. *Current Biology*, 21, 1070–1073. DOI: http://dx.doi.org/10.1016/j.cub.2011.05.017

Behari, M., Srivastava, A., Das, R. et al. 2001. Risk factors of Parkinson's disease in Indian patients. *Journal of the Neurological Sciences*, 190, 49–55. DOI: http://dx.doi.org/10.1016/S0022-510X(01)00578-0

Bekoff, M., Sherman, P. 2004. Reflections on animal selves. *Trends in Ecology and Evolution*, 19, 176–180. DOI: http://dx.doi.org/10.1016/j.tree.2003.12.010

Bell, D. 2011. Does anthropogenic climate change violate human rights? *Critical Review of International Social and Political Philosophy*, 14, 99–124. DOI: http://dx.doi.org/10.1080/13698230.2011.529703

Bell, D., Thompson, N., Deckers, J., et al. 2005. *Deliberating the environment. Scientists and the socially excluded in dialogue.* Newcastle University: Centre for Rural Economy.

Belshe, R. 2005. The origins of pandemic influenza—lessons from the 1918 virus. *New England Journal of Medicine,* 353, 2209–2211. DOI: http://dx.doi.org/10.1056/NEJMp058281

Benzie, I., Wachtel-Galor, S. 2010. Vegetarian diets and public health: biomarker and redox connections. *Antioxidants & Redox Signaling,* 13, 1575–1591. DOI: http://dx.doi.org/10.1089/Ars.2009.3024

Bergqvist, J., Gunnarson, S. 2013. Finfish aquaculture: Animal welfare, the environment, and ethical implications. *Journal of Agricultural and Environmental Ethics,* 26, 75–99. DOI: http://dx.doi.org/10.1007/s10806-011-9346-y

Bermúdez, J. 2003. *Thinking without words.* Oxford: Oxford University Press. DOI: http://dx.doi.org/10.1093/acprof:oso/9780195159691.001.0001

Berndsen, M., van der Pligt, J. 2005. Risks of meat: the relative impact of cognitive, affective and moral concerns. *Appetite,* 44, 195–205. DOI: http://dx.doi.org/10.1016/j.appet.2004.10.003

Berners-Lee, M., Hoolohan, C., Cammack, H. et al. 2012. The relative greenhouse gas impacts of realistic dietary choices. *Energy Policy,* 43, 184–190. DOI: http://dx.doi.org/10.1016/j.enpol.2011.12.054

Bernstein A., Sun Q., Hu F. et al. 2010. Major dietary protein sources and risk of coronary heart disease in women. *Circulation,* 122, 876–883. DOI: http://dx.doi.org/10.1161/CIRCULATIONAHA.109.915165

Birch, C., Cobb, J. 1984. *The liberation of life. From the cell to the community.* Second edition. Cambridge: Cambridge University Press.

Bonten, M., Willems, R., Weinstein, R. 2001. Vancomycin-resistant enterococci: Why are they here, and where do they come from? *Lancet Infectious Diseases,* 314–325. DOI: http://dx.doi.org/10.1016/S1473-3099(01)00145-1

Booth, S., Tucker, K., Chen, H. et al. 2000. Dietary vitamin K intakes are associated with hip fracture but not with bone mineral density in elderly men and women. *American Journal of Clinical Nutrition,* 71, 1201–1208.

Bouillon, R., Verlinden, L. 2014. Does a better vitamin D status help to reduce cardiovascular risks and events?. *Endocrine,* 47, 662–663. DOI: http://dx.doi.org/10.1007/s12020-014-0429-1

Braithwaite, V. 2010. Do fish feel pain. Oxford: Oxford University Press.

Brambell, R. 1965. *Report of the technical committee to enquire into the welfare of animals kept under intensive livestock husbandry systems.* London: Her Majesty's Stationery Office.

Brennan, A. 2003. Humanism, racism, and speciesism. *Worldviews. Global Religions, Culture, and Ecology,* 7, 274–302. DOI: http://dx.doi.org/10.1163/156853503322709146

Broom, D. 1990. Effects of handling and transport on laying hens. *World's Poultry Science Journal,* 46, 48–50. DOI: http://dx.doi.org/10.1079/WPS19900009

Bryman, A. 2008. *Social research methods*. Third edition. Oxford: Oxford University Press.

Buchmann, S., Nabhan, G. 1996. The pollination crisis. *The Sciences*, 36, 22–27. DOI: http://dx.doi.org/10.1002/j.2326-1951.1996.tb03254.x

Burckhardt, P. 2013. The negative effect of a high-protein—low-calcium diet. In P. Burckhardt, B. Dawson-Hughes, C. Weaver (eds.). *Nutritional influences on bone health*. London: Springer, 125–131. DOI: http://dx.doi.org/10.1007/978-1-4471-2769-7_12, DOI: http://dx.doi.org/10.1007/978-1-4471-2769-7

Burckhardt, P. 2015. Vitamin A and bone health. In: M. Holick, J. Nieves (eds.) *Nutrition and bone health*. New York: Springer, 409–421. DOI: http://dx.doi.org/10.1007/978-1-4939-2001-3_26

Burkholder, J., Glasgow, H. 2001. History of toxic Pfiesteria in North Carolina estuaries from 1991 to the present. *BioScience*, 51, 827–841. DOI: http://dx.doi.org/10.1641/0006-3568(2001)051[0827:HOTPIN]2.0.CO;2

Burkholder, J., Libra, B., Weyer, P. et al. 2007. Impacts of waste from concentrated animal feeding operations on water quality. *Environmental Health Perspectives*, 115, 308–312. DOI: http://dx.doi.org/10.1289/ehp.8839

Calvez, J., Poupin, N., Chesneau, C. et al. 2012. Protein intake, calcium balance and health consequences. *European Journal of Clinical Nutrition*, 66, 281–295. DOI: http://dx.doi.org/10.1038/ejcn.2011.196

Campbell, A., Matthews, S. 2014. Lactose intolerance. In: E. Lammert, M. Zeeb (eds.). *Metabolism of human diseases. Organ physiology and pathophysiology*. Vienna: Springer, 143–148. DOI: http://dx.doi.org/10.1007/978-3-7091-0715-7_23

Caney, S. 2008. Human rights, climate change, and discounting. *Environmental Politics*, 17, 536–555. DOI: http://dx.doi.org/10.1080/09644010802193401

Carey, J., Fulweiler, R. 2015. Human appropriation of biogenic silicon-the increasing role of agriculture. *Functional Ecology*. On-line first. DOI: http://dx.doi.org/10.1111/1365-2435.12544

Carlsson-Kanyama, A., González, A. 2009. Potential contributions of food consumption patterns to climate change. *American Journal of Clinical Nutrition*, 89S, 1704S–1709S. DOI: http://dx.doi.org/10.3945/ajcn.2009.26736AA

Carmody, R., Wrangham, R. 2009. The energetic significance of cooking. *Journal of Human Evolution*, 57, 379–391. DOI: http://dx.doi.org/10.1016/j.jhevol.2009.02.011

Carruthers, P. 1992. *The animal issue: Moral theory in practice*. Cambridge: Cambridge University Press. DOI: http://dx.doi.org/10.1017/CBO9780511597961

Catton, W. 1980. *Overshoot: the ecological basis of revolutionary change*. Urbana and Chicago: University of Illinois Press.

Catts, O., Zurr, I. 2013. Disembodied livestock: The promise of a semi-living Utopia. *Parallax*, 19, 101–113. DOI: http://dx.doi.org/10.1080/13534645.2013.752062

Chan, J., Gann, P., Giovannucci, E. 2005. Role of diet in prostate cancer development and progression. *Journal of Clinical Oncology*, 23, 8152–8160. DOI: http://dx.doi.org/10.1200/JCO.2005.03.1492

Chandroo, K., Duncan, I., Moccia, R. 2004. Can fish suffer?: Perspectives on sentience, pain, fear and stress. *Applied Animal Behaviour Science*, 86, 225–250. DOI: http://dx.doi.org/10.1016/j.applanim.2004.02.004

Charles, N., Kerr, M. 1988. *Women, food, and families*. Manchester: Manchester University Press.

Chen, B., Ho, C., Huang, N. 2009. Threats from farmed animals to food and human security. *Asia Pacific Journal of Clinical Nutrition*, 18, 549–551.

Chen, D., Abler, D. 2014. Demand growth for animal products in the BRIIC Countries. *Agribusiness*, 30, 85–97. DOI: http://dx.doi.org/10.1002/agr.21368

Childs, C., Romeu-Nadal, M., Burdge, G. et al. 2008. Gender differences in the n-3 fatty acid content of tissues. *Proceedings of the Nutrition Society*, 67, 19–27. DOI: http://dx.doi.org/10.1017/S0029665108005983

Chitnis, A., Rawls, D., Moore, J. 2000. Origin of HIV type 1 in colonial French Equatorial Africa?. *AIDS Research and Human Retroviruses*, 16, 5–8. DOI: http://dx.doi.org/10.1089/088922200309548

Chiu, C., Wu, T., Su, L. et al. 2002. The emergence in Taiwan of fluoroquinolone resistance in Salmonella enterica serotype choleraesuis. *New England Journal of Medicine*, 346, 413–419. DOI: http://dx.doi.org/10.1056/NEJMoa012261

Christman, J. 2008. The Gilgamesh complex: The quest for death transcendence and the killing of animals. *Society and Animals*, 16, 297–315. DOI: http://dx.doi.org/10.1163/156853008X357649

Christophersen, O., Haug, A. 2011. Animal products, diseases and drugs: a plea for better integration between agricultural sciences, human nutrition and human pharmacology. *Lipids In Health and Disease*, 10, 16. DOI: http://dx.doi.org/10.1186/1476-511X-10-16

Clements, K. 1995. *Why vegan. The ethics of eating and the need for change.* Second edition. London: Heretic Books.

Climate Change Act 2008, Chapter 27, London: The Stationery Office Limited.

Cochrane, A. 2009. Do animals have an interest in liberty?. *Political Studies*, 57, 660–679. DOI: http://dx.doi.org/10.1111/j.1467-9248.2008.00742.x

Cochrane, A. 2012. *Animal rights without liberation. Applied ethics and human obligations*. New York: Columbia University Press.

Cochrane, A. 2013. From human rights to sentient rights. *Critical Review of International Social and Political Philosophy*, 16, 655–675. DOI: http://dx.doi.org/10.1080/13698230.2012.691235

Cole, D., Cole, R., Gaydos, S. et al. 2009. Aquaculture: Environmental, toxicological, and health issues. *International Journal of Hygiene and Environmental Health*, 212, 369–377. DOI: http://dx.doi.org/10.1016/j.ijheh.2008.08.003

Cole, M., Morgan, K. 2011. Vegaphobia: derogatory discourses of veganism and the reproduction of speciesism in UK national newspapers. *British*

Journal of Sociology, 62, 134–153. DOI: http://dx.doi.org/10.1111/j.1468-4446.2010.01348.x

Compassion in World Farming. 2007. *Global Warning: Climate change and farmed animals' welfare*. Godalming: Compassion in World Farming.

Comstock, G. 2000. *Vexing nature? On the ethical case against agricultural biotechnology*. Boston: Kluwer Academic Publishers.

Cooper, R., Fehily, A., Pickering, J. et al. 2010. Honey, health and longevity. *Current aging science*, 3, 239–241. DOI: http://dx.doi.org/10.2174/1874609811003030239

Cordain, L., Miller, J., Eaton, S. et al. 2000. Plant-animal subsistence ratios and macronutrient energy estimations in worldwide hunter-gatherer diets. *American Journal of Clinical Nutrition*, 71, 682–692.

Cordell, D., Drangert, J., White, S. 2009. The story of phosphorus. Global food security and food for thought. *Global Environmental Change*, 19, 292–305. DOI: http://dx.doi.org/10.1016/j.gloenvcha.2008.10.009

Cottingham, J. 1986. Partiality, favouritism and morality. *The Philosophical Quarterly*, 36, 357–373. DOI: http://dx.doi.org/10.2307/2220190

Council Directive 1999/74/EC of 19 July 1999 laying down minimum standards for the protection of laying hens. *Official Journal of the European Union*, L 203/53, 53–57.

Council Directive 2007/43/EC of 28 June 2007 laying down minimum rules for the protection of chickens kept for meat production. *Official Journal of the European Union*, L 182/19, 19–28.

Council Directive 2008/120/EC of 18 December 2008 laying down minimum standards for the protection of pigs. *Official Journal of the European Union*, L 47/5, 5–13.

Council Directive 2010/63/EU of 22 September 2010 on the protection of animals used for scientific purposes. *Official Journal of the European Union*, L 276/33, 33–79.

Council for Agricultural Science and Technology. 1999. *Animal agriculture and global food supply. Task Force Report No.135*. Ames: Council for Agricultural Science and Technology.

Craig, W. 2009. Health effects of vegan diets. *American Journal of Clinical Nutrition*, 89S, 1627S–1633S. DOI: http://dx.doi.org/10.3945/ajcn.2009.26736N

Crary, A. 2011. A brilliant perspective: Diamondian ethics. *Philosophical Investigations*, 34, 331–352. DOI: http://dx.doi.org/10.1111/j.1467-9205.2011.01454.x

Crawford, M., Wang, Y., Lehane, C. et al. 2010. Fatty-acid ratios in free-living and domestic animals. In: F. De Meester, S. Zibadi, R. Watson (eds.). *Modern dietary fat intakes in disease promotion*. New York: Humana Press, 95–108. DOI: http://dx.doi.org/10.1007/978-1-60327-571-2_6

Crook, R., Walters, E. 2011. Nociceptive behavior and physiology of molluscs: animal welfare implications. *ILAR Journal*, 52, 185–195. DOI: http://dx.doi.org/10.1093/ilar.52.2.185

Crowe, F., Key, T., Allen, N. et al. 2009. The association between diet and serum concentrations of IGF-I, IGFBP-1, IGFBP-2, and IGFBP-3 in the European Prospective Investigation into Cancer and Nutrition. *Cancer Epidemiology Biomarkers and Prevention*, 18, 1333–1340. DOI: http://dx.doi.org/10.1158/1055-9965.EPI-08-0781

Crowe, F., Steur, M., Allen, N. et al. 2010. Plasma concentrations of 25hydroxyvitamin D in meat eaters, fish eaters, vegetarians and vegans: results from the EPIC—Oxford study. *Public Health Nutrition*, 14, 340–346. DOI: http://dx.doi.org/10.1017/S1368980010002454

Crowe, F., Appleby, P., Allen, N. et al. 2011. Diet and risk of diverticular disease in Oxford cohort of European Prospective Investigation into Cancer and Nutrition (EPIC): prospective study of British vegetarians and non-vegetarians. *British Medical Journal*, 343:d4131.

Crowe, F., Appleby, P., Travis, R. et al. 2013. Risk of hospitalization or death from ischemic heart disease among British vegetarians and nonvegetarians: results from the EPIC-Oxford cohort study. *The American Journal of Clinical Nutrition*, 97, 597–603.

Dahl-Jørgensen, K., Joner, G., Hanssen, K. 1991. Relationship between cows' milk consumption and incidence of IDDM in childhood. *Diabetes Care*, 14, 1081–1083. DOI: http://dx.doi.org/10.2337/diacare.14.11.1081

Daniels, N. 1979. Wide reflective equilibrium and theory acceptance in ethics. *Journal of Philosophy*, 76, 256–282. DOI: http://dx.doi.org/10.2307/2025881

Darlington, D. 2010. *Growing sustainability*. Chorlton: Vegan-organic Network.

Darwin, C. 1859. *On the origin of species by means of natural selection, or the preservation of favoured races in the struggle for life*. London: Murray.

Darwin, C. 1881. *The formation of vegetable mould, through the action of worms, with observations on their habits*. London: John Murray. DOI: http://dx.doi.org/10.5962/bhl.title.107559

Darwin, C., Darwin, F. 1880. *The power of movement in plants*. London: John Murray. DOI: http://dx.doi.org/10.5962/bhl.title.102319

Daszak, P., Plowright, R., Epstein, J. et al. 2006. The emergence of Nipah and Hendra virus: pathogen dynamics across a wildlife-livestock-human continuum. In: S. Collinge, C. Ray (eds.). *Disease ecology: community structure and pathogen dynamics*, Oxford: Oxford University Press, 186–201. DOI: http://dx.doi.org/10.1093/acprof:oso/9780198567080.003.0013

Davey, G., Spencer, E., Appleby, P. et al. 2003. EPIC-Oxford: lifestyle characteristics and nutrient intakes in a cohort of 33 883 meat-eaters and 31 546 non meat-eaters in the UK. *Public Health Nutrition*, 6, 259–268. DOI: http://dx.doi.org/10.1079/PHN2002430

Davis, B., Kris-Etherton, P. 2003. Achieving optimal essential fatty acid status in vegetarians: current knowledge and practical implications. *American Journal of Clinical Nutrition*, 78S, 640S–646S.

Davis, B., Melina, V. 2014. Becoming vegan. Comprehensive edition. The complete reference to plant-based nutrition. Summertown: Book Publishing Company.

Davis, J., Sonesson, U., Baumgartner, D. et al. 2010. Environmental impact of four meals with different protein sources: Case studies in Spain and Sweden. *Food Research International*, 43, 1874–1884. DOI: http://dx.doi.org/10.1016/j.foodres.2009.08.017

Davis, S. 2003. The least harm principle may require that humans consume a diet containing large herbivores, not a vegan diet. *Journal of Agricultural and Environmental Ethics*, 16, 387–394. DOI: http://dx.doi.org/10.1023/A:1025638030686

Davis, S. 2008. What would the world be like without animals for food, fiber, and labor? Are we morally obligated to do without them?. *Poultry Science*, 87, 392–394. DOI: http://dx.doi.org/10.3382/ps.2007-00401

de Lau, L., Breteler, M. 2006. Epidemiology of Parkinson's disease. *Lancet Neurology*, 5, 525–535. DOI: http://dx.doi.org/10.1016/S1474-4422(06)70471-9

De Schutter, O. 2011. The right of everyone to enjoy the benefits of scientific progress and the right to food: from conflict to complementarity. *Human Rights Quarterly*, 33, 304–350. DOI: http://dx.doi.org/10.1353/hrq.2011.0020

de Visser, C., Schreuder, R., Stoddard, F. 2014. The EU's dependency on soya bean import for the animal feed industry and potential for EU produced alternatives. *OCL*, 21, D407. DOI: http://dx.doi.org/10.1051/ocl/2014021

DeAngelo, B., De la Chesnaye, F., Beach, R. et al. 2006. Methane and nitrous oxide mitigation in agriculture. *Energy Journal* (Special issue 3), 89–108.

Dechet, A., Scallan, E., Gensheimer, K. et al. 2006. Outbreak of multidrug-resistant Salmonella enterica serotype Typhimurium Definitive Type 104 infection linked to commercial ground beef, northeastern United States, 2003-2004. *Clinical Infectious Diseases*, 42, 747–752. DOI: http://dx.doi.org/10.1086/500320

Deckers, J. 2005a. Why current UK legislation on embryo research is immoral. How the argument from lack of qualities and the argument from potentiality have been applied and why they should be rejected. *Bioethics*, 19, 251–271. DOI: http://dx.doi.org/10.1111/j.1467-8519.2005.00440.x

Deckers, J. 2005b. Are scientists right and non-scientists wrong? Reflections on discussions of GM. *Journal of Agricultural and Environmental Ethics*, 18, 451–478. DOI: http://dx.doi.org/10.1007/s10806-005-0902-1

Deckers, J. 2007. Are those who subscribe to the view that early embryos are persons irrational and inconsistent? A reply to Brock. *Journal of Medical Ethics*, 33, 102–106. DOI: http://dx.doi.org/10.1136/jme.2006.016311

Deckers, J. 2009. Vegetarianism, sentimental or ethical?. *Journal of Agricultural and Environmental Ethics*, 22, 573–597. DOI: http://dx.doi.org/10.1007/s10806-009-9176-3

Deckers, J. 2010. What policy should be adopted to curtail the negative global health impacts associated with the consumption of farmed animal products?.

Res Publica, 16, 57–72. DOI: http://dx.doi.org/10.1007/s11158-010-9117-z, DOI: http://dx.doi.org/10.1007/s11158-010-9128-9

Deckers, J. 2011a. Negative 'GHIs', the right to health protection, and future generations. *Journal of Bioethical Inquiry*, 8, 165–176. DOI: http://dx.doi.org/10.1007/s11673-011-9295-1

Deckers, J. 2011b. Could some people be wronged by contracting swine flu? A case discussion on the links between the farmed animals' sector and human disease. *Journal of Medical Ethics*, 37, 354–356. DOI: http://dx.doi.org/10.1136/jme.2010.040089

Deckers, J. 2011c. Does the consumption of farmed animal products cause human hunger?. *Journal of Hunger and Environmental Nutrition*, 6, 353–377. DOI: http://dx.doi.org/10.1080/19320248.2011.597836

Deckers, J. 2011d. Should Whiteheadians be vegetarians? A critical analysis of the thoughts of Hartshorne and Dombrowski. *Journal of Animal Ethics*, 1, 195–209. DOI: http://dx.doi.org/10.5406/janimalethics.1.2.0195

Deckers, J. 2011e. Should Whiteheadians be vegetarians? A Critical Analysis of the Thoughts of Whitehead, Birch, Cobb, and McDaniel. *Journal of Animal Ethics*, 1, 80–92. DOI: http://dx.doi.org/10.5406/janimalethics.1.1.0080

Deckers, J. 2013a. Obesity, public health, and the consumption of animal products. Ethical concerns and political solutions. *Journal of Bioethical Inquiry*, 10, 29–38. DOI: http://dx.doi.org/10.1007/s11673-012-9411-x

Deckers, J. 2013b. In defence of the vegan project. *Journal of Bioethical Inquiry*, 10, 187–195. DOI: http://dx.doi.org/10.1007/s11673-013-9428-9

DeGrazia, D. 1996. *Taking animals seriously: Mental life and moral status.* New York: Cambridge University Press. DOI: http://dx.doi.org/10.1017/CBO9781139172967

DeLeeuw, J., Galen, L., Aebersold, C. et al. 2007. Support for animal rights as a function of belief in evolution, religious fundamentalism, and religious denomination. *Society and Animals*, 15, 353–363. DOI: http://dx.doi.org/10.1163/156853007X235528

Department of Climate Change and Energy Efficiency. 2011. *Securing a clean energy future. The Australian Government's climate change plan.* Canberra: Department of Climate Change and Energy Efficiency.

Department of Climate Change and Energy Efficiency. 2012. *The carbon farming initiative handbook.* Canberra: Department of Climate Change and Energy Efficiency.

Devendra, C. 2007. Small farm systems to feed hungry Asia. *Outlook on Agriculture*, 36, 7–20. DOI: http://dx.doi.org/10.5367/000000007780223641

Dewell, A., Weidner, G., Sumner, M. et al. 2008. A very low-fat vegan diet increases intake of protective dietary factors and decreases intake of pathogenic dietary factors. *Journal of the American Dietetic Association*, 108, 347–356. DOI: http://dx.doi.org/10.1016/j.jada.2007.10.044

Diamond, C. 1978. Eating meat and eating people. *Philosophy*, 53, 465–479. DOI: http://dx.doi.org/10.1017/S0031819100026334

Diamond, C. 1991. The importance of being human. In: D. Cockburn (ed.). *Human Beings*. Cambridge: Cambridge University Press, 35–59. DOI: http://dx.doi.org/10.1017/CBO9780511752186.003

Dietz, T., Rosa, E., York, R. 2009. Environmentally efficient well-being: rethinking sustainability as the relationship between human well-being and environmental impacts. *Human Ecology Review*, 16, 114–123.

Dillard, J. 2008. Slaughterhouse nightmare: Psychological harm suffered by slaughterhouse employees and the possibility of redress through legal reform. *Georgetown Journal on Poverty Law & Policy*, 15, 391–408.

Dohoo, I., DesCoteaux, L., Leslie, K. et al. 2003. A meta-analysis review of the effects of recombinant bovine somatotropin: 2. Effects on animal health, reproductive performance, and culling. *Canadian Journal of Veterinary Research*, 67, 252.

Dombrowski, D. 1988. *Hartshorne and the metaphysics of animal rights*. Albany: State University of New York Press.

Dombrowski, D. 2006. Is the argument from marginal cases obtuse? *Journal of Applied Philosophy*, 23, 223–232. DOI: http://dx.doi.org/10.1111/j.1468-5930.2006.00334.x

Donaldson, M. 2000. Metabolic vitamin B-12 status on a mostly raw vegan diet with follow-up using tablets, nutritional yeast, or probiotic supplements. *Annals of Nutrition and Metabolism*, 44, 229–234. DOI: http://dx.doi.org/10.1159/000046689

Douglas, I. 2009. Climate change, flooding and food security in south Asia. *Food Security*,1, 127–136. DOI: http://dx.doi.org/10.1007/s12571-009-0015-1

Duffy, G., Moriarty, E. 2003. Cryptosporidium and its potential as a food-borne pathogen. *Animal Health Research Reviews*, 4, 95–107. DOI: http://dx.doi.org/10.1079/AHR200357

Dwyer, J. 2009. How to connect bioethics and environmental ethics: Health, sustainability, and justice. *Bioethics*, 23, 497–502. DOI: http://dx.doi.org/10.1111/j.1467-8519.2009.01759.x

Ebbeling, C., Leidig, M. , Feldman, H. et al. 2007. Effects of a low-glycemic load vs low-fat diet in obese young adults. *JAMA: The Journal of the American Medical Association*, 297, 2092–2102. DOI: http://dx.doi.org/10.1001/jama.297.19.2092

Ehrlich, P., Ehrlich, A. 1997. The population explosion: why we should care and what we should do about it. *Environmental Law*, 27, 1187–1208.

Eisner, T., Camazine, S. 1983. Spider leg autotomy induced by prey venom injection: An adaptive response to "pain"?. *Proceedings of the National Academy of Sciences*, 80, 3382–3385. DOI: http://dx.doi.org/10.1073/pnas.80.11.3382

Elferink, E., Nonhebel, S. 2007. Variations in land requirements for meat production. *Journal of Cleaner Production*, 15, 1778–1786. DOI: http://dx.doi.org/10.1016/j.jclepro.2006.04.003

Elferink, E., Nonhebel, S., Schoot Uiterkamp, A. 2007. Does the Amazon suffer from BSE prevention? *Agriculture, Ecosystems and Environment*, 120, 467–469. DOI: http://dx.doi.org/10.1016/j.agee.2006.09.009

Elwood, R., Barr, S., Patterson, L. 2009. Pain and stress in crustaceans? *Applied Animal Behaviour Science*, 118, 128–136. DOI: http://dx.doi.org/10.1016/j.applanim.2009.02.018

Emhan, A., Yildiz, A., Yasin, B. et al. 2012. Psychological symptom profile of butchers working in slaughterhouse and retail meat packing business: A comparative study. *Kafkas Universitesi Veteriner Fakultesi Dergisi*, 18, 319–322.

Engler, M., Defoor, P., King, C., et al. 2014. The impact of bovine respiratory disease: the current feedlot experience. *Animal Health Research Reviews*, 15, 126–129. DOI: http://dx.doi.org/10.1017/S1466252314000139

Escalera-Zamudio, M., Cobián-Güemes, G., de los Dolores Soto-del Río, M. et al. 2012. Characterization of an influenza A virus in Mexican swine that is related to the A/H1N1/2009 pandemic clade. *Virology*, 433, 176–182. DOI: http://dx.doi.org/10.1016/j.virol.2012.08.003

Eshel, G., Martin, P. 2006. Diet, energy, and global warming. *Earth Interactions*, 10, 1–17. DOI: http://dx.doi.org/10.1175/EI167.1

Eshel G., Martin, P. 2009. Geophysics and nutritional science: Toward a novel, unified paradigm. *American Journal of Clinical Nutrition*, 89S,1710S–1716S. DOI: http://dx.doi.org/10.3945/ajcn.2009.26736BB

European Commission. 2007. *Limiting global climate change to 2 degrees Celsius—The way ahead for 2020 and beyond*. 2007. Available at: http://eur-lex.europa.eu/LexUriServ/LexUriServ.do?uri=CELEX:52007DC0002: EN:NOT. (Accessed 26 August 2010.)

European Commission. 2011. *Food: from farm to fork statistics*. Luxembourg: Publications Office of the European Union.

European Commission. 2012. The Common Agricultural Policy. A partnership between Europe and farmers. Luxembourg: Publications Office of the European Union.

European Commission. 2015. Myths and facts. http://ec.europa.eu/budget/explained/myths/myths_en.cfm#9of15. (Accessed 15 February 2016.)

Fairlie, S. 2010. *Meat: A Benign Extravagance*. East Meon: Permanent Publications.

Farm Animal Welfare Council. 2009. *Farm animal welfare in Great Britain: Past, present and future*. London: Farm Animal Welfare Council. https://www.gov.uk/government/publications/fawc-report-on-farm-animal-welfare-in-great-britain-past-present-and-future (Accessed 15 January 2015.)

Farouk, M., Al-Mazeedi, H., Sabow, A. et al. 2014. Halal and Kosher slaughter methods and meat quality: A review. *Meat Science*, 98, 505–519. DOI: http://dx.doi.org/10.1016/j.meatsci.2014.05.021

Ferber, D. 2002. Livestock feed ban preserves drug's power. *Science*, 295, 27–28. DOI: http://dx.doi.org/10.1126/science.295.5552.27a

Fernandez-Duque, E., Valeggia, C., Maldonado, H. 1992. Multitrial inhibitory avoidance learning in the crab Chasmagnathus. *Behavioral and neural biology*, 57, 189–197. DOI: http://dx.doi.org/10.1016/0163-1047(92)90136-R

Feskanich, D., Weber, P., Willett, W. et al. 1999. Vitamin K intake and hip fractures in women: a prospective study. *American Journal of Clinical Nutrition*, 69, 74–79.

Feskanich D., Willett W., Colditz G. 2003. Calcium, vitamin D, milk consumption, and hip fractures: a prospective study among postmenopausal women. *American Journal of Clinical Nutrition*, 77, 504–511.

Fessler, D., Navarrete, C. 2003. Meat is good to taboo: Dietary proscriptions as a product of the interaction of psychological mechanisms and social processes. *Journal of Cognition and Culture*, 3, 1–40. DOI: http://dx.doi.org/10.1163/156853703321598563

Fetissenko, M. 2011. Beyond morality. Developing a new rhetorical strategy for the animal rights movement. *Journal of Animal Ethics*, 1, 150–175. DOI: http://dx.doi.org/10.5406/janimalethics.1.2.0150

Fey, P., Safranek, T., Rupp, M. et al. 2000. Ceftriaxone-resistant Salmonella infection acquired by a child from cattle. *New England Journal of Medicine*, 42, 1242–1249. DOI: http://dx.doi.org/10.1056/NEJM200004273421703

Fieldhouse, P. 1986. *Food and nutrition: Customs and culture.* London: Croom Helm.

Finks, S., Airee, A., Chow, S. et al. 2012. Key articles of dietary interventions that influence cardiovascular mortality. *Pharmacotherapy: The Journal of Human Pharmacology and Drug Therapy*, 32, e54–e87. DOI: http://dx.doi.org/10.1002/j.1875-9114.2011.01087.x

Finley, C., Barlow, C., Halton, T. et al. 2010. Glycemic index, glycemic load, and prevalence of the metabolic syndrome in the cooper center longitudinal study. *Journal of the American Dietetic Association*, 110, 1820–1829. DOI: http://dx.doi.org/10.1016/j.jada.2010.09.016

Fitzgerald, A. 2010. A social history of the slaughterhouse: From inception to contemporary implications. *Human Ecology Review*, 17, 58–69.

Foley, J. Ramankutty, N., Brauman, K. et al. 2011. Solutions for a cultivated planet. *Nature*, 478, 337–342. DOI: http://dx.doi.org/10.1038/nature10452

Fontana, L., Klein, S., Holloszy, J. 2006. Long-term low-protein, low-calorie diet and endurance exercise modulate metabolic factors associated with cancer risk. *American Journal of Clinical Nutrition*, 84, 1456–1462.

Food and Agriculture Organization of the United Nations. 2004. *What is agrobiodiversity?.* Rome: FAO. http://www.fao.org/docrep/007/y5609e/y5609e02.htm (Accessed 10 May 2016.)

Food and Agriculture Organization of the United Nations. 2014. *FAOSTAT online statistical service.* Rome, FAO. http://faostat.fao.org/ (Accessed 6 January 2015.)

Food and Agriculture Organization of the United Nations. 2015. *Food and Agriculture Organization of the United Nations Statistics Division.* http://faostat3.fao.org/home/E (Accessed 6 January 2015.)

Food and Agriculture Organization of the United Nations, World Health Organization, United Nations University. 2001. *Human energy requirements. Report of a joint Food and Agriculture Organization/World Health Organization/United Nations University Expert Consultation.* Rome: FAO.

Forster, P., Ramaswamy, V., Artaxo, P. et al. 2007. Changes in atmospheric constituents and in radiative forcing. In: S. Solomon, D. Qin, M. Manning et al. (eds.). *Climate change 2007: The physical science basis. Contribution of Working Group I to the Fourth Assessment Report of the Intergovernmental Panel on Climate Change.* Cambridge and New York: Cambridge University Press, 129–234.

Fox, N., Ward, K. 2008. Health, ethics and environment: A qualitative study of vegetarian motivations. *Appetite,* 50, 422–429. DOI: http://dx.doi.org/10.1016/j.appet.2007.09.007

Francione, G. 2008. *Animals as persons: Essays on the abolition of animal exploitation.* New York: Columbia University Press.

Francione, G. 2010a. The abolition of animal exploitation. In: G. Francione, R. Garner (eds.). *The animal rights debate: Abolition or regulation?* New York: Columbia University Press, 1–102.

Francione, G. 2010b. Animal welfare and the moral value of nonhuman animals. *Law, Culture and the Humanities,* 6, 24–36. DOI: http://dx.doi.org/10.1177/1743872109348989

Franklin, A. 1999. *Animals & modern cultures: A sociology of human-animal relations in modernity.* London: Sage.

Fredeen, A. 2006. Use of rbST and implications for cow health in the dairy industry. In: T. Morris, M. Keilty (eds.). *Alternative health practices for livestock,* Iowa: Blackwell, 164–170. DOI: http://dx.doi.org/10.1002/9780470384978.ch12

Friedrich, B. 2006. Effective advocacy. Stealing from the corporate playbook. In: P. Singer (ed.). *In defense of animals: The second wave,* Malden: Blackwell, 187–195.

Fung, T., Schulze, M., Manson, J. et al. 2004. Dietary patterns, meat intake, and the risk of type 2 diabetes in women. *Archives of Internal Medicine,* 164, 2235–2240. DOI: http://dx.doi.org/10.1001/archinte.164.20.2235

Fung, T., van Dam, R., Hankinson, S. et al. 2010. Low-carbohydrate diets and all-cause and cause-specific mortality: two cohort studies. *Annals of Internal Medicine,* 153, 289–298. DOI: http://dx.doi.org/10.7326/0003-4819-153-5-201009070-00003

Fürst, M., McMahon, D., Osborne, J. et al. 2014. Disease associations between honeybees and bumblebees as a threat to wild pollinators. *Nature,* 506, 364–366. DOI: http://dx.doi.org/10.1038/nature12977

Ganmaa, D., Sato, A. 2005. The possible role of female sex hormones in milk from pregnant cows in the development of breast, ovarian and corpus uteri cancers. *Medical Hypotheses,* 65, 1028–1037. DOI: http://dx.doi.org/10.1016/j.mehy.2005.06.026

Garcia-Graells, C., Antoine, J., Larsen, J. et al. 2012. Livestock veterinarians at high risk of acquiring methicillin-resistant Staphylococcus aureus ST398. *Epidemiology and infection*, 140, 383–389. DOI: http://dx.doi.org/10.1017/S0950268811002263

Garcia-Migura, L., Pleydell, E., Barnes, S. et al. 2005. Characterization of vancomycin-resistant Enterococcus faecium from broiler poulty and pig farms in England and Wales. *Clinical Microbiology*, 43, 3283–3289. DOI: http://dx.doi.org/10.1128/JCM.43.7.3283-3289.2005

Gardiner, S. 2001. The real tragedy of the commons. *Philosophy and Public Affairs*, 30, 387–416. DOI: http://dx.doi.org/10.1111/j.1088-4963.2001.00387.x

Garnett, T. 2008. *Cooking up a storm: Food, greenhouse gas emissions and our changing climate*. University of Surrey: Food Climate Research Network, Centre for Environmental Strategy.

Garnett, T. 2009. Livestock-related greenhouse gas emissions: Impacts and options for policy makers. *Environmental Science and Policy*, 12, 491–503. DOI: http://dx.doi.org/10.1016/j.envsci.2009.01.006

Gear, J., Fursdon, P., Nolan, D. et al. 1979. Symptomless diverticular disease and intake of dietary fiber. *Lancet*, 313, 511–514. DOI: http://dx.doi.org/10.1016/S0140-6736(79)90942-5

Geppert, J., Kraft, V., Demmelmair, H. et al. 2005. Docosahexaenoic acid supplementation in vegetarians effectively increases omega-3 index: a randomized trial. *Lipids*, 40, 807–814. DOI: http://dx.doi.org/10.1007/s11745-005-1442-9

Gerbens-Leenes, P., Nonhebel, S., Ivens, W. 2002. A method to determine land requirements relating to food consumption patterns. *Agriculture Ecosystems and Environment*, 90, 47–58. DOI: http://dx.doi.org/10.1016/S0167-8809(01)00169-4

Gerber, P., Steinfeld, H., Henderson, B., et al. 2013. *Tackling climate change through livestock – A global assessment of emissions and mitigation opportunities*. Rome: FAO.

Gibbs, H., Ruesch, A., Achard, F. et al. 2010. Tropical forests were the primary sources of new agricultural land in the 1980s and 1990s. *Proceedings of the National Academy of Sciences*, 107, 16732–16737. DOI: http://dx.doi.org/10.1073/pnas.0910275107

Gilbert, M., Bos, M., Duim, B. et al. 2012. Livestock-associated MRSA ST398 carriage in pig slaughterhouse workers related to quantitative environmental exposure. *Occupational and Environmental Medicine*, 69, 472–478. DOI: http://dx.doi.org/10.1136/oemed-2011-100069

Gill, M., Smith, P., Wilkinson, J. 2010. Mitigating climate change: the role of domestic livestock. *Animal*, 4, 323–333. DOI: http://dx.doi.org/10.1017/S1751731109004662

Giovanni, G. 2009. A diet for dopaminergic neurons?. Birth, life and death of dopaminergic neurons in the substantia nigra. *Journal of Neural Transmission. Supplementa*, 73, 317–331.

Gjerris, M., Gamborg, C., Röcklingsberg, H. 2011. The price of responsibility: Ethics of animal husbandry in a time of climate change. *Journal of Agricultural and Environmental Ethics*, 24, 331–350. DOI: http://dx.doi.org/10.1007/s10806-010-9270-6

Global Environmental Change and Human Health. 2007. *Science plan and implementation strategy. Earth system science partnership (DIVERSITAS, IGBP, IHDP, and WCRP) report no.4; Global environmental change and human health report no.1.* http://www.gechh.unu.edu/FINAL_GECHH_SP_UPDATED.pdf (Accessed 26 December 2012.)

Goldburg, R., Naylor, R. 2005. Future seascapes, fishing, and fish farming. *Frontiers in Ecology and the Environment*, 3, 21–28. DOI: http://dx.doi.org/10.1890/1540-9295(2005)003[0021:FSFAFF]2.0.CO;2

González, A., Frostell, B., Carlsson-Kanyama, A. 2011. Protein efficiency per unit energy and per unit greenhouse gas emissions: Potential contribution of diet choices to climate change mitigation. *Food Policy*, 36, 562–570. DOI: http://dx.doi.org/10.1016/j.foodpol.2011.07.003

Gonzalez, C., Riboli, E. 2006. Diet and cancer prevention: where we are, where we are going. *Nutrition and cancer*, 56, 225–231. DOI: http://dx.doi.org/10.1207/s15327914nc5602_14

Goodland, R. 1997. Environmental sustainability in agriculture: Diet matters. *Ecological Economics*, 23, 189–200. DOI: http://dx.doi.org/10.1016/S0921-8009(97)00579-X

Goodland, R., Pimentel, D. 2000. Sustainability and integrity in the agriculture sector. In: D. Pimentel, L. Westra, R. Noss (eds.). *Ecological integrity: Integrating environment, conservation and health*. Washington DC: Island Press, 121–137.

Goodland, R., Anhang, J. 2009. Livestock and climate change. What if the key actors in climate change are … cows, pigs, and chickens? *WorldWatch*, November/December, 10–19.

Goodland, R., Anhang, J. 2012. Comment to the editor. Livestock and greenhouse gas emissions. The importance of getting the numbers right, by Herrero et al. [Anim. Feed Sci. Technol.166–167, 779–782]. *Animal Feed Science and Technology*, 172, 252–256. DOI: http://dx.doi.org/10.1016/j.anifeedsci.2011.12.028

Gorringe, T. 2011. Rise Peter! Kill and eat: A response to John Barclay. *The Expository Times*, 123, 63–69. DOI: http://dx.doi.org/10.1177/0014524611418576

Goulson, D. 2003. Effects of introduced bees on native ecosystems. *Annual Review of Ecology, Evolution, and Systematics*, 34, 1–26. DOI: http://dx.doi.org/10.1146/annurev.ecolsys.34.011802.132355

Goulson, D., Sparrow, K. 2009. Evidence for competition between honeybees and bumblebees; effects on bumblebee worker size. *Journal of Insect Conservation*, 13, 177–181. DOI: http://dx.doi.org/10.1007/s10841-008-9140-y

Grace, D. 2015. Zoonoses of poverty: Measuring and managing the multiple burdens of zoonoses and poverty. In: A. Sing (ed.). *Zoonoses-Infections affecting humans and animals.* Dordrecht: Springer, 1127–1137. DOI: http://dx.doi.org/10.1007/978-94-017-9457-2_46

Graham, D., Knapp, C., Christensen, B. et al. 2016. Appearance of β-lactam resistance genes in agricultural soils and clinical isolates over the 20th century. *Scientific Reports,* 6, 21550; DOI: http://dx.doi.org/10.1038/srep21550

Grandin, T. 2014. *Recommended captive bolt stunning techniques for cattle.* http://www.grandin.com/humane/cap.bolt.tips.html (Accessed 10 May 2016).

Gray, C., Sellon, R., Freeman, L. 2004. Nutritional adequacy of two vegan diets for cats. *Journal of the American Veterinary Medical Association,* 225, 1670–1675. DOI: http://dx.doi.org/10.2460/javma.2004.225.1670

Griffin, D. 1998. *Unsnarling the world-knot: Consciousness, freedom, and the mind-body problem.* Berkeley: University of California Press.

Gruen, L. 2011. *Ethics and animals: An introduction.* Cambridge: Cambridge University Press. DOI: http://dx.doi.org/10.1017/CBO9780511976162

Gu, Y., Nieves, J., Stern, Y. et al. 2010. Food combination and Alzheimer disease risk: A protective diet. *Archives of Neurology,* 67, 699–706. DOI: http://dx.doi.org/10.1001/archneurol.2010.84

Gundersen, A. 1995. *The environmental promise of democratic deliberation.* Wisconsin: University of Wisconsin Press.

Gunderson, R. 2012. Meat and inequality: Environmental health consequences of livestock agribusiness. *Environmental Justice,* 5, 54–58. DOI: http://dx.doi.org/10.1089/env.2011.0010

Gutjahr, J. 2013. The reintegration of animals and slaughter into discourses of meat eating. In: H. Röcklinsberg, P. Sandin (eds.). *The ethics of consumption.* Wageningen: Wageningen Academic Publishers, 379–385. DOI: http://dx.doi.org/10.3920/978-90-8686-784-4_61

Haddad, E., Berk, L., Kettering, J. et al. 1999. Dietary intake and biochemical, hematologic, and immune status of vegans compared with nonvegetarians. *American Journal of Clinical Nutrition,* 70S, 586S–593S.

Hallberg, L., Rossander, L. 1982. Effect of different drinks on the absorption of non-heme iron from composite meals. *Human nutrition. Applied nutrition,* 36, 116.

Hallström, E., Carlsson-Kanyama, A., Börjesson, P. 2015. Environmental impact of dietary change: a systematic review. *Journal of Cleaner Production,* 91, 1–11. DOI: http://dx.doi.org/10.1016/j.jclepro.2014.12.008

Hanlon, P., McCartney, G. 2008. Peak oil: Will it be public health's greatest challenge? *Public Health,* 122, 647–652. DOI: http://dx.doi.org/10.1016/j.puhe.2008.03.020

Hardin, G. 1968. The tragedy of the commons. *Science,* 162, 1243–1248. DOI: http://dx.doi.org/10.1126/science.162.3859.1243

Hartshorne, C. 1972. The compound individual. In: C. Hartshorne (ed.). *Whitehead's Philosophy. Selected Essays, 1935-1970.* Lincoln: University of Nebraska Press, 41–46.

Hawthorne, M. 2013. *Bleating Hearts: The Hidden World of Animal Suffering.* Winchester: Changemakers Books.

Haya, K., Burridge, L., Chang, B. 2001. Environmental impact of chemical wastes produced by the salmon aquaculture industry. *Journal of Marine Science*, 58, 492–496. DOI: http://dx.doi.org/10.1006/jmsc.2000.1034

Haynes, R. 2008. *Animal welfare: competing conceptions and their ethical implications.* Dordrecht: Springer Science & Business Media. DOI: http://dx.doi.org/10.1007/978-1-4020-8619-9

He, F., Nowson, C., MacGregor, G. 2006. Fruit and vegetable consumption and stroke: meta-analysis of cohort studies. *Lancet*, 367, 320–326. DOI: http://dx.doi.org/10.1016/S0140-6736(06)68069-0, DOI: http://dx.doi.org/10.1016/S0140-6736(06)68731-X

Heaton, R., Randerson, P., Slater, F. 1999. The economics of growing short rotation coppice in the uplands of mid-Wales and an economic comparison with sheep production. *Biomass and Bioenergy*, 17, 59–71. DOI: http://dx.doi.org/10.1016/S0961-9534(99)00025-2

Hendrickson, M., James, H., Hefferman, W. 2008. Does the world need U.S. farmers even if Americans don't? *Journal of Agricultural and Environmental Ethics*, 21, 311–328. DOI: http://dx.doi.org/10.1007/s10806-008-9092-y

Hermans, D., Pasmans, F., Messens, W. et al. 2012. Poultry as a host for the zoonotic pathogen Campylobacter jejuni. *Vector-Borne and Zoonotic Diseases*, 12, 89–98. DOI: http://dx.doi.org/10.1089/vbz.2011.0676

Herrero, M., Gerber, P., Vellinga, T. et al. 2011. Livestock and greenhouse gas emissions: the importance of getting the numbers right. *Animal Feed Science and Technology*, 166–167, 779–782. DOI: http://dx.doi.org/10.1016/j.anifeedsci.2011.04.083

Hessler, K., Buchanan, A. 2002. Specifying the content of the human right to health care. In: R. Rhodes, R., Battin, M., Silvers, A. (eds.). *Medicine and Social Justice. Essays on the Distribution of Health Care*, Oxford: Oxford University Press, 84–96.

Hills, A. 2005. *Do animals have rights?* Cambridge: Icon Books.

Hindle, V., Lambooij, E., Reimert, H. et al. 2010. Animal welfare concerns during the use of the water bath for stunning broilers, hens, and ducks. *Poultry science*, 89, 401–412. DOI: http://dx.doi.org/10.3382/ps.2009-00297

Hocquette, A., Lambert, C., Sinquin, C. et al. 2015. Educated consumers don't believe artificial meat is the solution to the problems with the meat industry. *Journal of Integrative Agriculture*, 14, 273–284. DOI: http://dx.doi.org/10.1016/S2095-3119(14)60886-8

Hoedt, E., Evans, P., Denman, S. et al. 2015. Methane matters in animals and man: from beginning to end. *Microbiology Australia*, 36, 4–7. DOI: http://dx.doi.org/10.1071/MA15003

Hoekstra, A., Chapagain, A. 2007. Water footprints of nations: Water use by people as a function of their consumption pattern. *Water Resources Management*, 21, 35–48. DOI: http://dx.doi.org/10.1007/s11269-006-9039-x

Hoffman, L., Wiklund, E. 2006. Game and venison—Meat for the modern consumer. *Meat Science*, 74, 197–208. DOI: http://dx.doi.org/10.1016/j.meatsci.2006.04.005

Holick, M. 2007. Vitamin D deficiency. *New England Journal of Medicine*, 357, 266–281. DOI: http://dx.doi.org/10.1056/NEJMra070553

Holick, M., Biancuzzo, R., Chen, T. et al. 2008. Vitamin D2 Is as Effective as Vitamin D3 in Maintaining Circulating Concentrations of 25-Hydroxyvitamin D. *The Journal of Clinical Endocrinology and Metabolism*, 93, 677–681. DOI: http://dx.doi.org/10.1210/jc.2007-2308

Ho-Pham, L., Vu, B., Lai, T. et al. 2012. Vegetarianism, bone loss, fracture and vitamin D: a longitudinal study in Asian vegans and non-vegans. *European Journal of Clinical Nutrition*, 66, 75–82. DOI: http://dx.doi.org/10.1038/ejcn.2011.131

Hoppe, C., Molgaard, C., Michaelsen, K. 2006. Cow's milk and linear growth in industrialized and developing countries. *Annual Review of Nutrition*, 26, 131–173. DOI: http://dx.doi.org/10.1146/annurev.nutr.26.010506.103757

Hotchkiss, A., Rider, C., Blystone, C. et al. 2008. Fifteen years after 'Wingspread'—Environmental endocrine disruptors and human and wildlife health: Where we are today and where we need to go. *Toxicological Sciences*, 105, 235–259. DOI: http://dx.doi.org/10.1093/toxsci/kfn030

Hristov, A. 2012. Historic, pre-European settlement, and present-day contribution of wild ruminants to enteric methane emissions in the United States. *Journal of Animal Science*, 90, 1371–1375. DOI: http://dx.doi.org/10.2527/jas.2011-4539

Hu, F. 2003. Plant-based foods and prevention of cardiovascular disease: an overview. *The American Journal of Clinical Nutrition*, 78, 544S–551S.

Huang, J., Pray, C., Rozelle, S. 2002. Enhancing the crops to feed the poor. *Nature*, 418, 678–684. DOI: http://dx.doi.org/10.1038/nature01015

Huang, T., Yang, B., Zheng, J. et al. 2012. Cardiovascular disease mortality and cancer incidence in vegetarians: A meta-analysis and systematic review. *Annals of Nutrition and Metabolism*, 60, 233–240. DOI: http://dx.doi.org/10.1159/000337301

Huijsdens, X., van Dijke, B., Spalburg, E. et al. 2006. Community-acquired MRSA and pig farming. *Annals of Clinical Microbiology and Antimicrobials*, 5, 26–29. DOI: http://dx.doi.org/10.1186/1476-0711-5-26

Hume, D. 1978. *A treatise of human nature* (Second edition edited by L.A. Selby-Bigge). Oxford: Clarendon Press.

Huncharek, M., Muscat, J., Kupelnick, B. 2008. Dairy products, dietary calcium and vitamin D intake as risk factors for prostate cancer: A meta-analysis of 26,769 cases from 45 observational studies. *Nutrition and Cancer*, 60, 421–441. DOI: http://dx.doi.org/10.1080/01635580801911779

Hunt, J., Roughead, Z. 1999. Nonheme-iron absorption, fecal ferritin excretion, and blood indexes of iron status in women consuming controlled lactoovovegetarian diets for 8 wk. *American Journal of Clinical Nutrition*, 69, 944–952.

Hunt, J., Roughead, Z. 2000. Adaptation of iron absorption in men consuming diets with high or low iron bioavailability. *American Journal of Clinical Nutrition*, 71, 94–102.

Iannotti, L., Lutter, C., Bunn, D. et al. 2014. Eggs: the uncracked potential for improving maternal and young child nutrition among the world's poor. *Nutrition Reviews*, 72, 355–368. DOI: http://dx.doi.org/10.1111/nure.12107

Intergovernmental Panel on Climate Change. 2007a. *Climate change 2007: Synthesis report. Summary for policymakers*. http://www.ipcc.ch/pdf/ assessment-report/ar4/syr/ar4_syr_spm.pdf (Accessed 10 February 2013.)

Intergovernmental Panel on Climate Change. 2007b. *Climate change 2007: Synthesis report. Contribution of working groups I, II, and III to the Fourth Assessment Report of the Intergovernmental Panel on Climate Change*. [Core writing team: Pachauri, R. and Reisinger, A., (eds.)]. Geneva: Intergovernmental Panel on Climate Change.

Issatt, E. 2013. AquAdvantage or disadvantage: social and legal pros and cons of genetically modified fish. In: H. Röcklingsberg, P. Sandin (eds.). *The ethics of consumption*. Wageningen: Wageningen Academic Publishers, 299–304. DOI: http://dx.doi.org/10.3920/978-90-8686-784-4_48

Jamieson, D. 1990. Method and moral theory. In: P. Singer (ed.). *A companion to ethics*. Oxford: Blackwell, 476–487.

Janson, C. 2004. The effect of passive smoking on respiratory health in children and adults. *International Journal of Tuberculosis and Lung Disease*, 8, 510–516.

Jenkins, D., Wolever, T., Taylor, R. et al. 1981. Glycemic index of foods: a physiological basis for carbohydrate exchange. *American Journal of Clinical Nutrition*, 34, 362–366.

Jenkins D., Popovich D., Kendall C. et al. 1997. Effect of a diet high in vegetables, fruit, and nuts on serum lipids. *Metabolism* 46, 530–537. DOI: http:// dx.doi.org/10.1016/S0026-0495(97)90190-6

Jenkins D., Kendall C., Popovich D. et al. 2001. Effect of a very-high-fiber vegetable, fruit, and nut diet on serum lipids and colonic function. *Metabolism*, 50, 494–503. DOI: http://dx.doi.org/10.1053/meta.2001.21037

Jenkins, D., Kendall, C., Faulkner, D. et al. 2006. Assessment of the longer-term effects of a dietary portfolio of cholesterol-lowering foods in hypercholesterolemia. *American Journal of Clinical Nutrition*, 83, 582–591.

Jepson, J. 2008. A linguistic analysis of discourse on the killing of nonhuman animals. *Society and Animals*, 16, 127–148. DOI: http://dx.doi. org/10.1163/156853008X291426

Jha, A. 2013. First lab-grown hamburger gets full marks for 'mouth feel'. *The Guardian* (6 August). http://www.theguardian.com/science/2013/aug/05/ world-first-synthetic-hamburger-mouth-feel (Accessed 16 September 2015).

Joy, M. 2010. *Why we love dogs eat pigs and wear cows. An introduction to carnism*. San Francisco: Conari Press.

Joyce, A., Dixon, S., Comfort, J. et al. 2008. The cow in the room: public knowledge of the links between dietary choices and health and environmental impacts. *Environmental Health Insights*, 1, 31–34.

Juntti, H., Tikkanen, S., Kokkonen, J. et al. 1999. Cow's milk allergy is associated with recurrent otitis media during childhood. *Acta oto-laryngologica*, 119, 867–873. DOI: http://dx.doi.org/10.1080/00016489950180199

Kahleova, H., Pelikanova, T. 2015. Vegetarian diets in the prevention and treatment of type 2 diabetes. *Journal of the American College of Nutrition*, (ahead-of-print), 1–11.

Kalof, L., Dietz, T., Stern, P. et al. 1999. Social psychological and structural influences on vegetarian beliefs. *Rural Sociology*, 64, 500–511. DOI: http://dx.doi.org/10.1111/j.1549-0831.1999.tb00364.x

Kanaly, R., Manzanero, L., Macer, D. et al. 2009. *Energy flow, environment and ethical implications for meat production. Ethics and climate change in Asia and the Pacific (ECCAP) project, RUSHSAP*. Bangkok: UNESCO.

Kannus, P., Parkkari, J., Sievanen, H. et al. 1996. Epidemiology of hip fractures. *Bone*, 18S, 57S–63S. DOI: http://dx.doi.org/10.1016/8756-3282(95)00381-9

Karesh, W., Dobson, A., Lloyd-Smith, J. et al. 2012. Ecology of zoonoses: natural and unnatural histories. *Lancet*, 380, 1936–1945. DOI: http://dx.doi.org/10.1016/S0140-6736(12)61678-X

Kart, A., Bilgili, A. 2008. Ionophore antibiotics: toxicity, mode of action and neurotoxic aspect of carboxylic ionophores. *Journal of Animal and Veterinary Advances*, 7, 748–751.

Kasturirangan, R., Srinivasan K., Rao, S. 2014. Dark and dairy. *The Hindu*, (9 November).

Katan, M. 2009. Nitrate in foods: harmful or healthy? *American Journal of Clinical Nutrition*, 90, 11–12. DOI: http://dx.doi.org/10.3945/ajcn.2009.28014

Katan, M., Grundy, S., Jones, P. 2003. Efficacy and safety of plant stanols and sterols in the management of blood cholesterol levels. *Mayo Clinic Proceedings*, 78, 965–978. DOI: http://dx.doi.org/10.1016/S0025-6196(11)63144-3

Kawai, N., Kono, R., Sugimoto, S. 2004. Avoidance learning in the crayfish (Procambarus clarkii) depends on the predatory imminence of the unconditioned stimulus: a behavior systems approach to learning in invertebrates. *Behavioural Brain Research*, 150, 229–237. DOI: http://dx.doi.org/10.1016/S0166-4328(03)00261-4

Ka-Wai Hui, E. 2006. Reasons for the increase in emerging and re-emerging viral infectious diseases. *Microbes and infection*, 8, 905–916. DOI: http://dx.doi.org/10.1016/j.micinf.2005.06.032

Kearney, J., McElhone, S. 1999. Perceived barriers in trying to eat healthier—results of a pan-EU consumer attitudinal survey. *British Journal of Nutrition*, 81S, S133–S137. DOI: http://dx.doi.org/10.1017/S0007114599000987

Kearney, M., Kearney, J., Dunne, A. et al. 2000. Sociodemographic determinants of perceived influences on food choice in a nationally representative sample of Irish adults. *Public Health Nutrition*, 3, 219–226. DOI: http://dx.doi.org/10.1017/S1368980000000252

Kenyon, P., Barker, M. 1998. Attitudes towards meat-eating in vegetarian and non-vegetarian teenage girls in England—an ethnographic approach. *Appetite*, 30, 185–198. DOI: http://dx.doi.org/10.1006/appe.1997.0129

Key, T., Fraser, G., Thorogood, M. et al. 1999. Mortality in vegetarians and non-vegetarians: detailed findings from a collaborative analysis of 5 prospective studies. *American Journal of Clinical Nutrition*, 70(S), 516S–524S.

Key, T., Appleby, P., Rosell, M. 2006. Health effects of vegetarian and vegan diets. *Proceedings of the Nutrition Society*, 65, 35–41. DOI: http://dx.doi.org/10.1079/PNS2005481

Key, T., Appleby, P., Spencer, E. et al. 2009a. Cancer incidence in British vegetarians. *British Journal of Cancer*, 101, 192–197. DOI: http://dx.doi.org/10.1038/sj.bjc.6605098

Key, T., Appleby, P., Spencer, E. et al. 2009b. Mortality in British vegetarians: Results from the European Prospective Investigation into Cancer and Nutrition (EPIC-Oxford). *American Journal of Clinical Nutrition*, 89S,1613S–1619S. DOI: http://dx.doi.org/10.3945/ajcn.2009.26736L

Key, T., Appleby, P., Crowe, F. et al. 2014. Cancer in British vegetarians: updated analyses of 4998 incident cancers in a cohort of 32,491 meat eaters, 8612 fish eaters, 18,298 vegetarians, and 2246 vegans. *American Journal of Clinical Nutrition*, 100 S1, 378S–385S. DOI: http://dx.doi.org/10.3945/ajcn.113.071266

Keys, A. 1995. Mediterranean diet and public health: personal reflections. *American Journal of Clinical Nutrition*, 61S, 1321S–1323S.

Kheel, M. 2008. *Nature ethics. An ecofeminist perspective.* Lanham: Rowman & Littlefield.

Kirchmann, H., Thorvaldsson, G. 2000. Challenging targets for future agriculture. *European Journal of Agronomy*, 12, 145–161. DOI: http://dx.doi.org/10.1016/S1161-0301(99)00053-2

Kitzes, J., Wackernagel, M. 2009. Answers to common questions in ecological footprint accounting. *Ecological Indicators*, 9, 812–817. DOI: http://dx.doi.org/10.1016/j.ecolind.2008.09.014

Klimas, T., Vaiciukaite, J. 2008. Law of recitals in European Community legislation, *ILSA Journal of International & Comparative Law*, 15, 1–33.

Knight, A. 2011. *The costs and benefits of animal experiments.* New York: Palgrave Macmillan. DOI: http://dx.doi.org/10.1057/9780230306417

Knight, D., Ellio, W., Anderson, J. et al. 1992. The role of earthworms in managed permanent pastures in Devon, England. *Soil Biology and Biochemistry*, 24, 1511–1517. DOI: http://dx.doi.org/10.1016/0038-0717(92)90142-K

Knight, S., Vrij, A., Bard, K. et al. 2009. Science versus human welfare? Understanding attitudes toward animal use. *Journal of Social Issues*, 65, 463–483. DOI: http://dx.doi.org/10.1111/j.1540-4560.2009.01609.x

Koller, V., Fürhacker, M., Nersesyan, A. et al. 2012. Cytotoxic and DNA-damaging properties of glyphosate and Roundup in human-derived buccal epithelial cells. *Archives of Toxicology*, 86, 805–813. DOI: http://dx.doi.org/10.1007/s00204-012-0804-8

Korthals, M. 2012. Emotions, truths and meanings regarding cattle: Should we eat meat?. *Journal of Agricultural and Environmental Ethics*, 25, 625–629. DOI: http://dx.doi.org/10.1007/s10806-011-9334-2

Korzen, S., Sandøe, P., Lassen, J. 2011. Pure meat—Public perceptions of risk reduction strategies in meat production. *Food Policy*, 36, 158–165. DOI: http://dx.doi.org/10.1016/j.foodpol.2010.10.005

Kristensen, T. 1991. Sickness absence and work strain among Danish slaughterhouse workers: an analysis of absence from work regarded as coping behaviour. *Social Science & Medicine*, 32, 15–27. DOI: http://dx.doi.org/10.1016/0277-9536(91)90122-S

Laestadius, L. 2015. Public perceptions of the ethics of in-vitro meat: Determining an appropriate course of action. *Journal of Agricultural and Environmental Ethics*, 28, 991–1009. DOI: http://dx.doi.org/10.1007/s10806-015-9573-8

Laestadius, L., Caldwell, M. 2015. Is the future of meat palatable? Perceptions of in vitro meat as evidenced by online news comments. *Public Health Nutrition*, 18, 2457–2467. DOI: http://dx.doi.org/10.1017/S1368980015000622

Lakoff, G. 2004. *Don't think of an elephant! Know your values and frame the debate*. White River Junction: Chelsea Green Publishing.

Lal, R. 2009. Soil degradation as a reason for inadequate human nutrition. *Food Security*, 1, 45–57. DOI: http://dx.doi.org/10.1007/s12571-009-0009-z

Lamey, A. 2007. Food fight! Davis versus Regan on the ethics of eating beef. *Journal of Social Philosophy*, 38, 331–348. DOI: http://dx.doi.org/10.1111/j.1467-9833.2007.00382.x

Lang, T., Heasman, M. 2004. *Food wars. The global battle for mouths, minds, and markets*. London: Earthscan.

Lanou, A. 2009. Should dairy be recommended as part of a healthy vegetarian diet? Counterpoint. *American Journal of Clinical Nutrition*, 89S, 1638S–1642S. DOI: http://dx.doi.org/10.3945/ajcn.2009.26736P

Larsson, S., Orsini, N., Wolk, A. 2006. Milk, milk products and lactose intake and ovarian cancer risk: A meta-analysis of epidemiological studies, *International Journal of Cancer*, 118, 431–441. DOI: http://dx.doi.org/10.1002/ijc.21305

Lautensach, A. 2015. Sustainable health for all? The tension between human security and the right to health care. *Journal of Human Security*, 11, 5–18. DOI: http://dx.doi.org/10.12924/johs2015.11010005

Lay, D., Fulton, R., Hester, P. et al. 2011. Hen welfare in different housing systems. *Poultry Science*, 90, 278–294. DOI: http://dx.doi.org/10.3382/ps.2010-00962

Lea, E., Worsley, A. 2003. Benefits and barriers to the consumption of a vegetarian diet in Australia. *Public Health Nutrition*, 6, 505–511. DOI: http://dx.doi.org/10.1079/PHN2002452

Lea, E., Crawford, D., Worsley, A. 2006a. Consumers' readiness to eat a plant-based diet. *European Journal of Clinical Nutrition*, 60, 342–351. DOI: http://dx.doi.org/10.1038/sj.ejcn.1602320

Lea, E., Crawford, D., Worsley, A. 2006b. Public views of the benefits and barriers to the consumption of a plant-based diet. *European Journal of Clinical Nutrition*, 60, 828–837. DOI: http://dx.doi.org/10.1038/sj.ejcn.1602387

Legge, J. 1969. Learning to be a dutiful carnivore. *The British Vegetarian*, Jan/Feb, 59.

Lempainen, J., Tauriainen, S., Vaarala, O. et al. 2012. Interaction of enterovirus infection and cow's milk-based formula nutrition in type 1 diabetes-associated autoimmunity. *Diabetes/Metabolism Research and Reviews*, 28, 177–185. DOI: http://dx.doi.org/10.1002/dmrr.1294

Leonard, W. 2014. The global diversity of eating patterns: Human nutritional health in comparative perspective. *Physiology & Behavior*, 134, 5–14. DOI: http://dx.doi.org/10.1016/j.physbeh.2014.02.050

Lerner, H., Algers, B. 2013. Tail docking in the EU: a case of routine violation of an EU Directive. In: H. Röcklingsberg, P. Sandin (eds.). *The ethics of consumption*. Wageningen: Wageningen Academic Publishers, 374–378. DOI: http://dx.doi.org/10.3920/978-90-8686-784-4_60

Leung, A., LaMar, A., Xuemei, H. et al. 2011. Iodine status and thyroid function of Boston-area vegetarians and vegans. *Journal of Clinical Endocrinology and Metabolism*, 96, e1303–e1307. DOI: http://dx.doi.org/10.1210/jc.2011-0256

Levy, S., FitzGerald, G., Macone, A. 1976. Changes in intestinal flora of farm personnel after introduction of a tetracycline-supplemented feed on a farm. *New England Journal of Medicine*, 295, 583–588. DOI: http://dx.doi.org/10.1056/NEJM197609092951103

Lewens, T. 2012. Species, essence and explanation. *Studies in History and Philosophy of Science Part C: Studies in History and Philosophy of Biological and Biomedical Sciences*, 43, 751–757.

Lewis, S. 1994. An opinion on the global impact of meat consumption. *American Journal of Clinical Nutrition*, 59S, 1099S–1102S. DOI: http://dx.doi.org/10.1016/j.shpsc.2012.09.013

Li, D. 2011. Chemistry behind vegetarianism. *Journal of Agricultural and Food Chemistry*, 59, 777–784. DOI: http://dx.doi.org/10.1021/jf103846u

Lightowler, H. 2009. Assessment of iodine intake and iodine status in vegans. In: V. Preedy, G. Burrow, R. Watson. *Comprehensive handbook of iodine: nutritional, biochemical, pathological and therapeutic aspects*. Burlington: Academic Press, 429–436. DOI: http://dx.doi.org/10.1016/B978-0-12-374135-6.00045-5

Lin, O., Soon, M., Wu, S. et al. 2000. Dietary habits and right-sided colonic diverticulosis. *Diseases of the Colon & Rectum*, 43, 1412–1418. DOI: http://dx.doi.org/10.1007/BF02236638

Lindeberg, S., Eliasson, M., Lindahl, B. et al. 1999. Low serum insulin in traditional Pacific Islanders - The Kitava study. *Metabolism*, 48, 1216–1219. DOI: http://dx.doi.org/10.1016/S0026-0495(99)90258-5

Lindeberg, S., Jönsson, T., Granfeldt, Y. et al. 2007. A palaeolithic diet improves glucose tolerance more than a mediterranean-like diet in individuals with ischaemic heart disease. *Diabetologia*, 50, 1795–1807. DOI: http://dx.doi.org/10.1007/s00125-007-0716-y

Lines, J., Jones, T., Berry, P. et al. 2011. Evaluation of a breast support conveyor to improve poultry welfare on the shackle line. *Veterinary Record*, 168, 129. DOI: http://dx.doi.org/10.1136/vr.c5431

Lipton, M. 2001. Challenges to meet: food and nutrition security in the new millennium. *Proceedings of the Nutrition Society*, 60, 203–214. DOI: http://dx.doi.org/10.1079/PNS200084

Liu, S., Stampfer, M., Hu F. et al. 1999. Wholegrain consumption and risk of coronary heart disease: results from the nurses' health study. *American Journal of Clinical Nutrition*, 70, 412–419.

Liu, S., Willett, W., Stampfer, M. et al. 2000. A prospective study of dietary glycemic load, carbohydrate intake, and risk of coronary heart disease in U.S. women. *American Journal of Clinical Nutrition*, 71, 1455–1461.

Llorente, R. 2009. The moral framework of Peter Singer's Animal Liberation: An alternative to utilitarianism. *Ethical Perspectives*, 16, 61–80. DOI: http://dx.doi.org/10.2143/EP.16.1.2036278

Lloyd-Williams, F., O'Flaherty, M., Mwatsama, M. et al. 2008. Estimating the cardiovascular mortality burden attributable to the European Common Agricultural Policy on dietary saturated fats. *Bulletin of the World Health Organization*, 86, 535–541. DOI: http://dx.doi.org/10.2471/BLT.08.053728

Lock, K., Pomerleau, J. 2005. *Fruit and vegetable policy in the European Union: Its effects on the burden of cardiovascular disease*. Brussels: European Heart Network.

Lönnerdal, B. 2000. Dietary factors influencing zinc absorption. *Journal of Nutrition*, 130S, 1378S–1383S.

Loughnan, D. 2012. *Food shock: The truth about what we put on our plate—and what we can do to change it*. Wollombi, NSW: Exisle Publishing.

Ludwig, D. 2002. The glycemic index. Physiological mechanisms relating to obesity, diabetes, and cardiovascular disease. *JAMA: The Journal of the American Medical Association*, 287, 2414–2423. DOI: http://dx.doi.org/10.1001/jama.287.18.2414

Ma, G., Jin, Y., Piao, J. et al. 2005. Phytate, calcium, iron, and zinc contents and their molar ratios in foods commonly consumed in China. *Journal of Agricultural and Food Chemistry*, 53, 10285–10290. DOI: http://dx.doi.org/10.1021/jf052051r

Macdiarmid, J., Kyle, J., Horgan, G. et al. 2012. Sustainable diets for the future: can we contribute to reducing greenhouse gas emissions by eating a healthy diet?. *American Journal of Clinical Nutrition*, 96, 632–639. DOI: http://dx.doi.org/10.3945/ajcn.112.038729

MacDonald, M., Simon, J. 2011. *Cattle, soyanization, and climate change. Brazil's agricultural revolution*. New York: Brighter Green.

Macnaghten, P. 2004. Animals in their nature: A case study on public attitudes to animals, genetic modification, and 'nature'. *Sociology*, 38, 533–551. DOI: http://dx.doi.org/10.1177/0038038504043217

Majchrzak, D., Singer, I., Männer, M. et al. 2006. B-vitamin status and concentrations of homocysteine in Austrian omnivores, vegetarians and vegans. *Annals of Nutrition and Metabolism*, 50, 485–491. DOI: http://dx.doi.org/10.1159/000095828

Mancilla, A. 2009. Nonhuman animals in Adam Smith's moral theory. *Between the Species*, 13, 1–18. DOI: http://dx.doi.org/10.15368/bts.2009v13n9.2

Mann, N. 2000. Dietary lean red meat and human evolution. *European Journal of Nutrition*, 39, 71–79. DOI: http://dx.doi.org/10.1007/s003940050005

Manousos, O., Day, N., Tzonou, A. et al. 1985. Diet and other factors in the aetiology of diverticulosis: an epidemiological study in Greece. *Gut*, 26, 544–549. DOI: http://dx.doi.org/10.1136/gut.26.6.544

Marcus, E. 2001. *Vegan: The new ethics of eating*. Ithaca: McBooks Press.

Marlow, H., Hayes, W., Soret, S. et al. 2009. Diet and the environment: Does what you eat matter? *American Journal of Clinical Nutrition*, 5S, 1699S–1703S. DOI: http://dx.doi.org/10.3945/ajcn.2009.26736Z

Marsh, K. 2011. Nuts and diabetes. *Diabetes management: A journal for general practitioners and other health professionals*, 36, 16.

Marsh, K., Brand-Miller, J. 2011. Vegetarian Diets and Diabetes. *American Journal of Lifestyle Medicine*, 5, 135–143. DOI: http://dx.doi.org/10.1177/1559827610387393

Marshall, B., Levy, S. 2011. Food animals and antimicrobials: impacts on human health. *Clinical Microbiology Reviews*, 24, 718–733. DOI: http://dx.doi.org/10.1128/CMR.00002-11

Marvin, G. 2005. Sensing nature: Encountering the world in hunting. *Etnofoor*, 18, 15–26.

Marx, P., Li, Y., Lerche, N. et al. 1991. Isolation of a simian immunodeficiency virus related to human immunodeficiency virus type 2 from a west African pet sooty mangabey. *Journal of Virology*, 65, 4480–4485.

Mason, J., Finelli, M. 2006. Brave new farm?. In: P. Singer (ed). *In defense of animals: The second wave*. Malden: Blackwell, 104–122.

Materna, S., Cameron, R. 2008. The sea urchin genome as a window on function. *The Biological Bulletin*, 214, 266–273. DOI: http://dx.doi.org/10.2307/25470668

Matheny, G. 2003. Least harm: A defense of vegetarianism from Steven Davis's omnivorous proposal. *Journal of Agricultural and Environmental Ethics*, 16, 505–511. DOI: http://dx.doi.org/10.1023/A:1026354906892

Matthews, G. 2006. *Pesticides. Health, safety, and the environment*. Oxford: Blackwell, 2006.

May, T. 2014. Moral individualism, moral relationalism, and obligations to non-human animals. *Journal of Applied Philosophy*, 31, 155–168. DOI: http://dx.doi.org/10.1111/japp.12055

McCarty, M. 2001a. Upregulation of lymphocyte apoptosis as a strategy for preventing and treating autoimmune disorders: a role for whole-food vegan diets, fish oil and dopamine agonists. *Medical Hypotheses*, 57, 258–275. DOI: http://dx.doi.org/10.1054/mehy.2000.1318

McCarty, M. 2001b. Does a vegan diet reduce risk for Parkinson's disease? *Medical Hypotheses*, 57, 318–323. DOI: http://dx.doi.org/10.1054/mehy.2000.1321

McCarty, M. 2003a. A moderately low phosphate intake may provide health benefits analogous to those conferred by UV light—a further advantage of vegan diets. *Medical Hypotheses*, 61, 543–560. DOI: http://dx.doi.org/10.1016/S0306-9877(03)00228-7

McCarty, M. 2003b. Iatrogenic lipodystrophy in HIV patients—the need for very-low-fat diets. *Medical Hypotheses*, 61, 561–566. DOI: http://dx.doi.org/10.1016/S0306-9877(03)00230-5

McCarty, M. 2003c. A low-fat, whole-food vegan diet, as well as other strategies that down-regulate IGF-1 activity, may slow the human aging process. *Medical Hypotheses*, 60, 784–792. DOI: http://dx.doi.org/10.1016/S0306-9877(02)00235-9

McCarty, M. 2011. mTORC1 activity as a determinant of cancer risk—Rationalizing the cancer-preventive effects of adiponectin, metformin, rapamycin, and low-protein vegan diets. *Medical Hypotheses*, 77, 642–648. DOI: http://dx.doi.org/10.1016/j.mehy.2011.07.004

McCauley, D., Pinsky, M., Palumbi, S. et al. 2015. Marine defaunation: Animal loss in the global ocean. *Science*, 347, 1255641.1–1255641.7.

McCausland, C., O'Sullivan, S., Brenton, S. 2013. Trespass, animals and democratic engagement. *Res Publica*, 19, 205–221. DOI: http://dx.doi.org/10.1007/s11158-013-9214-x

McDonald, B. 2000. 'Once you know something, you can't not know it'. An empirical look at becoming vegan. *Society and Animals*, 8, 1–23. DOI: http://dx.doi.org/10.1163/156853000510961, DOI: http://dx.doi.org/10.1163/156853000X00011

McEvoy, C., Woodside J. 2010. Vegetarian and vegan diets: weighing the claims. In: T. Wilson, G. Bray, N. Temple et al. (eds.). *Nutrition and Health: Nutrition Guide for Physicians*. New York: Humana Press, 81–93. DOI: http://dx.doi.org/10.1007/978-1-60327-431-9_7

McMichael, A., Powles, J., Butler, C. et al. 2007. Food, livestock production, energy, climate change, and health. *Lancet*, 370, 1253–1263. DOI: http://dx.doi.org/10.1016/S0140-6736(07)61256-2

McPhail, E. 1998. *The evolution of consciousness*. Oxford: Oxford University Press. DOI: http://dx.doi.org/10.1093/acprof:oso/9780198503248.001.0001

Meek, R., Vyas, H., Piddock, L. 2015. Nonmedical uses of antibiotics: Time to restrict their use? *PLoS Biol*, 13, e1002266. DOI: http://dx.doi.org/10.1371/journal.pbio.1002266

Mekonnen, M., Hoekstra, A. 2012. A global assessment of the water footprint of farm animal products. *Ecosystems*, 15, 401–415. DOI: http://dx.doi.org/10.1007/s10021-011-9517-8

Melnik, B. 2011. Milk signalling in the pathogenesis of type 2 diabetes. *Medical Hypotheses*, 76, 553–559. DOI: http://dx.doi.org/10.1016/j.mehy.2010.12.017

Melnik, B. 2012. Dietary intervention in acne. Attenuation of increased mTORC1 signalling promoted by Western diet. *Dermato-Endocrinology*, 4, 20–32. DOI: http://dx.doi.org/10.4161/derm.19828

Menzies, D. 2011. The case for a worldwide ban on smoking in public places. *Current Opinion in Pulmonary Medicine*, 17, 116–122. DOI: http://dx.doi.org/10.1097/MCP.0b013e328341ce98

Messina, V., Mangels, A. 2001. Considerations in planning vegan diets: Children. *Journal of the American Dietetic Association*, 101, 661–669. DOI: http://dx.doi.org/10.1016/S0002-8223(01)00167-5

Messina, V., Mangels, R., Messina, M. 2004. *The dietitian's guide to vegetarian diets: issues and applications*. Second edition. Sudbury, MA: Jones and Bartlett Publishers.

Meyers, C. 2013. Why it is morally good to eat (certain kinds of) meat: The case for entomophagy. *Southwest Philosophy Review*, 29, 119–126. DOI: http://dx.doi.org/10.5840/swphilreview201329113

Milburn, J. forthcoming. The animal lovers' paradox? On the ethics of 'pet food'. In: C. Overall (ed.). *Pets and people*. Oxford: Oxford University Press.

Mill, J. 1859. *On liberty*. London: Parker.

Milligan, T. 2010. *Beyond animal rights. Food, pets and ethics*. London: Continuum.

Millward, D. 1999. The nutritional value of plant-based diets in relation to human amino acid and protein requirements. *Proceedings of the Nutrition Society*, 58, 249–260. DOI: http://dx.doi.org/10.1017/S0029665199000348

Millward, D., Garnett, T. 2010. Food and the planet: Nutritional dilemmas of greenhouse gas emission reductions through reduced intakes of meat and dairy foods. *Proceedings of the Nutrition Society*, 69, 103–118. DOI: http://dx.doi.org/10.1017/S0029665109991868

Milner, N. 2011. Taboo. In: T. Insoll (ed.). *The Oxford handbook of the archaeology of ritual and religion*. Oxford: Oxford University Press, 105–114. DOI: http://dx.doi.org/10.1093/oxfordhb/9780199232444.013.0009

Milton, K. 1999. Nutritional characteristics of wild primate foods: do the diets of our closest living relatives have lessons for us? *Nutrition*, 15, 488–498. DOI: http://dx.doi.org/10.1016/S0899-9007(99)00078-7

Moinard, C., Morisse, J., Faure, J. 1998. Effect of cage area, cage height and perches on feather condition, bone breakage and mortality of laying hens. *British Poultry Science*, 39, 198–202. DOI: http://dx.doi.org/10.1080/00071669889123

Mølbak, K., Baggesen, D., Aarestrup, F. et al. 1999. An outbreak of multidrug-resistant, quinolone-resistant Salmonella enterica serotype typhinurium DT104. *New England Journal of Medicine*, 341, 1420–1425. DOI: http://dx.doi.org/10.1056/NEJM199911043411902

Moran, D., Wackernagel, M., Kitzes, J. 2009. Trading spaces. Calculating embodied ecological footprints in international trade using a product land use matrix (PLUM). *Ecological Economics*, 68,1938–1951. DOI: http://dx.doi.org/10.1016/j.ecolecon.2008.11.011

Morton, J., Kerven, C. 2013. *Livelihoods and basic service support in the drylands of the Horn of Africa. Brief prepared by a Technical Consortium hosted by CGIAR in partnership with the FAO Investment Centre. Technical Consortium Brief 3.* Nairobi: International Livestock Research Institute.

Mozaffarian, D., Appel, L., Van Horn, L. 2011. Components of a cardioprotective diet. *New Insights*, 123, 2870–2891.

Mukuddem-Petersen, J., Oosthuizen, W., Jerling, J. 2005. A systematic review of the effects of nuts on blood lipid profiles in humans. *Journal of Nutrition*, 135, 2082–2089.

Naess, A. 1995. Self-realisation: An ecological approach to being in the world. In A. Drengson, Y. Inoue. 1995. *The deep ecology movement: An introductory anthology*. Berkeley: North Atlantic Books, 13–30.

Nagel, T. 1979. *Mortal Questions*. Cambridge: Cambridge University Press.

Nardella, C., Carracedo, A., Alimonti, A. et al. 2009. Differential requirement of mTOR in post-mitotic tissues and tumorigenesis. *Science Signaling*, 2, ra2. DOI: http://dx.doi.org/10.1126/scisignal.2000189

Naylor, R., Hardy, R., Bureau, D. et al. 2009. Feeding aquaculture in an era of finite resources. *Proceedings of the National Academy of Sciences of the United States of America*, 106, 15103–15110. DOI: http://dx.doi.org/10.1073/pnas.0905235106

Nepstad, D., Stickler, C., Almeida, O. 2006. Globalization of the Amazon soy and beef industries: Opportunities for conservation. *Conservation Biology*, 20, 1595–1603. DOI: http://dx.doi.org/10.1111/j.1523-1739.2006.00510.x

Nestle, M. 1999. Animal v. plant foods in human diets and health: is the historical record unequivocal? *Proceedings of the Nutrition Society*, 58, 211–218. DOI: http://dx.doi.org/10.1017/S0029665199000300

New, S. 2003. Intake of fruit and vegetables: implications for bone health. *Proceedings of the Nutrition Society*, 62, 889–899.

Niazi, S. 2014. In India, the world's first vegetarian city. *Worldcrunch* (5 October). http://www.worldcrunch.com/culture-society/in-india-the-world-039-s-first-vegetarian-city/india-palitana-food-meat-fish-gujarat/c3s17132/ (Accessed 17 February 2016.)

Norat, T., Dossus, L., Rinaldi, S. et al. 2007. Diet, serum insulin-like growth factor-I and IGF-binding protein-3 in European women. *European Journal of Clinical Nutrition*, 61, 91–98. DOI: http://dx.doi.org/10.1038/sj.ejcn.1602494

Nordgren, A. 2012. Ethical issues in mitigation of climate change: The option of reduced meat production and consumption. *Journal of Agricultural and Environmental Ethics*, 25, 563–584. DOI: http://dx.doi.org/10.1007/s10806-011-9335-1

Norouzy, A., Razavi, A., Sanders, T. et al. 2011. Vegan diet improves cardiovascular risk factors compared to omnivore diet. *Clinical Nutrition Supplements*, 6, 18. DOI: http://dx.doi.org/10.1016/S1744-1161(11)70044-8

Norris, J., Messina, V. 2011. *Vegan for life: Everything you need to know to be healthy and fit on a plant-based diet*. Cambridge, MA: Da Capo Lifelong Books.

Norton, M. 2015. The chicken or the iegue: Human-animal relationships and the Columbian exchange. *The American Historical Review*, 120, 28–60. DOI: http://dx.doi.org/10.1093/ahr/120.1.28

Nuffield Council on Bioethics. 2005. *The ethics of research involving animals*. London: Nuffield Council on Bioethics.

Nussbaum, M. 2004. Beyond "compassion and humanity." Justice for nonhuman animals. In M. Nussbaum, C. Sunstein (eds.). *Animal rights. Current debates and new directions*. Oxford: Oxford University Press, 299–320.

Nussbaum, M. 2006. *Frontiers of justice: disability, nationality, species membership*. Cambridge, MA: Harvard University Press.

Oliveira, G. 2015. The geopolitics of Brazilian soybeans. *The Journal of Peasant Studies*, (ahead-of-print), 1–25.

O'Neill, B. 2010. A scientific review of the reported effects of vegan nutrition on the occurrence and prevalence of cancer and cardio-vascular disease. *Bioscience Horizons*, 3,197–212. DOI: http://dx.doi.org/10.1093/biohorizons/hzq022

Orlich, M., Singh, P., Sabaté, J. et al. 2013. Vegetarian dietary patterns and mortality in Adventist Health Study 2. *JAMA Internal Medicine*, 173, 1230–1238. DOI: http://dx.doi.org/10.1001/jamainternmed.2013.6473

Ostfeld, R. 2009. Biodiversity loss and the rise of zoonotic pathogens. *Clinical Microbiology and Infection*, 15, 40–43. DOI: http://dx.doi.org/10.1111/j.1469-0691.2008.02691.x

Packer, M. [Mark]. 1996. The aesthetic dimension of ethics and law: Some reflections on harmless offence. *American Philosophical Quarterly*, 33, 57–74.

Packer, M. [Mike]. 2009. Algal capture of carbon dioxide; biomass generation as a tool for greenhouse gas mitigation with reference to New Zealand energy strategy and policy. *Energy Policy*, 37, 3428–3437. DOI: http://dx.doi.org/10.1016/j.enpol.2008.12.025

Palmer, C. 2010. *Animal ethics in context*. New York: Columbia University Press.

Pan, A., Sun, Q., Bernstein, A. et al. 2011. Red meat consumption and risk of type 2 diabetes: 3 cohorts of US adults and an updated meta-analysis. *American Journal of Clinical Nutrition*, 94, 1088–1096. DOI: http://dx.doi.org/10.3945/ajcn.111.018978

Park, Y., Subar. A., Hollenbeck, A. et al. 2011. Dietary fiber intake and mortality in the NIHAARP diet and health study. *Archives of Internal Medicine*, 171, 1061–1068. DOI: http://dx.doi.org/10.1001/archinternmed.2011.18

Parry, M., Canziani, O., Pultikof, J. et al. (eds.) 2007. *Climate change 2007: Impacts, adaptation, and vulnerability. Contribution of Working Group II to the Fourth Assessment Report of the Intergovernmental Panel on Climate Change.* Cambridge: Cambridge University Press.

Peeters, M., Honoré, C., Huet, T. et al. 1989. Isolation and partial characterization of an HIV-related virus occurring naturally in chimpanzees in Gabon. *Aids*, 3, 625–630. DOI: http://dx.doi.org/10.1097/00002030-198910000-00001

Pelletier, N., Tyedmers, P. 2010. Forecasting potential global environmental costs of livestock production 2000—2050. *Proceedings of the National Academy of Sciences*, 107, 18371–18374. DOI: http://dx.doi.org/10.1073/pnas.1004659107

Pendergrast, N. 2016. Environmental concerns and the mainstreaming of veganism. In: T. Raphaely, D. Marinova (eds.). *Impacts of meat consumption on health and environmental sustainability.* IGI Global, 106–123. DOI: http://dx.doi.org/10.4018/978-1-4666-9553-5.ch006

Penning de Vries, F., Van Keulen, H., Rabbinge, R. 1995. Natural resources and limits of food production in 2040. In: J. Bouma (ed.). *Eco-regional approaches for sustainable land use and food production.* Dordrecht: Kluwer, 65–88. DOI: http://dx.doi.org/10.1007/978-94-011-0121-9_5

Pennisi, E. 2008. "Simple animal"'s genome proves unexpectedly complex. *Science*, 321, 1028–1029. DOI: http://dx.doi.org/10.1126/science.321.5892.1028b

Pershin, Y., La Fontaine, S., Di Ventra, M. 2009. Memristive model of amoeba learning. *Physical Review E*, 80, 021926. DOI: http://dx.doi.org/10.1103/PhysRevE.80.021926

Peters, C., Wilkins, J., Fick, G. 2007. Testing a complete-diet model for estimating the land resource requirements of food consumption and agricultural carrying capacity: The New York State example. *Renewable Agriculture and Food Systems*, 22, 145–153. DOI: http://dx.doi.org/10.1017/S1742170507001767

Pettersen, B., Anousheh, R., Fan, J. et al. 2012. Vegetarian diets and blood pressure among white subjects: results from the Adventist Health Study-2 (AHS-2). *Public Health Nutrition*, 15, 1909–1916. DOI: http://dx.doi.org/10.1017/S1368980011003454

Phaniraja, K., Panchasara, H. 2009. Indian draught animals power. *Veterinary World*, 2, 404–407.

Piccoli, G., Clari, R., Vigotti, F. et al. 2015. Vegan—vegetarian diets in pregnancy: danger or panacea? A systematic narrative review. *BJOG: An International Journal of Obstetrics & Gynaecology*, 122, 623–633. DOI: http://dx.doi.org/10.1111/1471-0528.13280

Pimentel, D., Pimentel, M. 2008. *Food, energy, and society*. Third edition. Boca Raton: CRC Press.

Plous, S. 1993. Psychological mechanisms in the human use of animals. *Journal of Social Studies*, 49, 11–52. DOI: http://dx.doi.org/10.1111/j.1540-4560.1993.tb00907.x

Pluimers, J., Blonk, H. 2011. *Methods for quantifying the environmental and health impacts of food consumption patterns*. Gouda: Blonk Environmental Consultants.

Pollan, M. 2006. *The omnivore's dilemma. The search for a perfect meal in a fast-food world*. London: Penguin Press.

Popkin, B. 2009. Reducing meat consumption has multiple benefits for the world's health. *Archives of Internal Medicine*, 169, 543. DOI: http://dx.doi.org/10.1001/archinternmed.2009.2

Popkin, B., Du, S. 2003. Dynamics of the nutrition transition toward the animal foods sector in China and its implications: A worried perspective. *Journal of Nutrition*, 133S, 3898S–3906S.

Popovich, D., Jenkins, D., Kendall, C. et al. 1997. The western lowland gorilla diet has implications for the health of humans and other hominoids. *Journal of Nutrition*, 127, 2000–2005.

Post, M. 2012. Cultured meat from stem cells: Challenges and prospects. *Meat Science*, 92, 297–301. DOI: http://dx.doi.org/10.1016/j.meatsci.2012.04.008

Post, M. 2014. An alternative animal protein source: cultured beef. *Annals of the New York Academy of Sciences*, 1328, 29–33. DOI: http://dx.doi.org/10.1111/nyas.12569

Povey, R., Wellens, B., Conner, M. 2001. Attitudes towards following meat, vegetarian and vegan diets: an examination of the role of ambivalence. *Appetite*, 37, 15–26. DOI: http://dx.doi.org/10.1006/appe.2001.0406

Powlson, D., Addiscott, T., Benjamin, N. et al. 2008. When does nitrate become a risk for humans? *Journal of Environmental Quality*, 37, 291–295. DOI: http://dx.doi.org/10.2134/jeq2007.0177

Price, L., Koch, B., Hungate, B. 2015. Ominous projections for global antibiotic use in food-animal production. *Proceedings of the National Academy of Sciences*, 112, 5554–5555. DOI: http://dx.doi.org/10.1073/pnas.1505312112

Proctor, H. 2012. Animal sentience: Where are we and where are we heading?. *Animals*, 2, 628–639. DOI: http://dx.doi.org/10.3390/ani2040628

Qin, L., He, K., Xu, J. 2009. Milk consumption and circulating insulin-like growth factor-I level: a systematic literature review. *International Journal of Food Sciences and Nutrition*, 60S, 330S–340S. DOI: http://dx.doi.org/10.1080/09637480903150114

Randolph, T., Schelling, E., Grace, D. et al. 2007. Role of livestock in human nutrition and health for poverty reduction in developing countries. *Journal of Animal Science*, 85, 2788–2800. DOI: http://dx.doi.org/10.2527/jas.2007-0467

Rawls, J. 1971. *A theory of justice*. Cambridge, Massachusetts: Cambridge University Press.

Raz, J. 2010. Human rights without foundations, in S. Besson, J. Tasioulas (eds.). *The philosophy of international law.* Oxford: Oxford University Press, 321–337.

Rees, W. 2003. A blot on the land. *Nature,* 421, 898. DOI: http://dx.doi.org/10.1038/421898a

Rees, W. 2006a. Ecological footprints and bio-capacity: Essential elements in sustainability assessment. In J. Dewulf, H. Van Langenhove (eds.). *Renewables-Based Technology: Sustainability Assessment.* Chichester: John Wiley & Sons, 143–158. DOI: http://dx.doi.org/10.1002/0470022442.ch9

Rees, W. 2006b. Why conventional economic logic won't protect biodiversity. In: D. Lavigne (ed.). *Gaining ground: In pursuit of ecological sustainability.* Guelph and Limerick: International Fund for Animal Welfare and the University of Limerick, 207–226.

Rees, W. 2008. Human nature, eco-footprints and environmental injustice. *Local Environment: The International Journal of Justice and Sustainability,* 13, 658–701.

Regan, T. 1983. *The case for animal rights.* Berkeley: University of California Press.

Regan, T. 1997. The rights of humans and other animals. *Ethics and Behavior,* 7, 103–111. DOI: http://dx.doi.org/10.1207/s15327019eb0702_2

Regan, T. 2004. *The case for animal rights.* New edition. Berkeley: University of California Press.

Regulation (EC) No 999/2001 of the European Parliament and of the Council of 22 May 2001 laying down rules for the prevention, control and eradication of certain transmissible spongiform encephalopathies. *Official Journal of the European Union,* L 147/1, 1–40.

Reijnders, L., Soret, S. 2003. Quantification of the environmental impact of different dietary protein choices. *American Journal of Clinical Nutrition,* 78S, 664S–668S.

Rifkin, J. 1993. *Beyond beef. The rise and fall of the cattle culture.* New York: Plume.

Rissanen, T., Voutilainen, S., Virtanen, J. et al. 2003. Low intake of fruits, berries and vegetables is associated with excess mortality in men: the Kuopio Ischaemic Heart Disease Risk Factor (KIHD) Study. *Journal of Nutrition,* 133, 199–204.

Rizzo, N., Jaceldo-Siegl, K., Sabaté, J. et al. 2013. Nutrient profiles of vegetarian and nonvegetarian dietary patterns. *Journal of the Academy of Nutrition and Dietetics,* 113, 1610–1619. DOI: http://dx.doi.org/10.1016/j.jand.2013.06.349

Rollin, B. 1995. *The Frankenstein syndrome: Ethical and social issues in the genetic engineering of animals.* New York: Cambridge University Press. DOI: http://dx.doi.org/10.1017/CBO9781139172806

Rose, J., Arlinghaus, R., Cooke, S. et al. 2014. Can fish really feel pain? *Fish and Fisheries,* 15, 97–133. DOI: http://dx.doi.org/10.1111/faf.12010

Rothgerber, H., Mican, F. 2014. Childhood pet ownership, attachment to pets, and subsequent meat avoidance. The mediating role of empathy toward animals. *Appetite*, 79, 11–17. DOI: http://dx.doi.org/10.1016/j.appet.2014.03.032

Roubenoff, R. 2000. Acquired immunodeficiency syndrome wasting, functional performance, and quality of life. *The American Journal of Managed Care*, 6, 1003–1016.

Royal Society. 2009. *Reaping the benefits: Science and the sustainable intensification of global agriculture.* London: Royal Society.

Ruby, M., Heine, S. 2011. Meat, morals, and masculinity. *Appetite*, 56, 447–450. DOI: http://dx.doi.org/10.1016/j.appet.2011.01.018

Ruby, M., Heine, S. 2012. Too close to home. Factors predicting meat avoidance. *Appetite*, 59, 47–52. DOI: http://dx.doi.org/10.1016/j.appet.2012.03.020

Ruger, J. 2006. Toward a theory of a right to health: capability and incompletely theorized agreements. *Yale Journal of Law & The Humanities*, 18.

Sabaté, J. 2003. The contribution of vegetarian diets to health and disease: a paradigm shift? *American Journal of Nutrition*, 78S, 502S–507S.

Sabaté, J., Oda, K., Ros, E. 2010. Nut consumption and blood lipid levels: a pooled analysis of 25 intervention trials. *Archives of internal medicine*, 170, 821–827. DOI: http://dx.doi.org/10.1001/archinternmed.2010.79

Sacks, F., Appel, L., Moore, T. et al. 1999. A dietary approach to prevent hypertension: A review of the dietary approaches to stop hypertension (DASH) study. *Clinical Cardiology*, 22S, 1106S–1110S. DOI: http://dx.doi.org/10.1002/clc.4960221503

Safran Foer, J. 2009. *Eating animals.* London: Hamish Hamilton.

Saigusa, T., Tero, A., Nakagaki, T. et al. 2008. Amoebae anticipate periodic events. *Physical Review of Letters*, 100, 1–4. DOI: http://dx.doi.org/10.1103/PhysRevLett.100.018101

Salas-Salvadó, J., Martinez-Gonzalez, M., Bullo, M. et al. 2011. The role of diet in the prevention of type 2 diabetes. *Nutrition, Metabolism and Cardiovascular Diseases*, 21, B32–B48. DOI: http://dx.doi.org/10.1016/j.numecd.2011.03.009

Sanders, T. 1999. The nutritional adequacy of plant-based diets. *Proceedings of the Nutrition Society*, 58, 265–269. DOI: http://dx.doi.org/10.1017/S0029665199000361

Sanders, T., Gleason, K., Griffen, B. et al. 2006. Influence of an algal triacylglycerol containing docosahexaenoic acid (22:6n-3) and docosapentaenoic acid (22:5n-6) on cardiovascular risk factors in healthy men and women. *British Journal of Nutrition*, 95, 525–531. DOI: http://dx.doi.org/10.1079/BJN20051658

Sandøe, P., Nielsen, B., Christensen, L. et al. 1999. Staying good while playing God – The ethics of breeding farm animals. *Animal Welfare*, 8, 313–328.

Sandøe, P., Hocking, P., Förkman, B. et al. 2014. The blind hens' challenge: Does it undermine the view that only welfare matters in our dealings with animals?. *Environmental Values*, 23, 727–742. DOI: http://dx.doi.org/10.31 97/096327114X13947900181950

Saunders, A., Davis, B., Garg, M. 2012a. Omega-3 polyunsaturated fatty acids and vegetarian diets. *Medical Journal of Australia Open*, 1S, 22S–26S. DOI: http://dx.doi.org/10.5694/mjao11.11507

Saunders, A., Craig, W., Baines, S. 2012b. Zinc and vegetarian diets. *Medical Journal of Australia Open*, 1S, 17S–21S. DOI: http://dx.doi.org/10.5694/ mjao11.11493

Savolainen, P., Leitner, T., Wilton, A. et al. 2004. A detailed picture of the origin of the Australian dingo, obtained from the study of mitochondrial DNA. *Proceedings of the National Academy of Sciences of the United States of America*, 101, 12387–12390. DOI: http://dx.doi.org/10.5694/mjao11.11507

Scarborough, P., Noaham, K., Clarke, D. et al. 2012a. Modelling the impact of a healthy diet on cardiovascular disease and cancer mortality. *Journal of Epidemiology and Community Health*, 66, 420–426. DOI: http://dx.doi. org/10.1136/jech.2010.114520

Scarborough, P., Allender, S., Clarke, D. et al. 2012b. Modelling the health impact of environmentally sustainable dietary scenarios in the UK. *European Journal of Clinical Nutrition*, 66, 710–715. DOI: http://dx.doi.org/10.1038/ejcn.2012.34

Schecter, A., Cramer, P., Boggess, K. et al. 1997. Levels of dioxins, dibenzo-furans, PCB and DDE congeners in pooled food samples collected in 1995 at supermarkets across the United States. *Chemosphere*, 34, 1437–1447. DOI: http://dx.doi.org/10.1016/S0045-6535(97)00440-2

Schedler, G. 2005. Does ethical meat eating maximize utility? *Social theory and practice*, 31, 499–511. DOI: http://dx.doi.org/10.5840/soctheorpract200531422

Schmidt, J., Crowe, F., Appleby, P. et al. 2013. Serum uric acid concentrations in meat eaters, fish eaters, vegetarians and vegans: A cross-sectional analysis in the EPIC-Oxford Cohort. *PloS one*, 8(2), e56339. DOI: http://dx.doi. org/10.1371/journal.pone.0056339

Schmidt, K. 2011. Concepts of animal welfare in relation to positions in animal ethics. *Acta Biotheoretica*, 59, 153–171. DOI: http://dx.doi.org/10.1007/ s10441-011-9128-y

Scruton, R. 2000. *Animal rights and wrongs*. Third edition. London: Metro.

Seneff, S., Wainwright, G., Mascitelli, L. 2011. Nutrition and Alzheimer's disease: The detrimental role of a high carbohydrate diet. *European Journal of Internal Medicine*, 22, 134–140. DOI: http://dx.doi.org/10.1016/j.ejim. 2010.12.017

Shapiro, J. 2007. Bacteria are small but not stupid: cognition, natural genetic engineering and socio-bacteriology. *Studies in History and Philosophy of Biological and Biomedical Sciences*, 38, 807–819. DOI: http://dx.doi. org/10.1016/j.shpsc.2007.09.010

Sharma, N., Rho, G., Hong, Y. 2012. Bovine mastitis: An Asian perspective. *Asian Journal of Animal and Veterinary Advances*, 7, 454–476. DOI: http:// dx.doi.org/10.3923/ajava.2012.454.476

Shaw, R., Cantley, L. 2006. Ras, PI(3)K and mTOR signalling controls tumour cell growth. *Nature*, 441, 424–430. DOI: http://dx.doi.org/10.1038/nature04869

Shellnhuber, H., Cramer, W., Nakicenovic, N. et al. (eds.) 2006. *Avoiding dangerous climate change*. Cambridge: Cambridge University Press.

Sherwin, C. 2001. Can invertebrates suffer? Or, how robust is the argument-by-analogy? *Animal Welfare*, 10S, 103S–118S. DOI: http://dx.doi.org/10.10 80/00071668.2010.502518

Sherwin, C., Richards, G., Nicol, C. 2010. A comparison of the welfare or layer hens in four housing systems in the UK. *British Poultry Science*, 51, 488–499.

Shields, S., Park, S., Mohan Raj, A. 2010. A critical review of electrical water-bath stun systems for poultry slaughter and recent developments in alternative technologies. *Journal of Applied Animal Welfare Science*, 13, 281–299. DOI: http://dx.doi.org/10.1080/10888705.2010.507119

Shine, K., Sturges, W. 2007. Atmospheric science. CO_2 is not the only gas. *Science*, 315, 1804–1805. DOI: http://dx.doi.org/10.1126/science.1141677

Siener, R., Hönow, R., Voss, S. et al. 2006. Oxalate content of cereals and cereal products. *Journal of Agricultural and Food Chemistry*, 54, 3008–3011. DOI: http://dx.doi.org/10.1021/jf052776v

Simoons, F. 1994. *Eat not this flesh. Food avoidances from prehistory to the present*. Wisconsin: University of Wisconsin Press.

Simopoulos, A. 2002. The importance of the ratio of omega-6/omega-3 essential fatty acids. *Biomedicine and Pharmacotherapy*, 56, 365–379. DOI: http://dx.doi.org/10.1016/S0753-3322(02)00253-6

Sims, L., Domenech, J., Benigno, C. et al. 2005. Origin and evolution of highly pathogenic H5N1 avian influenza in Asia. *Veterinary Record*, 157, 159–164. DOI: http://dx.doi.org/10.1136/vr.157.6.159

Singer, P. 1975. *Animal liberation*. New York: New York Review/Random House.

Singer, P. 1987. Animal liberation or animal rights. *The Monist*, 70, 3–14. DOI: http://dx.doi.org/10.5840/monist19877018

Singer, P. 1990. *Animal liberation*. Second Edition. London: Jonathan Cape.

Singer, P. 1995. *Rethinking life and death. The collapse of our traditional ethics*. Oxford: Oxford University Press.

Singer, P. 2006. Introduction. In P. Singer (ed.). *In defense of animals. The second wave*. Oxford: Blackwell Publishing, 1–12. DOI: http://dx.doi.org/10.1177/0725513606068771

Singer, P. 2009. *The life you can save. Acting now to end world poverty*. London: Picador.

Singhal, A., Lucas, A. 2004. Early origins of cardio-vascular disease: is there a unifying hypothesis? *Lancet*, 363, 1642–1645. DOI: http://dx.doi.org/10.1016/S0140-6736(04)16210-7

Smil, V. 2001. *Enriching the earth: Fritz Haber, Carl Bosch, and the transformation of world food production*. Cambridge, MA: MIT.

Smil, V. 2002. Eating meat: Evolution, patterns, and consequences. *Population and Development Review*, 28, 599–639. DOI: http://dx.doi.org/10.1111/j.1728-4457.2002.00599.x

Smil, V. 2005. Losing the links between livestock and land. *Science*, 310, 1621–1622. DOI: http://dx.doi.org/10.1126/science.1117856

Smil, V. 2011. Nitrogen cycle and world food production. *World Agriculture*, 2, 1.

Smith, A. 1982. *The theory of moral sentiments*. Indianapolis: Liberty Fund.

Smith, J., Boyd, K. (eds.) 1991. *Lives in the balance. The ethics of using animals in biomedical research. (Report of a working party of the Institute of Medical Ethics)*. Oxford: Oxford University Press.

Smith, K., Besser, J., Hedberg, C. et al. 1999. Quinolone-resistant Campylobacter jejuni infections in Minnesota, 1992—1998. *New England Journal of Medicine*, 340, 1525–1532. DOI: http://dx.doi.org/10.1056/NEJM199905203402001

Smith, P. 2014. Do grasslands act as a perpetual sink for carbon? *Global change biology*, 20, 2708–2711.

Smith, P., Martino, D., Cai, Z. et al. 2007. Agriculture. In: B. Metz, O. Davidson, P. Bosch et al. (eds.). *Climate change 2007: Mitigation. Contribution of working group III to the Fourth Assessment Report of the Intergovernmental Panel on Climate Change*. Cambridge and New York: Cambridge University Press, 497–540.

Smith, T., Pearson, N. 2011. The emergence of Staphylococcus aureus ST398. *Vector-Borne and Zoonotic Diseases*, 11, 327–339. DOI: http://dx.doi.org/10.1089/vbz.2010.0072

Sobal, J. 2005. Men, meat, and marriage. Models of masculinity. *Food and Foodways*, 13, 135–158. DOI: http://dx.doi.org/10.1080/07409710590915409

Sørensen, T., Blom, M., Monnet, D. et al. 2001. Transient intestinal carriage after ingestion of antibiotic-resistant Enterococcus faecium from chicken and pork. *New England Journal of Medicine*, 345, 1161–1166. DOI: http://dx.doi.org/10.1056/NEJMoa010692

Spencer, E., Appleby, P., Davey, G. et al. 2003. Diet and body mass index in 38 000 EPIC-Oxford meat-eaters, fish-eaters, vegetarians and vegans. *International Journal of Obesity*, 27, 728–734. DOI: http://dx.doi.org/10.1038/sj.ijo.0802300

Stacey, T., Dunn-Emke, M., Weidner, G. et al. 2005. Nutrient adequacy of a very low-fat vegan diet. *Journal of the American Dietetic Association*, 105, 1442–1446. DOI: http://dx.doi.org/10.1016/j.jada.2005.06.028

Stefano, G., Cadet, P., Kream, R. et al. 2008. The presence of endogenous morphine signaling in animals. *Neurochemical research*, 33, 1933–1939. DOI: http://dx.doi.org/10.1007/s11064-008-9674-0

Stehfest, E., Bouwman, L., van Vuuren, D. et al. 2009. Climate benefits of changing diet. *Climatic Change*, 95, 83–102. DOI: http://dx.doi.org/10.1007/s10584-008-9534-6

Steiner, G. 2008. *Animals and the moral community: Mental life, moral status, and kinship*. New York: Columbia University Press.

Steiner, G. 2013. *Animals and the limits of postmodernism*. New York: Columbia University Press.

Steinfeld, H., Gerber, P., Wassenaar, T. et al. 2006. *Livestock's long shadow. Environmental issues and options*. Rome: FAO.

Stern, N. 2006. *The economics of climate change*. Cambridge: Cambridge University Press.

Stoll-Kleemann, S., O'Riordan, T. 2015. The sustainability challenges of our meat and dairy diets. *Environment: Science and Policy for Sustainable Development*, 57, 34–48. DOI: http://dx.doi.org/10.1080/00139157.2015.1025644

Sutcliffe, S., Giovannucci, E., Isaacs, W. et al. 2007. Acne and risk of prostate cancer. *International Journal of Cancer*, 121, 2688–2692. DOI: http://dx.doi.org/10.1002/ijc.23032

Takachi, R., Inoue, M., Ishihara, J. et al. 2008. Fruit and vegetable intake and risk of total cancer and cardio-vascular disease. Japan Public Health Center-based prospective study. *American Journal of Epidemiology*, 167, 59–70. DOI: http://dx.doi.org/10.1093/aje/kwm263

Tang, B., Eslick, G., Nowson, C. et al. 2007. Use of calcium or calcium in combination with vitamin D supplementation to prevent fractures and bone loss in people aged 50 years and older: a meta-analysis. *The Lancet*, 370, 657–666. DOI: http://dx.doi.org/10.1016/S0140-6736(07)61342-7

Taubenberger, J., Reid, A., Lourens, R. et al. 2005. Characterization of the 1918 influenza virus polymerase genes. *Nature*, 437, 889–893. DOI: http://dx.doi.org/10.1038/nature04230

Taylor, N., Main, D., Mendl, M. et al. 2010. Tail-biting: a new perspective. *The Veterinary Journal*, 186, 137–147. DOI: http://dx.doi.org/10.1016/j.tvjl.2009.08.028

Thompson, P. 2008. The opposite of human enhancement. Nanotechnology and the blind chicken problem. *Nanoethics*, 2, 305–316. DOI: http://dx.doi.org/10.1007/s11569-008-0052-9

Thorpe, D., Knutsen, S., Lawrence Beeson, W. et al. 2008. Effects of meat consumption and vegetarian diet on risk of wrist fracture over 25 years in a cohort of peri- and postmenopausal women. *Public Health Nutrition*, 11, 564–572. DOI: http://dx.doi.org/10.1017/S1368980007000808

Tonstad, S., Butler, T., Yan, R. et al. 2009. Type of vegetarian diet, body weight, and prevalence of type 2 diabetes. *Diabetes Care*, 32, 791–796. DOI: http://dx.doi.org/10.2337/dc08-1886

Torfadottir, J., Steingrimsdottir, L., Mucci, L. 2011. Milk intake in early life and risk of advanced prostate cancer. *American Journal of Epidemiology*, 175, 144–153. DOI: http://dx.doi.org/10.1093/aje/kwr289

Torres-Vélez, F., Brown, C. 2004. Emerging infections in animals--potential new zoonoses?. *Clinics in Laboratory Medicine*, 24, 825–838. DOI: http://dx.doi.org/10.1016/j.cll.2004.05.001

Trapp, C., Levin, S. 2012. Preparing to prescribe plant-based diets for diabetes prevention and treatment. *Diabetes Spectrum*, 25, 38–44. DOI: http://dx.doi.org/10.2337/diaspect.25.1.38

Trout, T. 2000. Environmental effects of irrigated agriculture. *Acta Horticulturae*, 537, 605–610. DOI: http://dx.doi.org/10.17660/ActaHortic.2000.537.71

Tucker, K., Hannan, M., Kiel, D. 2001. The acid-base hypothesis: diet and bone in the Framingham Osteoporosis Study. *European Journal of Nutrition*, 40, 231–237. DOI: http://dx.doi.org/10.1007/s394-001-8350-8

Tukker, A., Huppes, G., Guinée, J. et al. 2006. *Environmental impact of products (EIPRO): Analysis of the life cycle environmental impacts related to the final consumption of the EU25. European Commission technical report EUR 22284 EN.* Available at: http://ftp.jrc.es/EURdoc/eur22284en.pdf. (Accessed 24 December 2012.)

Tukker, A., Goldbohm, R., De Koning, A. et al. 2011. Environmental impacts of changes to healthier diets in Europe. *Ecological Economics*, 70, 1776–1788. DOI: http://dx.doi.org/10.1016/j.ecolecon.2011.05.00

Tuomisto, H., de Mattos, J. 2011. Environmental impacts of cultured meat production. *Environmental Science and Technology*, 45, 6117–6123. DOI: http://dx.doi.org/10.1021/es200130u

Turner, J. 2010. *Animal breeding, welfare and society.* London: Earthscan.

Turner-McGrievy, G., Jenkins, D., Barnard, N. et al. 2011. Decreases in dietary glycemic index are related to weight loss among individuals following therapeutic diets for type 2 diabetes. *Journal of Nutrition*, 141, 1469–1474. DOI: http://dx.doi.org/10.3945/jn.111.140921

Tuyttens, F., Vanhonacker, F., Verbeke, W. 2014. Broiler production in Flanders, Belgium: current situation and producers' opinions about animal welfare. *World's Poultry Science Journal*, 70, 343–354. DOI: http://dx.doi.org/10.1017/S004393391400035X

Twigg, J. 1983. Vegetarianism and the meanings of meat. In: A. Murcott (ed.). *The Sociology of Food and Eating.* Aldershot: Gower Publishing, 18–30.

Union of Concerned Scientists. 2001. *Hogging it: Estimates of antimicrobial abuse in livestock.* Boston: Union of Concerned Scientists.

United Nations Committee on Economic, Social and Cultural Rights. 1999. *The right to adequate food (Art. 11, E/C.12/1999/5).* Geneva: Office of the United Nations High Commissioner for Human Rights.

van Belkum, A., Melles, D., Peeters, J. et al. 2008. Methicillin-resistant and -susceptible Staphylococcus aureus sequence type 398 in pigs and humans. *Emerging Infectious Diseases*, 14, 479–483. DOI: http://dx.doi.org/10.3201/eid1403.070760, DOI: http://dx.doi.org/10.3201/eid1403.0760

van Cleef, B., Verkade, E., Wulf, M. et al. 2010. Prevalence of livestock-associated MRSA in communities with high pig-densities in The Netherlands. *Public Library of Science One*, 5, e9385. DOI: http://dx.doi.org/10.1371/journal.pone.0009385

Van den Bergh, J., Verbruggen, H. 1999. Spatial sustainability, trade and indicators: an evaluation of the "ecological footprint." *Ecological Economics*, 29, 61–72. DOI: http://dx.doi.org/10.1016/S0921-8009(99)00032-4

van der Kooi, M. 2010. The inconsistent vegetarian. *Society and Animals*, 18, 291–305. DOI: http://dx.doi.org/10.1163/156853010X510799

van der Pols, J., Bain, C., Gunnell, D. et al. 2007. Childhood dairy intake and adult cancer risk: 65-y follow-up of the Boyd Orr cohort. *American Journal of Clinical Nutrition*, 86, 1722–1729.

van Gelder, J., Kammeraat, K., Kroes, H. 2008. *Soy consumption for feed and fuel in the European Union. A research paper prepared for Milieudefensie (Friends of the Earth Netherlands).* Castricum: Profundo Economic Research.

van Popering, R. 2015. *Jain vegetarian laws in the city of Palitana: Indefensible legal enforcement or praiseworthy progressive moralism?* Linköping: Linköping University.

Van Winckel, M., Vande Velde, S., De Bruyne, R. et al. 2011. Clinical practice. Vegetarian infant and child nutrition. *European Journal of Pediatrics*, 170, 1489–1494. DOI: http://dx.doi.org/10.1007/s00431-011-1547-x

Vandevenne, F., Barão, A., Schoelynck, J. et al. 2013. Grazers: biocatalysts of terrestrial silica cycling. *Proceedings of the Royal Society of London B: Biological Sciences*, 280 (December), 1–9. DOI: http://dx.doi.org/10.1098/rspb.2013.2083

Varner, G. 2012. *Personhood, ethics, and animal cognition.* Oxford: Oxford University Press. DOI: http://dx.doi.org/10.1093/acprof:oso/9780199758784.001.0001

Vinagre, J., Vinagre, C., Pozzi, F. et al. 2013. Metabolism of triglyceride-rich lipoproteins and transfer of lipids to high-density lipoproteins (HDL) in vegan and omnivore subjects. *Nutrition, Metabolism and Cardio-vascular Diseases*, 23, 61–67. DOI: http://dx.doi.org/10.1016/j.numecd.2011.02.011

Vinnari, M., Tapio, P. 2012. Sustainability of diets: From concepts to governance. *Ecological Economics*, 74, 46–54. DOI: http://dx.doi.org/10.1016/j.ecolecon.2011.12.012

Vogel, G. 2010. For more protein, filet of cricket. *Science*, 327, 811. DOI: http://dx.doi.org/10.1126/science.327.5967.811

von Schacky, C. 2009. Cardio-vascular disease prevention and treatment. *Prostaglandins, Leukotrienes and Essential Fatty Acids*, 81, 193–198. DOI: http://dx.doi.org/10.1016/j.plefa.2009.05.009

Voss, A., Loeffen, F., Bakker, J. 2005. Methicillin-resistant Staphylococcus aureus in pig farming. *Emerging Infectious Diseases*, 11, 1965–1966. DOI: http://dx.doi.org/10.3201/eid1112.050428

Wackernagel, M., Rees, W. 1996. *Our ecological footprint: reducing human impact on the earth.* Gabriola Island, BC: New Society Publishers.

Waldmann, A., Koschizke, J., Leitzmann, C. et al. 2005. German vegan study: diet, life-style factors, and cardio-vascular risk profile. *Annals of Nutrition and Metabolism*, 49, 366–372. DOI: http://dx.doi.org/10.1159/000088888

Walker, P., Rhubart-Berg, P., McKenzie, S. 2005. Public health implications of meat production and consumption. *Public Health Nutrition*, 8, 348–356. DOI: http://dx.doi.org/10.1079/PHN2005727

Wallis, I. 2014. Is vegetarianism bad for the environment? *Australian Zoologist*, 1–10. DOI: http://dx.doi.org/10.7882/az.2014.034

Waltz, E. 2016. GM salmon declared fit for dinner plates. *Nature biotechnology*, 34, 7–9. DOI: http://dx.doi.org/10.1038/nbt0116-7a

Wang, Q., Bailey, C., Ng, C. et al. 2011. Androgen receptor and nutrient signaling pathways coordinate the demand for increased amino acid transport during prostate cancer progression. *Cancer Research*, 71, 7525–7536. DOI: http://dx.doi.org/10.1158/0008-5472.CAN-11-1821

Wardle, J., Steptoe, A. 2003. Socioeconomic differences in attitudes and beliefs about healthy lifestyles. *Journal of Epidemiology and Community Health*, 57, 440–443. DOI: http://dx.doi.org/10.1136/jech.57.6.440

Wardle, J., Haase, A., Steptoe, A. et al. 2004. Gender differences in food choice: the contribution of health beliefs and dieting. *Annals of Behavioral Medicine*, 27, 107–116. DOI: http://dx.doi.org/10.1207/s15324796abm2702_5

Waters, C., Bassler, B. 2005. Quorum sensing: cell-to-cell communication in bacteria. *Annual Review of Cell and Developmental Biology*, 21, 319–346. DOI: http://dx.doi.org/10.1146/annurev.cellbio.21.012704.131001

Webb, P. 2010. Medium- to long-run implications of high food prices for global nutrition. *Journal of Nutrition*, 140S, 143S–147S. DOI: http://dx.doi.org/10.3945/jn.109.110536

Weber, C. , Matthews, H. 2008. Food-miles and the relative climate impacts of food choices in the United States. *Environmental Science and Technology*, 42, 3508–3513. DOI: http://dx.doi.org/10.1021/es702969f

Webster, J. 2013. *Animal husbandry regained: The place of farm animals in sustainable agriculture*. Abingdon: Routledge.

Weidema, B., Wesnaes, M., Hermansen, J. et al. 2008. *Environmental improvement potentials of meat and dairy products*. European Commission, DG JRC, Institute for Prospective Technological Studies. Technical report EUR 23491 EN. Luxembourg: Office for Official Publications of the European Communities.

Weis, T. 2013. The meat of the global food crisis. *Journal of Peasant Studies*, 40, 65–85. DOI: http://dx.doi.org/10.1080/03066150.2012.752357

Weiss, R., McMichael, A. 2004. Social and environmental risk factors in the emergence of infectious diseases. *Nature Medicine*, 10, S70–S76. DOI: http://dx.doi.org/10.1038/nm1150

Wexler, B. 2006. *Brain and culture: neurobiology, ideology and social change*. Cambridge, MS: Bradford Books, MIT Press.

Whitaker, D., Macrae, A., Burrough, E. 2004. Disposal and disease rates in British dairy herds between April 1998 and March 2002. *The Veterinary Record*, 155, 43–47. DOI: http://dx.doi.org/10.1136/vr.155.2.43

White, B., Borras, S., Hall, R. et al. 2012. The new enclosures: critical perspectives on corporate land deals. *Journal of Peasant Studies*, 39, 619–647. DOI: http://dx.doi.org/10.1080/03066150.2012.691879

Whitehead, A. 1978. *Process and Reality. An Essay in Cosmology (Corrected edition by David Griffin and Donald Sherburne)*. New York: The Free Press.

Willett, W., Manson, J., Liu, S. 2002. Glycemic index, glycemic load, and risk of type 2 diabetes. *The American Journal of Clinical Nutrition*, 76, 274S–280S.

Williams, C., Burge, G. 2006. Long-chain n-3 PUFA: plant v. marine sources. *Proceedings of the Nutrition Society*, 65,17–36. DOI: http://dx.doi.org/10.1079/PNS2005473

Williams, N. 2008. Affected ignorance and animal suffering: Why our failure to debate factory farming puts us at moral risk. *Journal of Agricultural and Environmental Ethics*, 21, 371–384. DOI: http://dx.doi.org/10.1007/s10806-008-9087-8

Wirdefeldt, K., Adami, H., Cole, P. et al. 2011. Epidemiology and etiology of Parkinson's disease: a review of the evidence. *European Journal of Epidemiology*, 26, 1S–58S. DOI: http://dx.doi.org/10.1007/s10654-011-9581-6

Wirsenius, S., Hedenus, F. 2010. Policy strategies for a sustainable food system: Options for protecting the climate. In: J. D'Silva, J. Webster (eds.). *The meat crisis: Developing more sustainable production and consumption*. London: Earthscan, 237–253.

Wirsenius, S., Hedenus, F., Mohlin, K. 2011. Greenhouse gas taxes on animal food products: Rationale, tax scheme and climate mitigation effects. *Climatic Change*, 108, 159–184. DOI: http://dx.doi.org/10.1007/s10584-010-9971-x

Wolfe, C. 2010. *What is posthumanism?* Minneapolis: University of Minnesota Press.

Wolfson, D., Sullivan, M. 2004. Foxes in the hen house: Animals, agribusiness and the law: A modern American fable, In M. Nussbaum, C. Sunstein (eds.). *Animal rights. Current debates and new directions*. Oxford: Oxford University Press, 205–233.

Woo, K., Kwok, T., Celermajer, D. 2014. Vegan diet, subnormal vitamin B-12 status and cardiovascular health. *Nutrients*, 6, 3259–3273. DOI: http://dx.doi.org/10.3390/nu6083259

Woolhouse, M., Gowtage-Sequeria, S. 2005. Host range and emerging and re-emerging pathogens. *Emerging Infectious Diseases*, 11, 1842–1847. DOI: http://dx.doi.org/10.3201/eid1112.050997

World Bank. 2008. *World development report 2008: Agriculture for development*. Washington DC: World Bank.

World Bank. 2009. *Global economic prospects 2009*. Washington DC: World Bank.

World Cancer Research Fund and American Institute for Cancer Research. 2007. *Food, nutrition, physical activity, and the prevention of cancer: a global perspective*. Washington DC: AICR.

World Health Organization. 2010. Pandemic (H1N1) 2009 - update 112. http://www.who.int/csr/don/2010_08_06/en/index.html (Accessed 10 May 2016.)

World Health Organization. 2012. *Influenza at the human-animal interface. Summary and assessment as of 17 December 2012.* http://www.who.int/influenza/human_animal_interface/Influenza_Summary_IRA_HA_interface_17Dec12updated.pdf (Accessed 6 January 2015.)

World Water Assessment Programme. 2009. *The United Nations world water development report 3: Water in a changing world.* Paris: Unesco Publishing, and London: Earthscan.

World Wildlife Fund. 2012. *Living planet report 2012.* Gland: World Wildlife Fund.

Yang, S., Li, X., Zhang, W. et al. 2012. Chinese lacto-vegetarian diet exerts favorable effects on metabolic parameters, intima-media thickness, and cardio-vascular risks in healthy men. *Nutrition in Clinical Practice*, 27, 392–398. DOI: http://dx.doi.org/10.1177/0884533611436173

Ziegler, E. 2011. Consumption of cow's milk as a cause of iron deficiency in infants and toddlers. *Nutrition Reviews*, 69, 37S–42S. DOI: http://dx.doi.org/10.1111/j.1753-4887.2011.00431.x

Zoncu, R., Efeyan, A., Sabatini, D. 2011. mTOR: from growth signal integration to cancer, diabetes and ageing. *Nature Reviews Molecular Cell Biology*, 12, 21–35. DOI: http://dx.doi.org/10.1038/nrm3025

Printed in March 2023
by Rotomail Italia S.p.A., Vignate (MI) - Italy